Magnetic Resonance Imaging of the Thorax

Magnetic Resonance Imaging of the Thorax

by

Miriam Sperber, M.D.

Head, Thoracic Division
Department of Radiology
University Hospital
Antwerpen, Belgium

Marc C. Kaiser, M.D.

Staff Radiologist, MRI Section
Department of Radiology
Free University Hospital
Amsterdam, The Netherlands

with contribution by

Professor J. Struyven

Department of Radiology
Hospital Erasme
Belgium

WARREN H. GREEN, INC.
St. Louis, Missouri, U.S.A.

Published by

WARREN H. GREEN, INC.
8356 Olive Boulevard
St. Louis, Missouri 63132, U.S.A.

ISBN No. 87527-375-0

Printed in the United States of America

To the memory of our mothers:
Fanny Frenkel
and
Olga Kaiser

Also to the spirit of friendship, collegiality and love of learning which makes scientific work a rewarding experience.

Miriam Sperber
Marc C. Kaiser

Acknowledgments

We would like to thank the whole staff of the Radiology Department at the Free University Hospital of Amsterdam under the direction of Professor J. Valk for their participation in the diagnostic MRI work that was used in part in the preparation of this book. We also are very grateful to our technicians Adrie, Karin, Marga, Willy and Ronald for their patience and devotion during the technical performance of the MRI examinations. We are indebted to Miss Galia Sperber for her secretarial help in the preparation of the manuscript.

Contents

Magnetic Resonance Imaging of the Thorax

I

Introduction

The last 10 to 15 years have seen the introduction and vertiginous development of new imaging technologies. Among them, computerized tomography and magnetic resonance imaging are without doubt the ones which have revolutionized modern radiology. As a result of their extended clinical use, an enormous amount of information emerged to supplement the data available from conventional radiographic studies.

Although it became inevitable to compare MRI to CT in the study of various pathological conditions, in most cases it seems too early to arrive at a final statement. The evolution of MRI systems and the advancement in the understanding of MR imaging clinical benefits are still promoting new conclusions.

In the study of the thorax, the major differences between the two modalities are a result of the lack of ionizing radiation to the patient during MR examination and the obviated need for the use of contrast materials with MRI. It is essential to understand that although both investigative methods allow multiplanar visualization of body tissue, there are major differences in the grey scale ordering of the tissues. In CT it is constant and well established on a range of Hounsfield numbers, and in MRI it varies widely even for the same tissue. There is an obvious need therefore, while attempting to interpret MR images, to clearly note and understand the technical conditions under which the examination has been performed.

This book is designed to help the diagnostic radiologist as well as the clinician involved in the study and treatment of pulmonary and cardiac disorders, to become familiar with the presentations of the various abnormalities on MR images. While radiology has become increasingly interventional as well as diagnostic, a multitude of modalities are available for the study of the various thoracic organs. Practitioners and radiologists are continuously struggling with the need for the selection of an optimal imaging technique.

By offering detailed descriptions of the magnetic resonance findings in various conditions (i.e., diffuse lung diseases, cardiac abnormalities or bronchogenic carcinoma) the present text offers up-dated information on magnetic resonance imaging of the thorax. It serves as a guide to the understanding of the advantages, as well as the limitations of this modality, when compared to other existing techniques.

This book contains discussions and suggestions on preferable examination techniques in various specific clinical conditions. In addition, numerous photographs were carefully selected to illustrate and exemplify a wide variety of pathology.

The authors express their hope that this book will prove to be of interest to radiologists, trainees and specialists, as well as to various clinicians dealing with the treatment of pulmonary and cardiac disorders. The text facilitates an understanding of the fundamentals of MR imaging of the thorax, and works toward promoting a realistic and appropriate use of this exciting diagnostic modality.

Miriam Sperber, M.D.
Marc C. Kaiser, M.D.

2

Technical Considerations

One of the main advantages of Magnetic Resonance Imaging (MRI) over CT-scanning is its capability to provide high resolution sagittal and coronal images which are far superior to CT reconstructed images performed upon whole series of contiguous axial CT slices. MRI displays small differences in tissue density with unequalized clarity without subjecting the patient to ionizing radiation. All parts of the body may be investigated by MRI in the transverse, sagittal, coronal, or oblique planes without having to move the patient who remains in the supine position during the entire examination. The thoracic cage and the whole intrathoracic contents may noninvasively be investigated during one visit to the Radiology Department and contrast injections are not required to visualize the cardiovascular system.

Until now MRI has mainly found application in neuroradiology, the musculoskeletal system, the gynecological and urogenital systems. Gated MRI has been reported by several authors (1-6) to be mostly accurate for imaging the cardiovascular system and it seems to bear a great potential for the evaluation of cardiac function (3, 5). Reports about MRI studies of the thoracic cage, the lungs and mediastinum are still scarce (1, 2, 4, 6, 7-12).

For proper understanding of MR images it is essential to acquaint oneself with the physical principles of MRI which have been explained in detail (2). In this chapter, we will attempt to outline the most important technical details of magnetic resonance imaging in a summarized form permitting easier understanding of diagnostic pathways with MRI as applied to the chest.

MRI investigation systems mainly consist of:

1. A magnetic field of high strength having a homogeneous character. Actually the vast majority of magnets used are superconductive magnets which operate at a field strength ranging from 0.5 to 2.0 Tesla and which have no resistance to current flow at low temperatures. For this purpose the magnet is enveloped by a liquid helium environment at -269° Celsius (-454° F).

2. Gradient coils which are used during scanning to generate small gradient magnetic fields along the x, y, and z coordinate planes.

3. Radio frequency coils, transmitting or receiving radio waves of a predetermined frequency.

4. A computer system to analyze the signals measured and to process all the information obtained to reconstruct an image.

GENERATION AND DETECTION OF MR SIGNALS

The patient is placed in the strong, uniform magnetic field. The hydrogen nuclei (protons) in his body will preferentially align themselves along the long axis of the magnetic field. By the energy of short radio waves transmitted by the radio frequency coils the hydrogen protons will deviate from the plane of the magnetic field. By doing so, small amounts of energy will be released (Figure 2.1). These small energy pulses can be detected by receiving radio frequency coils and they constitute the basis for the MR imaging signal. As the body is composed of different tissue components containing a variable number of hydrogen nuclei, the intensity and frequency of signals received from different parts of the body is also extremely variable. The amplitude of MR signals depends to a large degree on the proton density, i.e., the number of nuclei per volume unit of a determined tissue. The difference in proton density determines the different white and gray levels in MRI. Contrast on MRI images is nevertheless mainly influenced by proton relaxation times (T_1 and T_2). The time period that begins with proton excitation by the radio frequency pulse and ends with their realignment within the main magnetic field is called relaxation time. T_1 relaxation time is the time needed for hydrogen protons that have been rotated 180° away from the plane of the magnetic field to return to their equilibrium plane. The time needed for the signal generated by hydrogen protons rotating in the transverse plane to decay and to disappear is called T_2 relaxation time. All factors capable of influencing or altering one or both of the relaxation times will also alter the quality and intensity of MR images (13). This principle is also at the basis of the application of paramagnetic contrast agents which are capable of modifying the relaxation times of tissues under investigation whereby tissue differentiation and contrast resolution may be optimalized. From

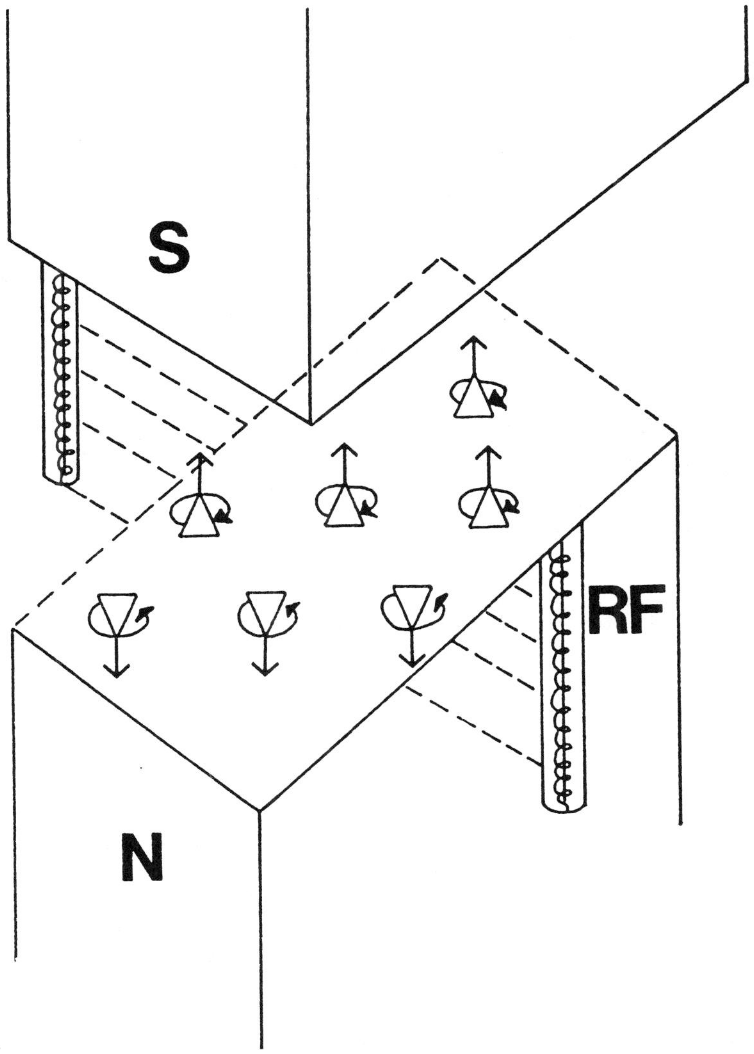

Figure 2.1. Diagram demonstrating alignment of hydrogen protons in strong uniform magnetic field. (S = south; N = north; RF = radio frequency). Slightly more protons get aligned in the direction of the magnetic field as it requires less energy to be aligned in this direction than in the opposite way. Precession (rotation) of hydrogen protons around the axis of the magnetic field is indicated.

commonly used contrast medium is Gadolinium-DTPA. By shortening proton relaxation times of tissues, these contrast agents permit the use of shorter pulse sequences to obtain high contrast images in MRI. This characteristic of paramagnetic substances is interesting also in patients suffering from cardiac or respiratory distress and which cannot be placed for long time intervals into the MRI device.

SCANNING TECHNIQUES

A pulse sequence defines the time and nature of the radio frequency excitation pulse that are beamed into the body. The time during which the radio wave pulse has to be applied depends on the angle through which one wants to move the hydrogen protons. The interval between the beginning of a pulse sequence and the start of the next pulse sequence is called "Time of Repetition" (TR). The time between the first 90° pulse and the moment at which a signal is returned from the object under study can be read out is named "Time to Echo" (TE). By playing on the choice of different TR and TE values, one may obtain images that depend on the T_1 and T_2 relaxations times of tissues (T_1 or T_2 weighted images):

1. Decreased TR values increase T_1 characteristics of MR images
2. Increased TR values reduce the T_1 influence of the image. It ensues that scanning times will be much longer, but the signal-to-noise ratio will be significantly improved.
3. Shortening TE values reinforces T_1 effect on images.
4. By long TE values more T_2 weighted images will be obtained.

With long TR values more hydrogen protons may recover between two pulses and are consequently excitable again when the next energy pulse arrives. Although adjacent tissues may have different relaxation times, their T_1 recovery may be complete, provided that the TR value is long enough. With short TR values, more hydrogen nuclei will recover in tissues having short T_1 relaxation times, more hydrogen nuclei will be available in these tissues by the time that the next energy pulse arrives. This structure will have a whiter appearance on MR images than tissues having a long T_1 relaxation time.

The wrong choice of pulse parameters reduces tissue contrast and could mask even large abnormalities (14).

Pulse sequences most commonly used in MRI are the saturation recovery (SR), the inversion recovery (IR) and above all the spin-echo (SE) techniques.

For our clinical studies we had at our disposition a Teslacon superconductive system operating at 0.6 Tesla. Multi-section spin-echo images were obtained with a 100 cm body coil, the patient being supine and breathing quietly. A 128 x 256 matrix was used. The total duration of the examination varied between 25 and 40 minutes.

We routinely started MRI studies of the chest by performing a spin-echo pulse sequence in the sagittal plane using a TR of 350 ms, a TE of 32 ms, a 1 cm slice thickness and 2 measurements (3.5 minutes). This way we obtained 5 sagittal images, the midline scan of this series was used as a "scout" for subsequent coronal and transverse scanning. After this 9 images in the coronal plane were performed with a TR 500 ms, TE 32 ms and 4 measurements (4.5 minutes). Moreover, a series of 14 transverse images was then generated with a TR 3000 ms, TE 32 ms, 2 measurements, a 1.5 cm slice thickness and 4 delayed echos (13.5 minutes). In all series performed, a 5 mm slice interval was used. Finally, in selected cases MR imaging was performed with cardiac gating. In post-pneumonectomy patients an additional series of transverse MR images was routinely done with cardiac gating. For this series we used a TR of 500 ms, TE 32 ms, 4 measurements and a 1 cm slice thickness. In fact, the pulse sequence repetition time (TR) is determined by the patient's heart rate, the radio frequency pulses being triggered by the R wave of the electrocardiogram (5). Following pneumonectomy, massive herniation of cardio-mediastinal structures into the postoperative hemithorax may occur. In an effort to optimalize differentiation between the various soft tissue components within the post-pneumonectomy space which at their turn, have to be separated from eventual pericardial pathology, it is important to reduce at maximum artifacts which may arise from cardiovascular beating. For these reasons we think that it is important to use cardiac gating in MRI investigation of the post-pneumonectomy chest or in any condition in which cardiovascular movement is liable to interfere with the quality of the imaging towards the establishment of an accurate diagnosis. Gating is not necessary in most MRI studies of noncardiovascular pathology.

We also have had some experience with respiratory gating in MR imaging of the chest (8). Our early results with this technique were disappointing. The respiratory cycle is subject to wide variations in the same patient and from patient to patient. This explains why the image obtained with respiratory gating may be worse than its ungated counterpart (2). Ways to overcome these shortcomings have been suggested (2), but we have not as yet had any experience with these experimental technique modifications. The main disadvantage is due to markedly increased scan time by respiratory gating, which is very cumbersome in patients suffering already from some degree of respiratory distress. For this reason, we actually disregard respiratory gating and we feel that it's value has to be reassessed at the moment when fundamental improvement of this technique will be achieved. In our experience, images with relatively short TR intervals (350-500 ms) provide the best spatial resolution and high contrast definition between normal

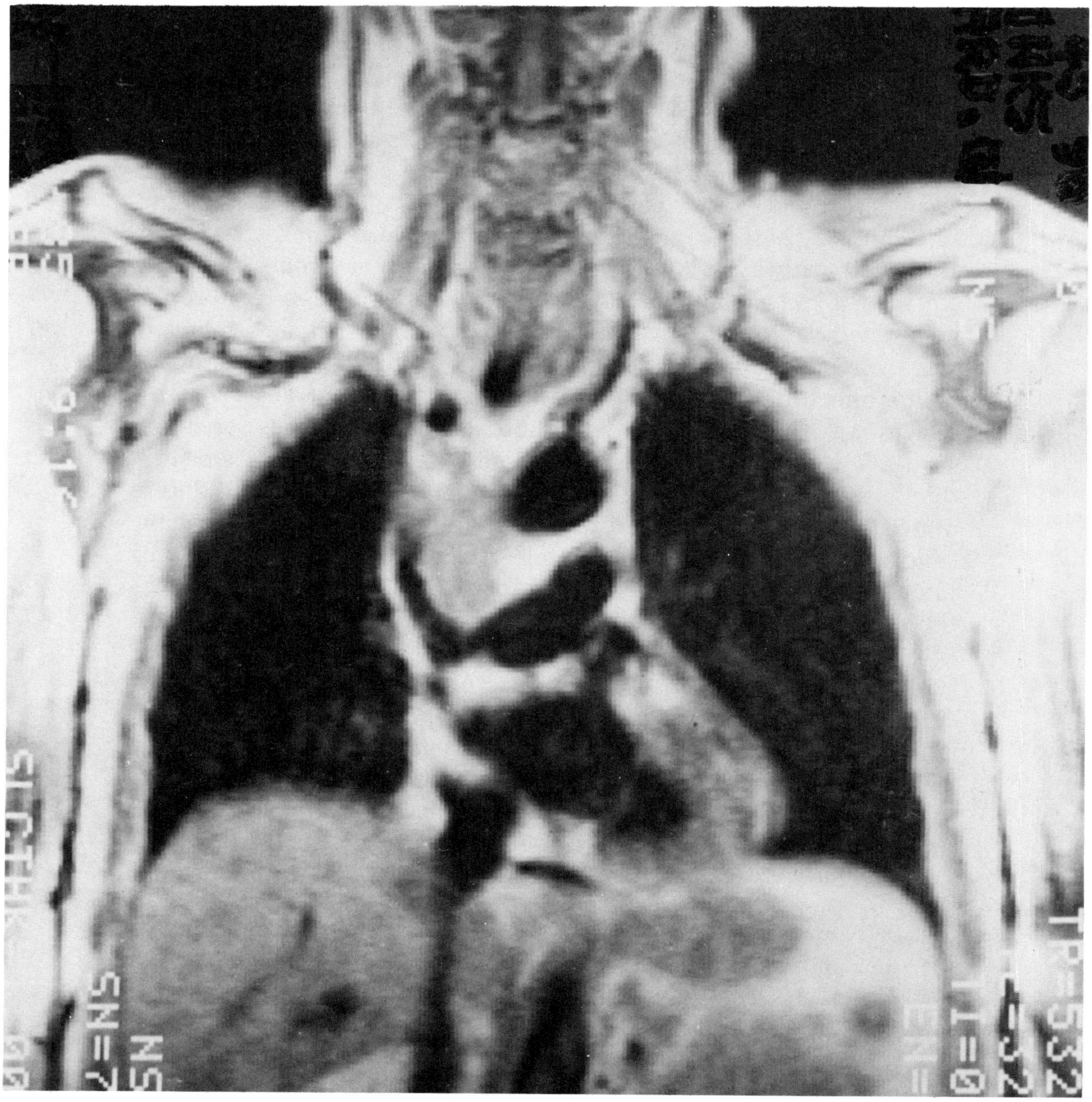

Figure 2.2. Coronal spin-echo MR image obtained with a TR 532 ms, a TE 32 ms and 4 measurements. A mediastinal mass is shown with intermediate signal intensity permitting easy differentiation from very low signal intensity structures due to vascular branches and from very high signal intensity due to mediastinal fat.

anatomical structures and pathological tissues. Especially in cases of mediastinal tumors, the low signal intensity of neoplasms may easily be differentiated from the high signal intensity of mediastinal fat (Figure 2.2). Nevertheless, if the main interest resides in the lungs, more T_2 weighted images are preferable (Figure 2.3).

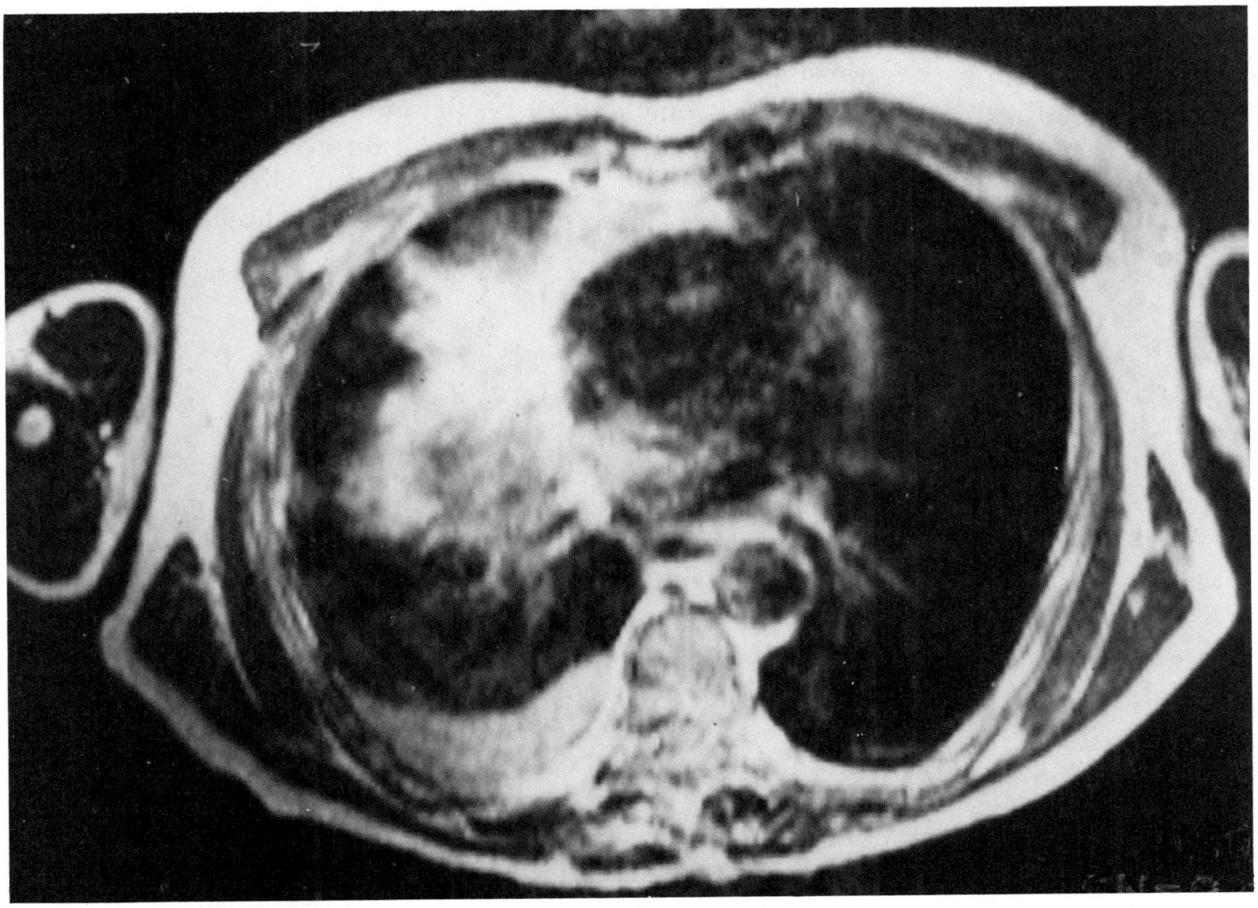

Figure 2.3. MRI always outlines both lungs as very low density structures. To permit optimal visualization of pulmonary pathology, technical parameters should be selected in such a way that the contrast difference between mass and surrounding lung is reinforced. This relatively T2 weighted image (TR 2000 ms, TE 32 ms, 2nd of 4 delayed echos) shows accurately an extensive high signal intensity area due to tumor pathology in the right lung.

Images obtained with long TR intervals produce significant differential change of the signal intensity of pathological tissues in a way that they may easily be separated from normal structures, but the signal contrast between tumor and mediastinal fat decreases. These pulse sequences are particularly valuable in patients in which the lungs and the pleural space have to be investigated simultaneously. Many of the lung disorders have prolonged T_2 relaxation times and are seen as areas of increased signal intensity.

Inversion recovery images do not supply incremental information in MRI of the chest (2). Furthermore, as they have reduced spatial resolution and require long data acquisition times, we excluded this sequence from the MRI examination scheme of thoracic pathology.

We think that MRI is going to develop and evolve at an increasing pace during the upcoming years. From this evolution, significant technical improvement may result and the diagnostic accuracy of MRI in pathology of the chest will improve proportionally. The use of surface coils for imaging mediastinal or focal pulmonary pathology is an interesting step in this direction.

CORONAL AND SAGITTAL IMAGING

The long axis of the body is contained in the coronal and sagittal planes. From this it becomes obvious that images performed in these planes necessarily contain more anatomical details per generated cut than transverse (axial) body slices. Furthermore, pathology is shown in the same plane as encountered by the surgeon during the operative approach. Due to the design of CT scanning systems, body investigations were mainly restricted to the transverse plane. Although it became possible to generate electronically coronal and sagittal CT reformated images based on whole series of contiguous axial slices, these images had still definitely lower spatial resolution than direct scans and the radiation penalty to patients was too high. For the prementioned reasons, some authors tried to overcome these shortcomings of CT scanning by introducing patient positioning variations and by recommending design modifications of CT imaging systems (15, 16). In order to allow complete CT examination of the body, important and expensive hardware modifications would have been required. Much larger gantry apertures and image reconstruction circles would be necessary to permit easy imaging in those planes as a routine technique.

An examination technique whereby the patient is introduced in a sitting position inside the gantry aperture has been described (Figure 2.4A) (16–20). Similarly, infants and small children were put in a lateral decubitus position on the table top device to perform direct coronal CT images of the body (Figure 2.4B and C) (17–19). This way direct coronal CT slices of relatively good quality were obtained, mainly in the region of the spine and paraspinal gutter (Figure 2.5). In small sized patients some parts of the chest, including the aorta, the trachea, the heart and the hilar structures, could also be shown in the coronal plane (Figures 2.6, 2.7, 2.8, and 2.9). Nevertheless, these techniques remained cumbersome and were too time consuming to be routinely used as a diagnostic procedure and could not be applied to a large number of patients.

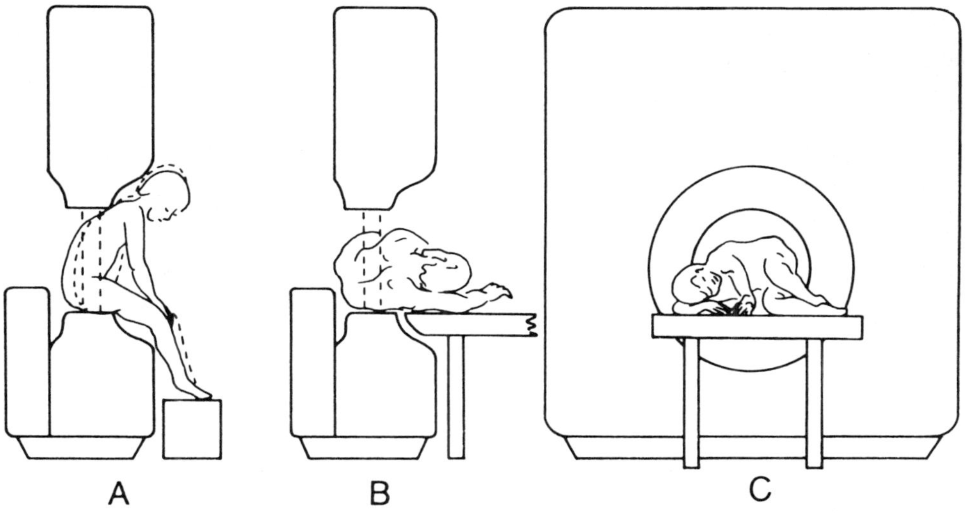

Figure 2.4. Diagram showing (A) sitting position and (B,C) lateral decubitus position for direct coronal body CT scanning (with permission reference 16).

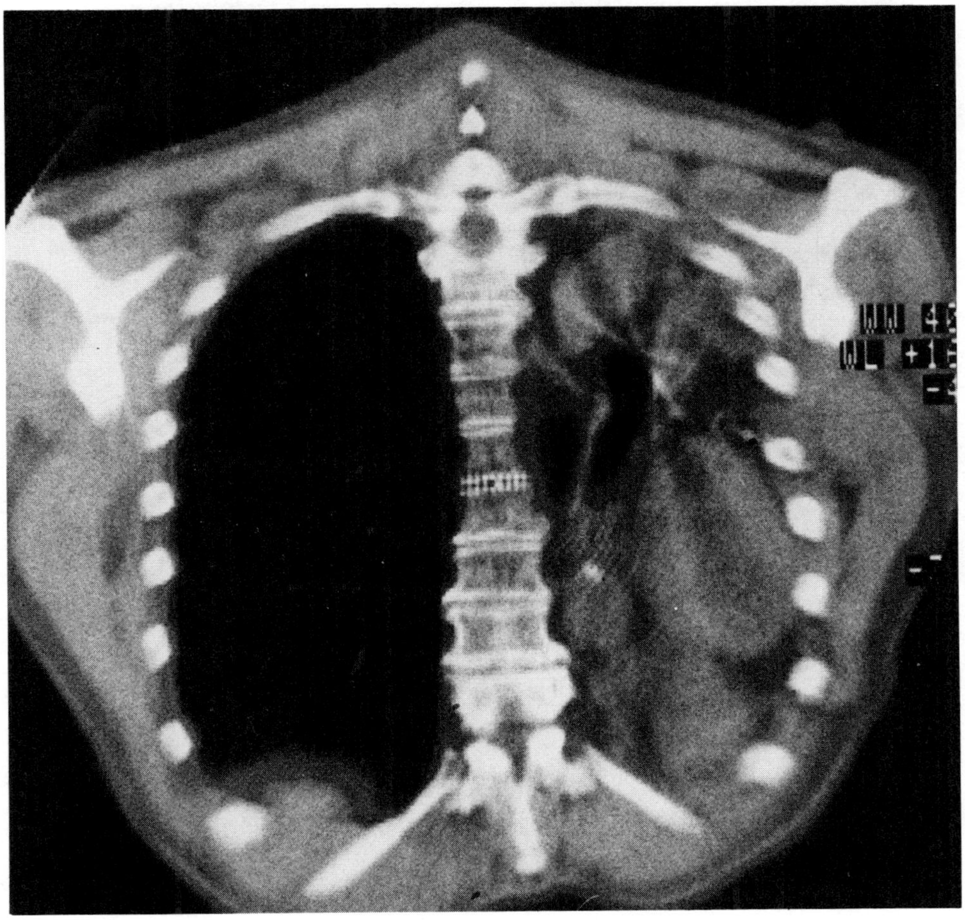

Figure 2.5. Direct coronal CT image through posterior portion of the thorax in a post-pneumonectomy patient. Massive intra-thoracic herniation of abdominal content demonstrated on the left side.

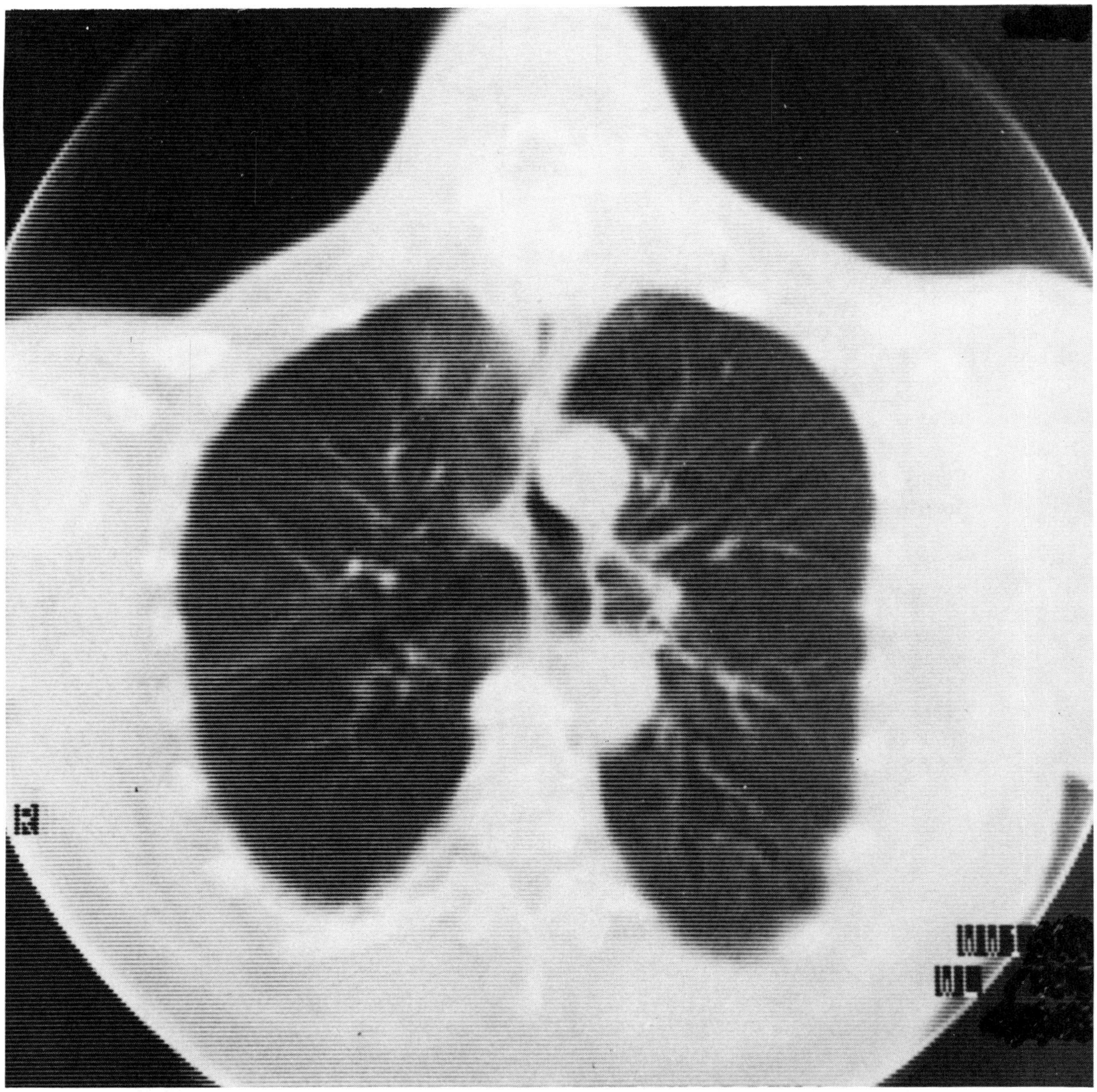

Figure 2.6. Direct coronal CT scan at a more anterior level in a different patient shows mid-mediastinal broncho-vascular structures.

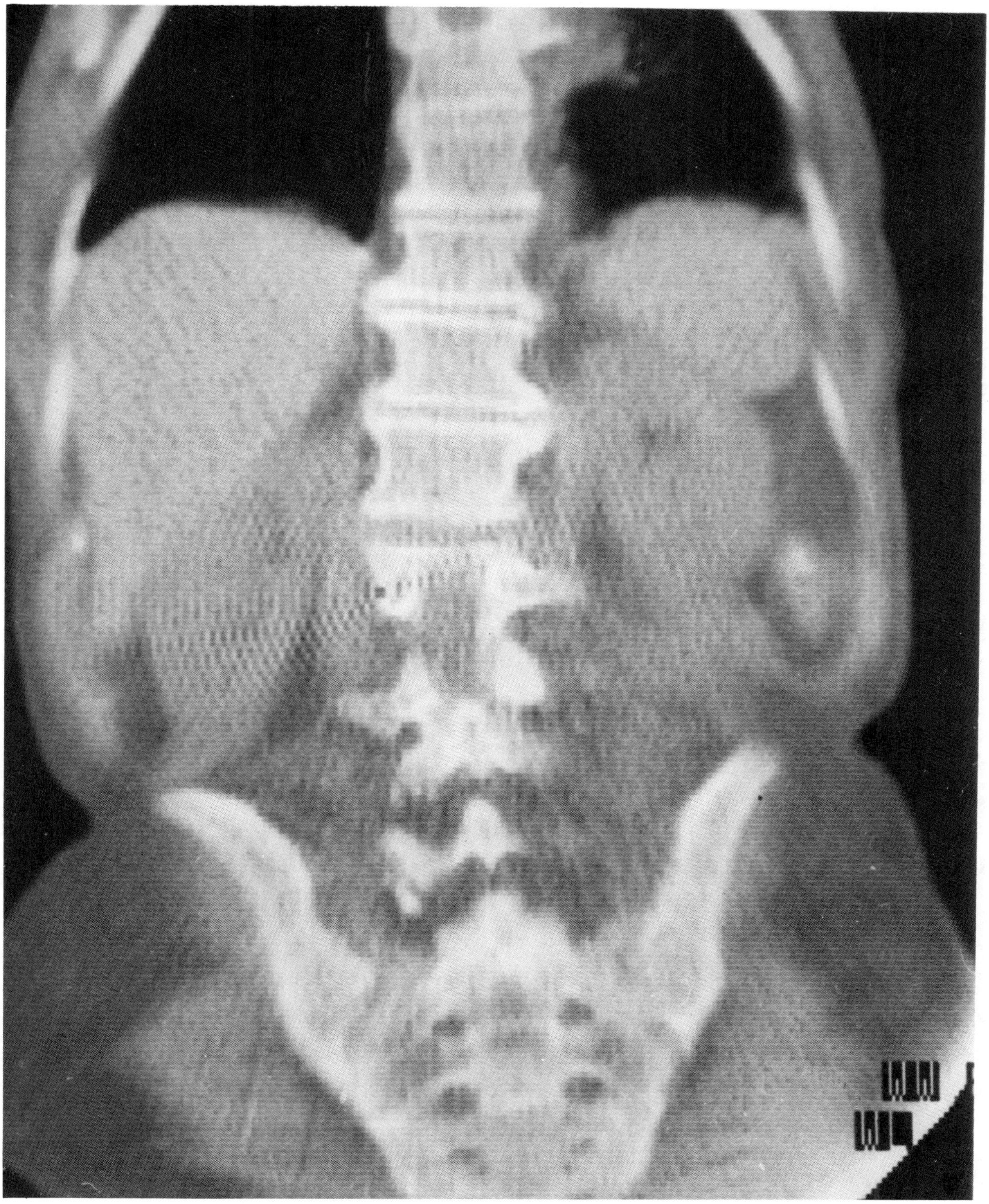

Figure 2.7. Direct coronal CT image outlines malignant infiltration of left costo-vertebral gutter descending into retroperitoneal space. The intra-abdominal organs are also well delineated (with permission reference 16).

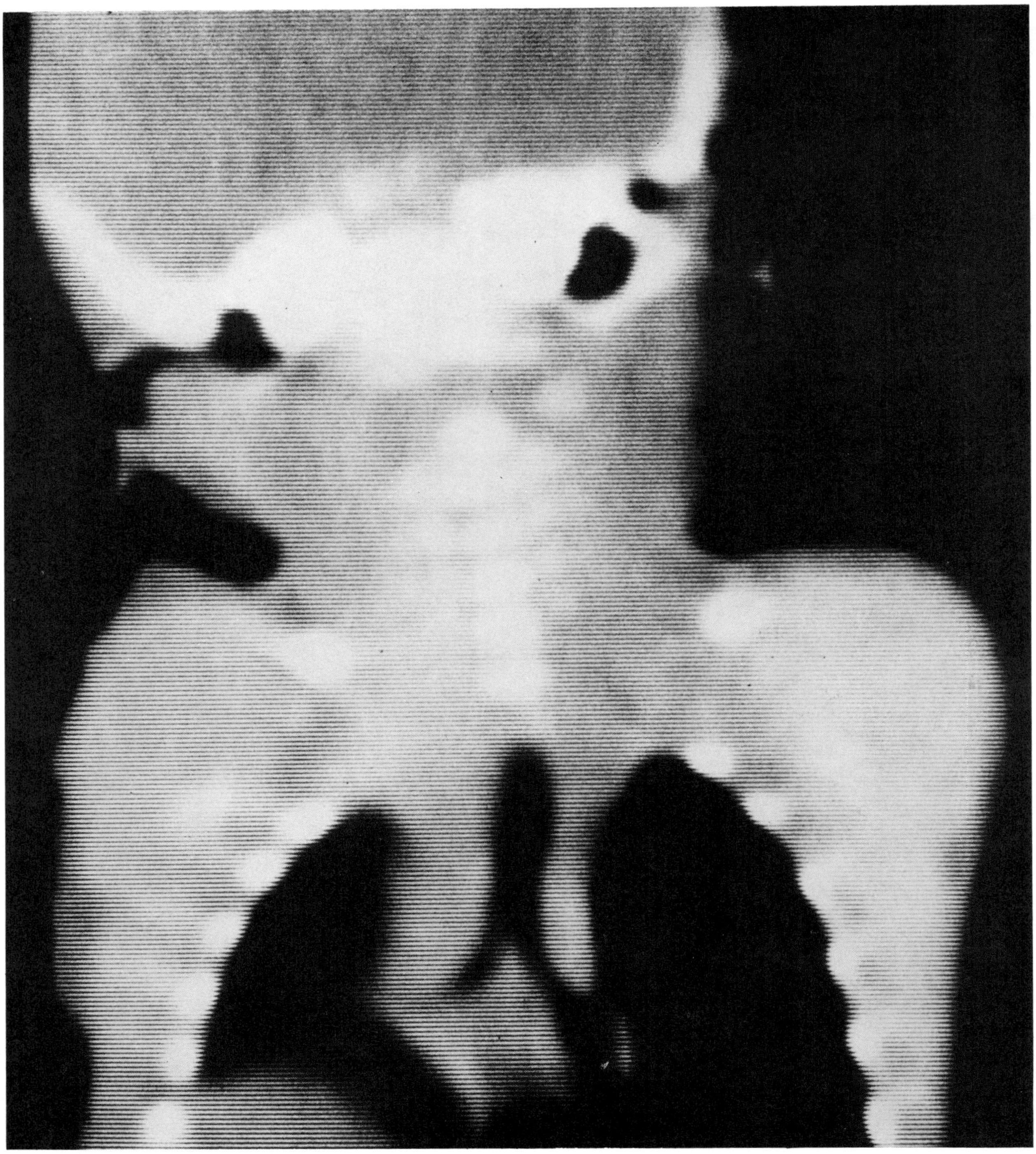

Figure 2.8. Direct coronal CT scan performed on an infant lying in lateral decubitus position on the table top device. A coronal slice through cranio-cervical region and upper thorax shows a hypoplastic lung on the right side, but a normal trachea and normal main bronchi were seen (with permission reference 19).

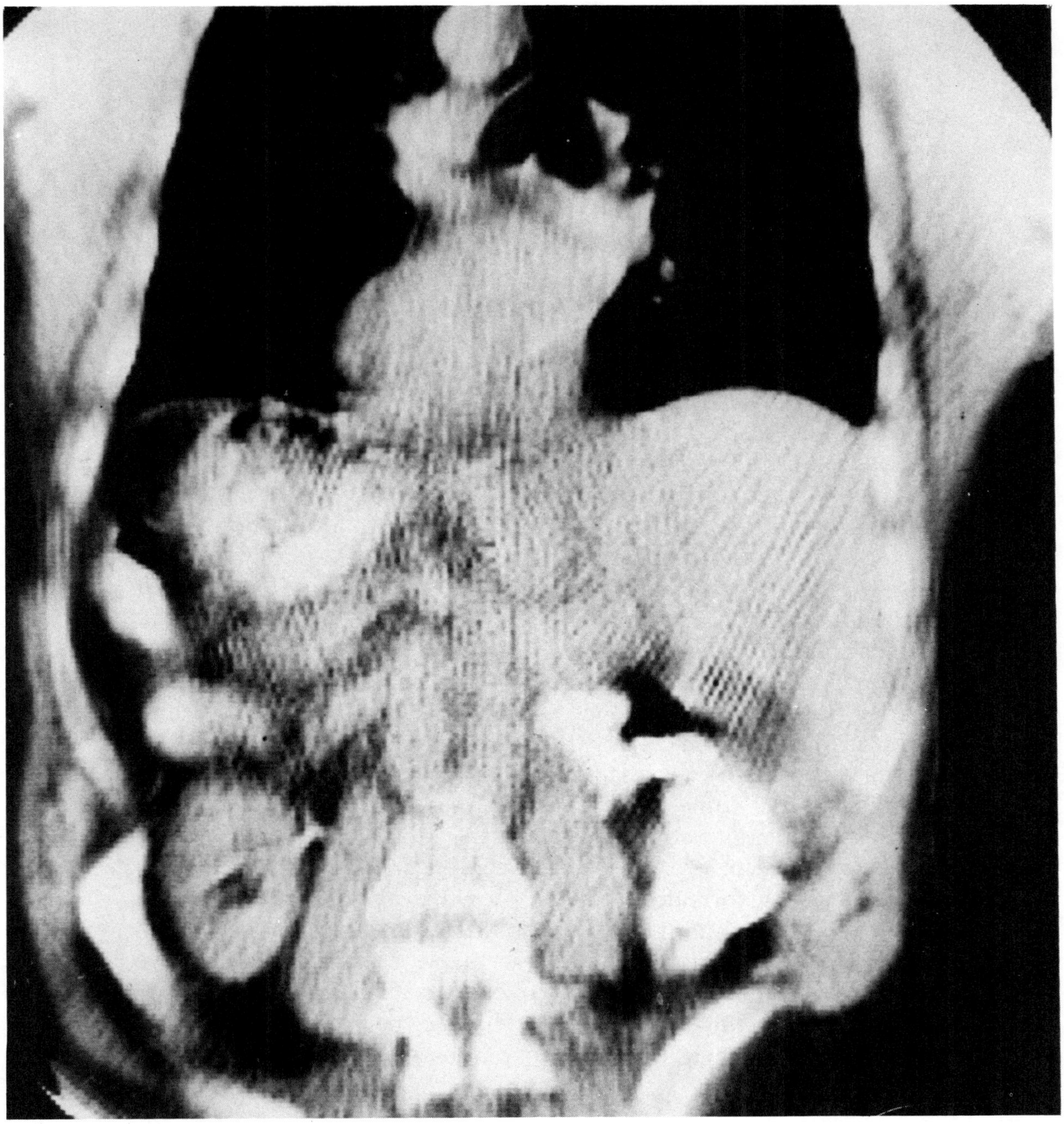

Figure 2.9. Direct coronal CT cut shows some segments of cardiovascular system, but complete examination of this area was impossible. A three-dimensional investigation of the anterior mediastinum and of the cardio-vascular system can only be achieved by MRI.

With the advent of MRI it became possible to investigate the whole body in any plane without having to move the patient. As a consequence, a three-dimensional representation of chest pathology became routinely available. For diagnostic evaluation of pulmonary or mediastinal pathology the most appropriate MRI investigation plane capable of outlining the topography of lesions to surrounding structures may be selected in a view to obtain additional information about their etiology. In our experience the relationship of pathological masses to neighboring bronchi and vessels is well shown on coronal and transverse MR images. Examinations in these two planes appear to be most valuable in the diagnostic work-up of mediastinal, paramediastinal and hilar pathology (11).

The vertical extent of coronal and sagittal MR images includes the entire thorax as well as the lower neck and upper abdomen. On these images, longer portions of the trachea and of the main vascular branches may be demonstrated. Sagittal imaging does not provide significant incremental information about hilar or mediastinal lesions. This may be explained by the fact that on these images it is difficult to understand the relation of a lesion to surrounding vessels or bronchi (12). However, in some cases the localization of subcarinal masses in comparison to the trachea or pulmonary arteries may be shown with further detail on sagittal images. Furthermore, coronal and sagittal images provided very useful information in cases where extensive pathology existed at the apex or base of the lungs. Extension of the disease in relation to the thoracic dome or to the diaphragmatic leaflets was more precisely shown and abnormalities in the subpleural, subphrenic or supraclavicular spaces were more accurately evaluated. However, as no unique information can be provided by sagittal or coronal MR imaging, we think that they should always be used in conjunction with imaging in the transverse plane. Moreover, we believe that three-dimensional imaging of chest pathology is most valuable whenever fine needle biopsy has to be carried out or for planning transtracheal needle biopsy in cases of subcarinal masses.

CARDIAC GATING

Motion degrades MR images. Motion artifacts may be due to:

1. Patient movement, either because the patient is anxious or claustrophobic, or because the patient badly understands the scan procedure.
2. Respiration, mainly in patients with respiratory distress or in patients having very irregular respiratory movements.
3. Cardiovascular movement.
4. Swallowing.

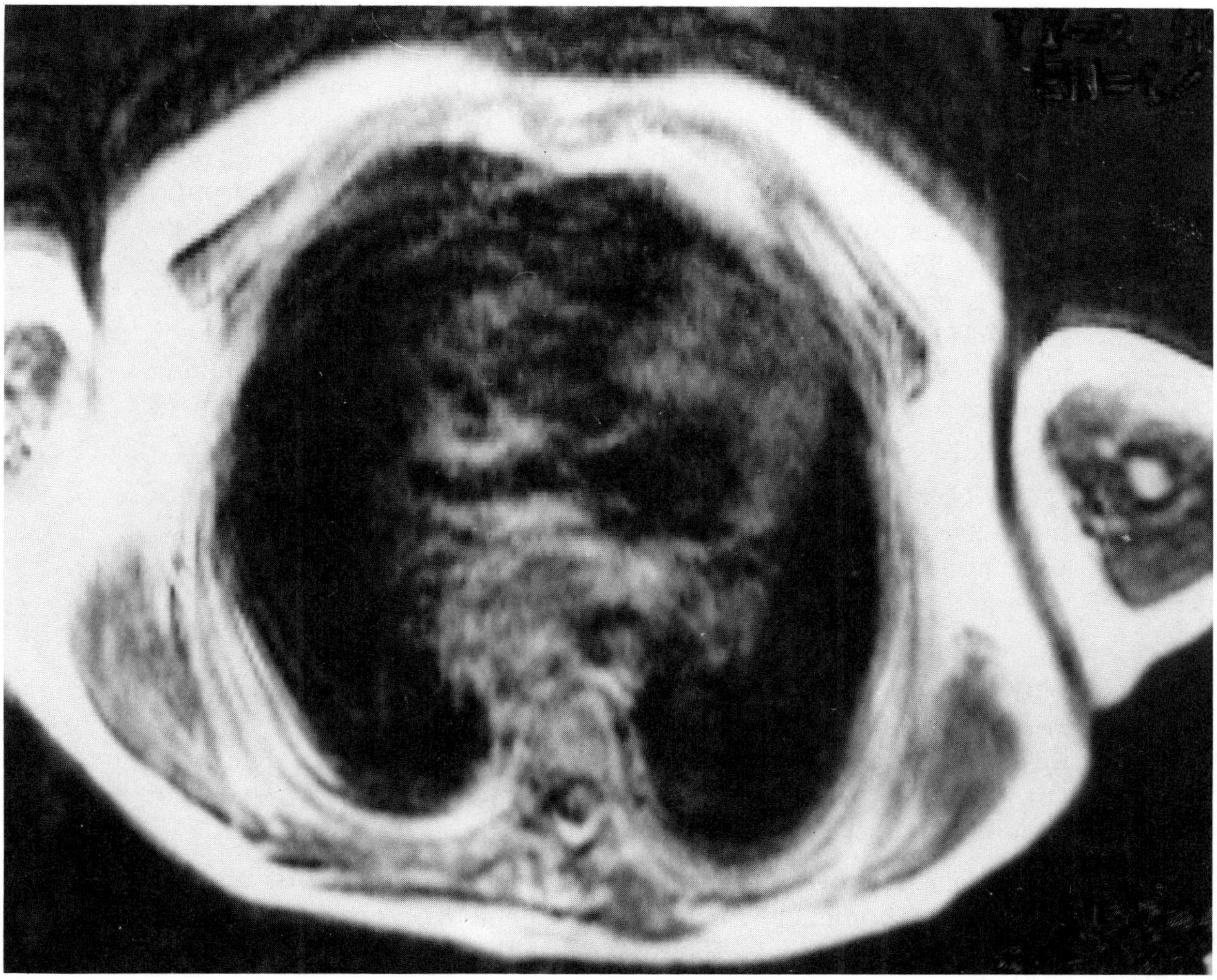

Figure 2.10. MRI examination of the chest performed without cardiac gating. Due to motion artifacts the images obtained were insufficiently diagnostic.

Motion may cause blurring on MR images (Figure 2.10), alternatively ghost images may be produced. Cardiac gating is not required in MRI studies of noncardiovascular pathology. Although reasonably good quality images of the cardiovascular system may be obtained without cardiac gating, most authors strongly recommend it in every situation where it is wanted to investigate the heart or the main vascular structures (6). Without gating, the best MR images are obtained with pulse sequences using short TR and TE parameters (2). But even with short TR and TE values, the images are not as good as if cardiac gating had been applied. On the other hand, it is quite obvious that cardiac gating has no influence on artifacts due to other origins and which also may degrade the MR images.

The main disadvantages of gating are that the scanning times are significantly increased and that the control of the choice of TR values is lost as the heart rate determines the TR value. Therefore, the number of pulse sequences that may be performed on the same patient may be limited by cardiac gating. In some cases, only a limited portion of the chest may be investigated during a pulse sequence as only a reduced number of slices can be obtained due to a low TR value. With a heart rate of 60/min, a radio frequency pulse is generated 60 times in a minute and the value of TR is 1.0 sec (1000 ms). With a heart rate of 75/min, the TR value is 0.8 sec (800 ms). The number of MR images that may be obtained from a single pulse sequence is obviously more limited due to relatively low TR values.

We reserved cardiac gating for patients with vascular lesions, lung masses (situated in the vicinity of the heart) and to post-pneumonectomy patients.

In order to obtain gated images, a signal at a fixed time of the cardiac cycle must be received to initiate the pulse sequence. With ECG gating, the radio frequency pulses are triggered by the R wave of the electrocardiogram. By choosing different time delays, images can be obtained at any period of the cardiac cycle (5). We choose a 5 ms delay after the peak of the R wave (end diastole) to initiate the imaging sequence.

For the above reasons cardiac gating seems to be of value in selected cases, namely in those in which cardiac or vascular movement can interfere with the making of the final diagnosis (Figure 2.11).

FLOW EFFECTS

MRI signals received from hydrogen nuclei in blood are dependent on the blood flow velocity. It has been stated that the signal intensity of flowing blood is inversely proportional to the percentage of moving hydrogen nuclei and to their velocity (3). If the flow of hydrogen nuclei is quick enough to propulse them through the scan slice being imaged in the time necessary to perform one data acquisition sequence, then their signal gets lost and blood will be demonstrated as a very low signal intensity structure (Figure 2.12). From experimental studies, it is known that when flow occurs at a velocity exceeding 10 to 15 cm/sec, almost no MRI signal results (21). Nuclei moving at a comparatively high velocity escape the imaged volume during the interval required for radio frequency and gradient pulse administration. This phenome-

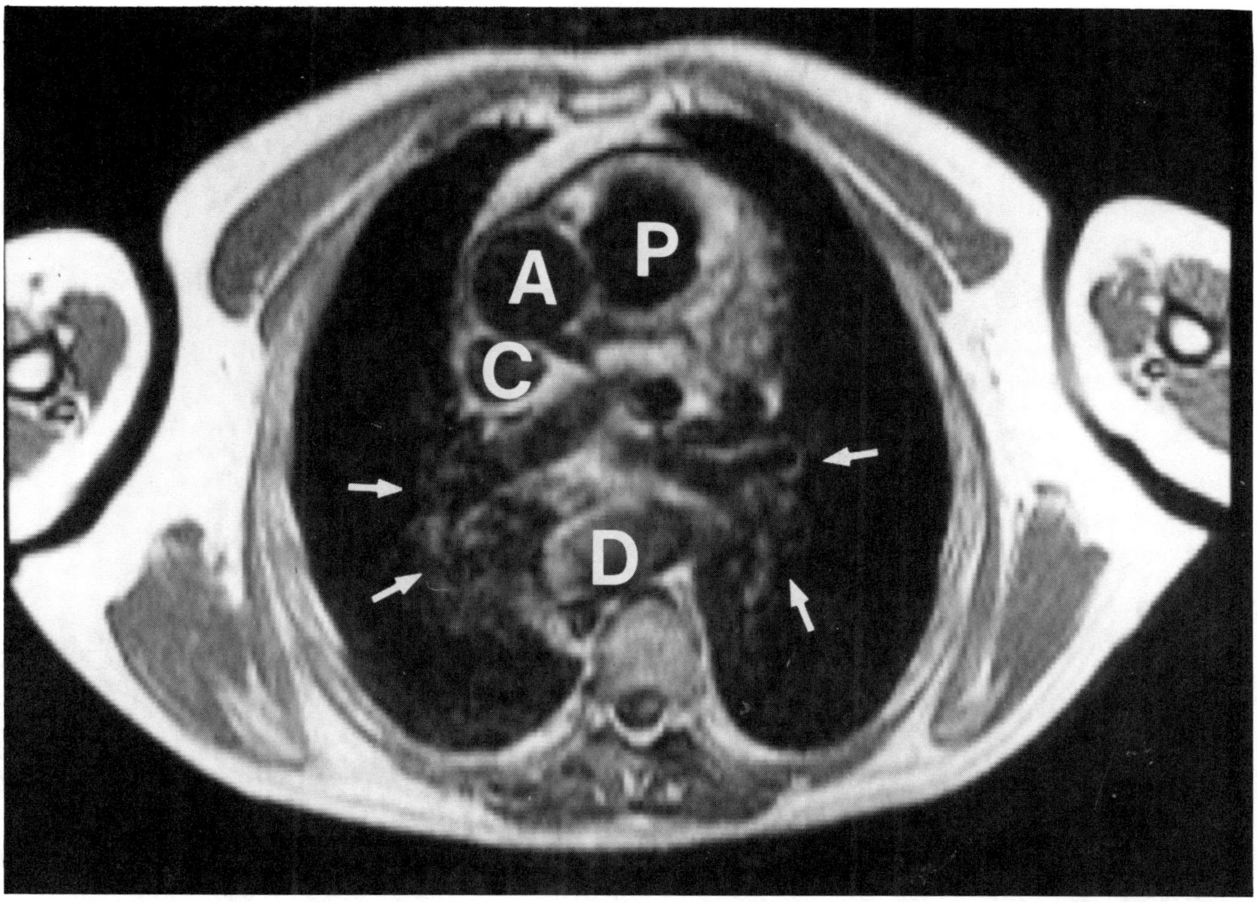

Figure 2.11. Same patient as in Figure 2.10. Transverse MRI with cardiac gating accurately shows cardiovascular, mediastinal and pulmonary structures (A = ascending aorta, P = main pulmonary artery, C = vena cava, D = descending aorta passing at anterior aspect of the spine towards the right side). Arrows point to bronchial distribution.

non explains why with spin-echo techniques the main mediastinal and pulmonary vessels are shown with superb anatomical detail. Contrast injections are not required as there is an intrinsic signal intensity difference between flowing blood and the wall of the vessel. Temporal parameters of imaging techniques may also influence to some extent the signals received from flowing blood. However, the signal emitted by the protons in blood has a more complex behavior. Under determined imaging conditions flowing blood may produce a high signal intensity. This effect has been termed "paradoxical enhancement." In occluded or thrombosed vessels, the stationary protons yield a MRI signal intensity related to the degree of magnetization they may reach between two radio frequency pulses. Slowly flowing blood may produce a higher signal intensity than stationary blood. This can be explained by the

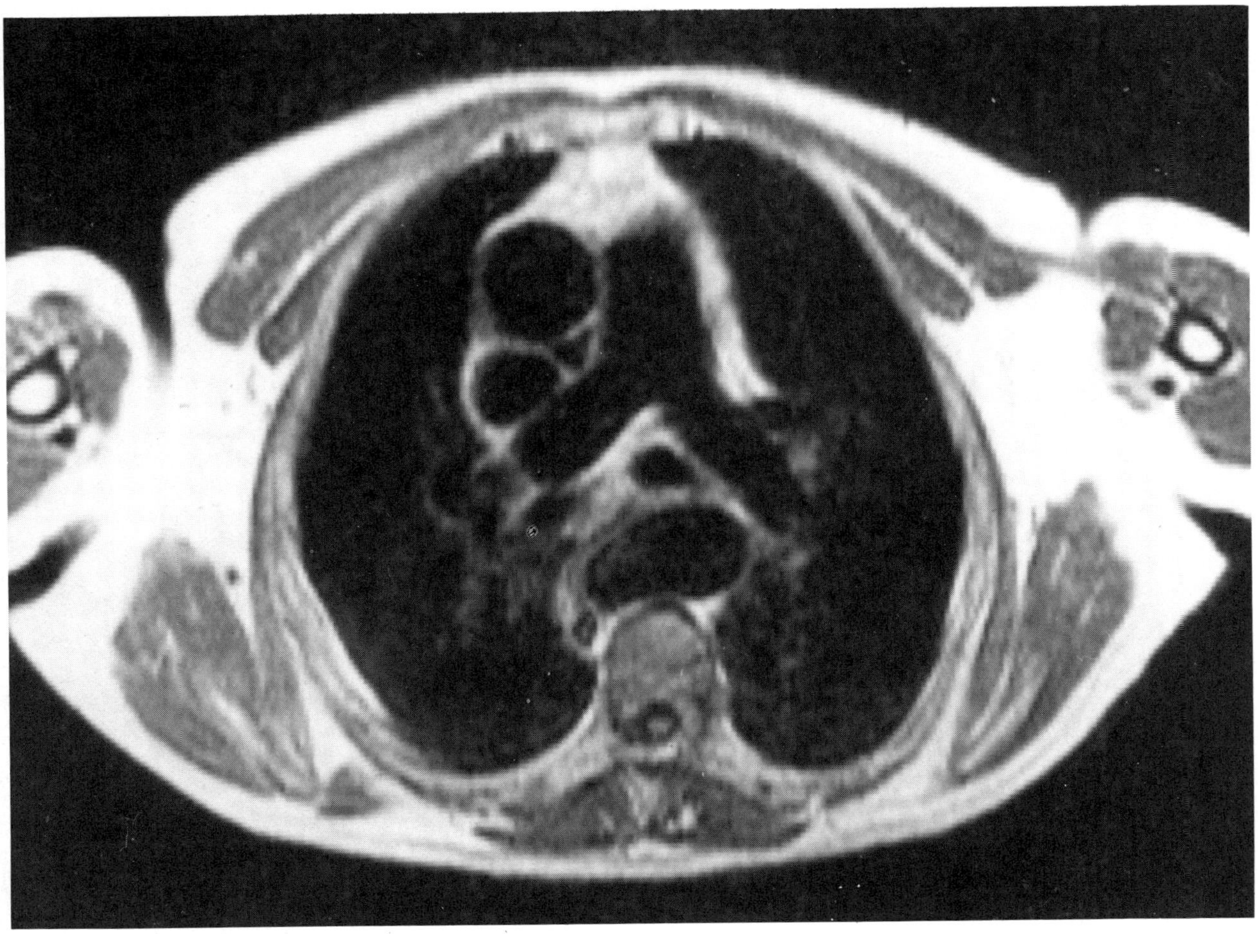

Figure 2.12. Vascular structures very well outlined due to low signal intensity of flowing blood.

fact that if blood flows into an area of the patient under investigation, the hydrogen nuclei arriving at the entrance level have not yet been exposed previously. At this first cross-sectional level they get fully magnetized and they produce a very high signal intensity that is even greater than that from stationary blood (Figure 2.13). Paradoxical enhancement exists whenever flowing blood produces, on an entrance image of a data acquisition sequence, a higher signal intensity than stationary blood (22).

By using different technical parameters, changes in signal intensity from vascular structures may be useful to recognize pathological alterations of blood flow. Slowly flowing blood may be distinguished from stationary blood by the signal intensity variation between the first and the following delayed echos. On the contrary, in cases of slowly flowing blood the signal intensity is usually increasing on the delayed echos.

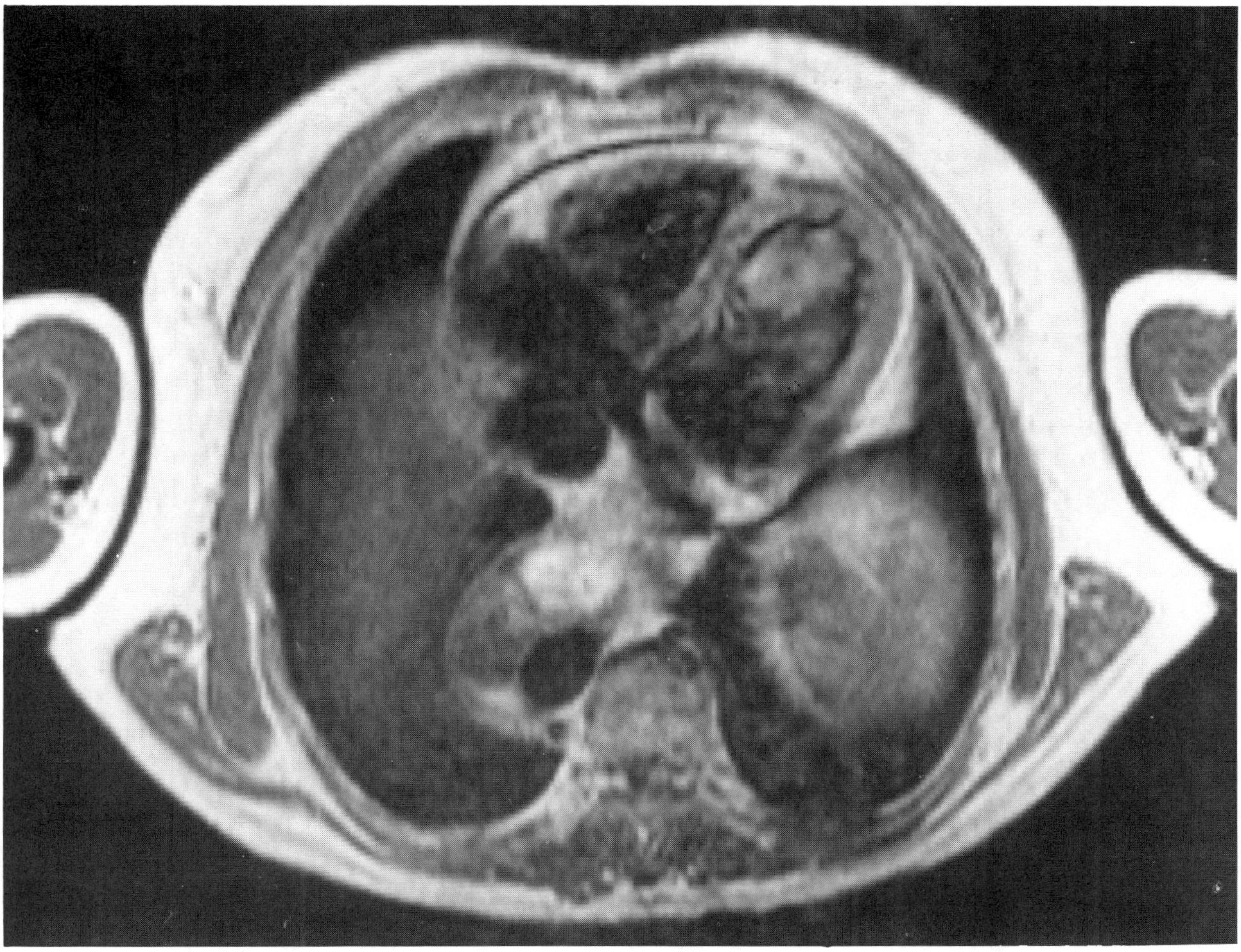

Figure 2.13. Same patient as in Figures 2.11 and 2.12. Obvious dissection of descending aorta outlined on the right side. Aortic pseudolumen contains a high signal intensity and a relatively low signal intensity area due to thrombosis and slowly flowing blood.

It has been stated that by using multi-section sequences, blood flow studies may be performed which allow distinction between arterial and venous blood flow movements (22). Although understanding of MR flow phenomena is still quite incomplete (for instance in cases of flow turbulences), we are, nevertheless, convinced that further advances in this field are likely to occur concomitantly with technical improvements which may be achieved during the upcoming years.

T_1 AND T_2 MEASUREMENTS

Various studies (4, 23, 24, 25) have tried to assess the practical value of T_1 and T_2 measurements. These studies have attempted to apply the principle to specific clinical conditions and find out whether particular measurements could have a diagnostic impact where tissue characterization is concerned.

In vitro and in vivo experiments demonstrated a quite prominent overlap of T_1 and T_2 values. In order to differentiate between malignant and benign lesions, no convincing standard values have been established to enable reliable identification of water, fat, soft tissue, etc. For example, T_2 relaxation time values have been found to be longer for acute inflammatory nodes when compared to those involved by lymphoma or metastases. However, the T_1 values showed overlap in these groups (26).

Studies employing spectroscopic evaluation have postulated that the most probable cause for the overlap in the T_1 and T_2 measurements in various conditions has to be found in the constantly changing water content of the tissues under study (27, 28).

While existent preliminary studies have been based on limited and uneven categories of patients (which makes statistical evaluation not entirely reliable), it is hoped that further technical improvements and larger studies will allow the solving of this particular diagnostic problem.

REFERENCES

1. Cohen AM: Magnetic resonance imaging of the thorax. *Radiol Clin N Am, 22:*829-846, 1984.

2. Cohen MD: Respiratory system and mediastinum. In: *Pediatric Magnetic Resonance Imaging.* Philadelphia: WB Saunders, 1986, pp. 18-33.

3. Higgins CB, Lanzer P, Herfkens R, Botvinik E, Lipton MJ: Cardiovascular system. In: *Clinical Magnetic Resonance Imaging.* San Francisco: Radiology Research and Education Foundation, 1983, pp. 159-184.

4. Ross JS, O'Donovan PB, Novoa R, Mehta A, Buonocore E, MacIntyre WJ, Golish JA, Ahmad M: Magnetic resonance of the chest: Initial experience with imaging and in vivo T1 and T2 calculations. *Radiology, 152:* 95-101, 1984.

5. Tscholakoff D, Higgins CB: Gated magnetic resonance imaging for assessment of cardiac function and myocardial infarction. *Radiol Clin N Am, 23:*449-457, 1985.

6. Webb WR: Magnetic resonance imaging of the chest. In: *Magnetic Resonance Annual 1986,* Kressel HY (Ed.). New York: Raven Press, 1986, pp. 161-176.

7. Aronberg DJ, Glazer HS, Sagel SS: MRI and CT of the mediastinum: Comparisons, controversies and pitfalls. *Radiol Clin N Am, 23:*439-448, 1985.

8. Ehman RL, McNamara MT, Pallack M, Hricak H, Higgins CB: Magnetic resonance imaging with respiratory gating: Techniques and advantages. *AJR, 143:*1175-1182, 1984.

9. O'Donovan PB, Ross JS, Sivak ED, O'Donnell JK, Meaney TF: Magnetic resonance imaging of the thorax: The advantages of coronal and sagittal planes. *AJR, 143:*1183-1188, 1984.

10. Webb WR, Gamsu G, Stark DD, Moore EH: Magnetic resonance imaging of the normal and abnormal pulmonary hila. *Radiology, 152:* 89-94, 1984.

11. Webb WR, Jensen BG, Gamsu G, Sollitto R, Moore EH: Coronal magnetic resonance imaging of the chest: Normal and abnormal. *Radiology, 153:*729-735, 1984.

12. Webb WR, Jensen BG, Gamsu G, Sollitto R, Moore EH: Sagittal MR imaging of the chest: Normal and abnormal. *J Comput Assist Tomogr, 9:* 471-479, 1985.

13. Cohen MD: Construction and interpretation of the magnetic resonance image. In: *Pediatric Magnetic Resonance Imaging.* Philadelphia: WB Saunders, 1986, pp. 4-14.

14. Young IR, Burl M, Bydder GM: Comparative efficiency of different pulse sequences in MR imaging. *J Comput Assist Tomgr, 10:*271-286, 1986.

15. Veiga-Pires JA, Kaiser MC: Preliminary report on a new mode of CT scanning of the thorax. *Comput Tomogr, 4:*139-143, 1980.

16. Veiga-Pires JA, Kaiser MC: Direct coronal mode (DCM) in whole-body CT scanning. *Brit J Radiol, 55:*75-78, 1982.

17. Kaiser MC, Martin DJ: Direct coronal images - a valuable addition to pediatric body CT scanning. *Pediatr Radiol, 12:*295-297, 1982.

18. Kaiser MC, Pettersson H, Harwood-Nash DC, Fitz CR, Armstrong E: Direct coronal CT of the spine in infants and children. *AJNR, 2:*465-466, 1981.

19. Kaiser MC, Veiga-Pires JA, Descamps P, Brihaye C: CT in the diagnostic work up of hypogenetic lung syndrome (HLS) in homozygotic twins. *Fortschr Röntgenstr, 144:*476-478, 1986.

20. Van Waes PFGM, Zonneveld FW: Direct coronal body Computed Tomography. *J Comput Assist Tomogr, 6:*58-66, 1982.

21. Axel L: Blood flow effects in magnetic resonance imaging. *AJR, 143:*1157-1166, 1984.

22. Kaufman L, Sheldon P, Norman D, Bank W, Newton TH: Nuclear magnetic resonance: Principles of blood flow imaging. *AJNR, 4:*1161-1166, 1983.

23. Damadian R, Zaner K, Hor D: Human tumors detected by nuclear magnetic resonance. *Proc Natl Acad Sci USA, 71:*1471-1473, 1979.

24. Lee JKT, Heiken JP, Ling D, *et al.*: Magnetic resonance imaging of abdominal and pelvic lymphadenopathy. *Radiology, 153:*181-188, 1984.

25. Dooms GC, Hricak H, Crooks LE, Higging CB: Magnetic resonance imaging of the lymph nodes: Comparison with CT. *Radiology, 153:*719-728, 1984.

26. Dooms GC, Hricak H, Moseley ME, Bottles K, Fisher M, Higgins CB: Characterization of lymphadenopathy by magnetic resonance relaxation times: Preliminary results. *Radiology, 155:*691-697, 1985.

27. Davis PL, Kaufman L, Crooks LE: Tissue characterization. In: *Clinical Magnetic Resonance Imaging 1983,* Margulis AR, Higgins CB, Kaufman L, and Crooks LE (Eds.). San Francisco: Radiology Research and Education Foundation, pp. 53-77.

28. Webb WR, Gamsu G: Chest. *Ibid.*, pp. 151-152.

Notes

3

Normal Thoracic Anatomy

The radiological image of the human thorax is compiled of numerous structures of various densities. The development of computed tomography over the past decade has allowed these structures to be accurately visualized, especially secondary to the three dimensional imaging ability of this modality.

With the development of MRI, an important addition has been provided to the viewing of the thorax, as MR is able to display anatomy in sagittal and coronal planes supplementary to the transaxial projection, without the need of reformating multiple slices or uncomfortable patient positioning, as in CT.

As explained previously in the chapter dealing with the physical principles of MRI, it is to be expected to receive minimal signal intensity from the pulmonary parenchyma as its density of protons is very low. Contrary to CT, peripheral pulmonary vessels and individual bronchi are seldom seen on MR images. Centrally located pulmonary vessels and bronchi can, however, be identified branching from the hilar region into the pulmonary parenchyma. Coronal images are useful in the depiction of the normal anatomy of this area as they permit visualization of longer sections of bronchi and vessels. While the bronchial and vascular walls produce a relatively high signal intensity on MR images, their inner content mostly gives a low signal intensity due to the low proton content of air and movement of flowing blood.

Starting from the top of the thoracic cavity at the level of the sternal notch in normal subjects, an MR transaxial section through the lung apexes will demonstrate (similar to CT) a number of major mediastinal vessels: the carotid arteries, the jugular veins and the subclavian arteries (Figure 3.1). On MR images, vessels extending to the neck are easily visualized and separated from adjacent fat, muscle and lymph nodes present in this area. The excellent contrast resolution and absence of streak artifacts make MRI a better modality than CT for the study of vascular structures at the thoracic inlet.

In this area, the trachea, although presenting the same low signal intensity as the vessels, can be easily identified by its size and central location. Anteriorly and laterally to the trachea extends the thyroid gland which can sometimes be recognized by its intermediate signal intensity, being less intense than fat and more intense than the air-filled trachea. The esophagus can be identified posteriorly to the trachea as a round structure which sometimes contains air within its lumen.

On both sides of the sternal notch are the medial heads of the clavicles, and posteriorly to them, the sternothyroid muscles can be seen. MRI is of limited value in the demonstration of bony structure, however, it has a great ability in delineating muscular anatomy.

In this area, as in various locations around the thoracic cage, muscle groups are recognized by their intermediate signal intensity, separated by adipose tissue of high signal intensity (Figure 3.2). The fascial tissue surrounding main muscular groups may be recognized sometimes on MR images by its low signal intensity. Also of low signal intensity are the cortical bone of the thoracic vertebrae along with their bodies and posterior elements (the same as the cortical bone of the thoracic ribs).

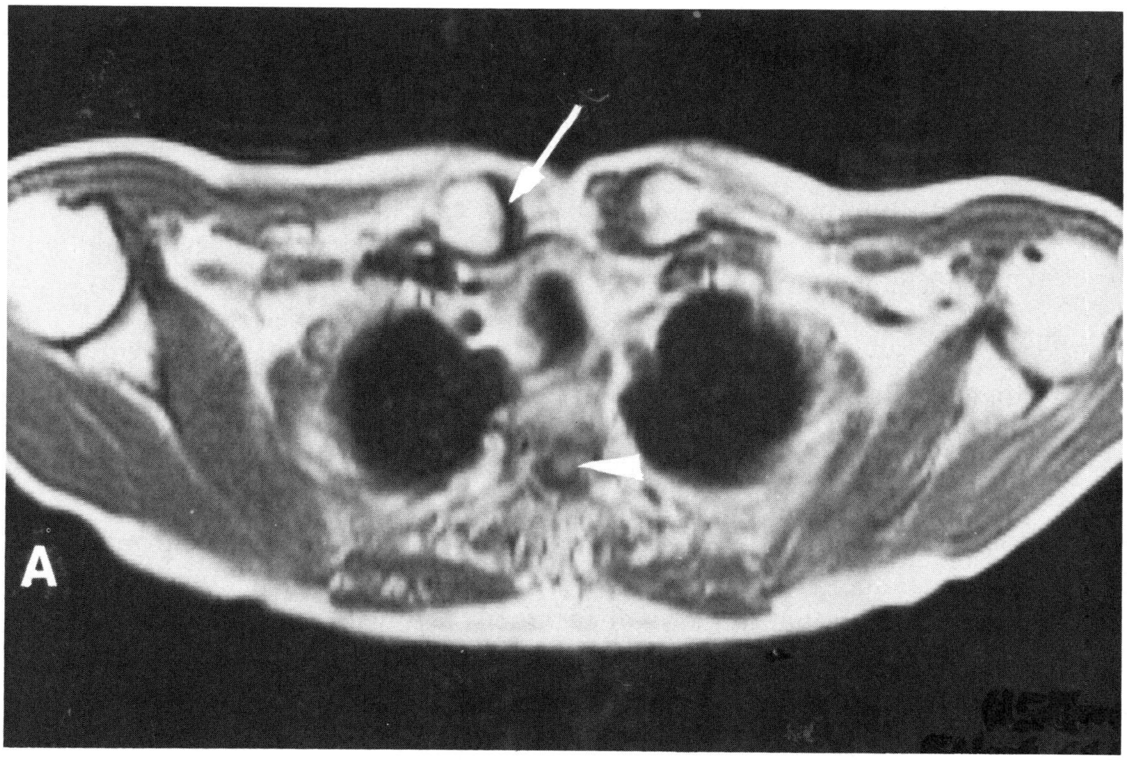

Figure 3.1 (A,B,C). CT and MRI similar transaxial sections at the level of the sternal notch demonstrate major mediastinal vessels, the carotid arteries (c), the jugular veins (jg) and the subclavian arteries (sc). The trachea (T) is recognized both on CT and MRI by its size and central location. On MRI section, the spinal cord (arrowhead) is seen surrounded by low signal intensity cerebrospinal fluid. Low signal cortical bone (long arrow) is surrounding high signal bone marrow.

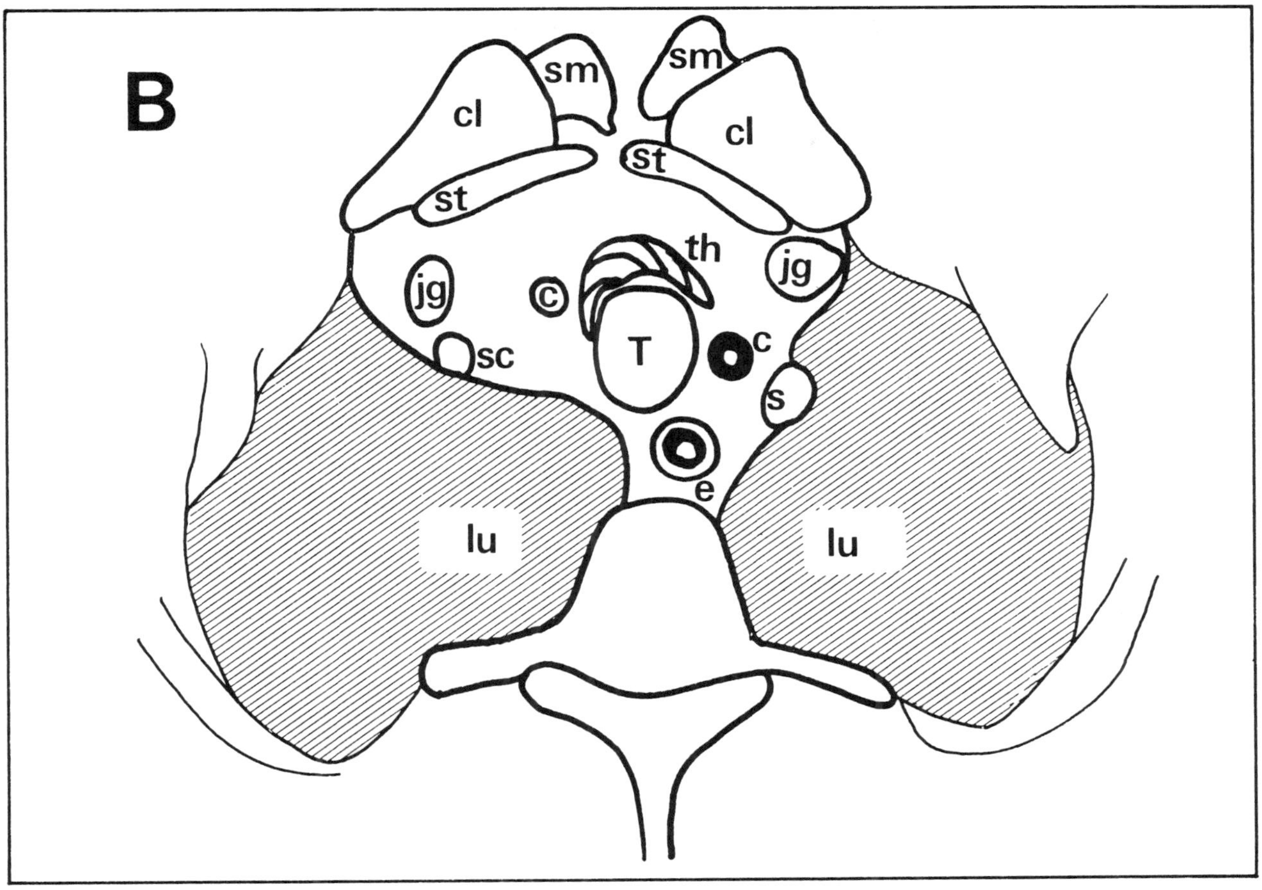
B
sm
sm
cl
cl
st
st
th
jg
jg
©
c
T
sc
s
e
lu
lu

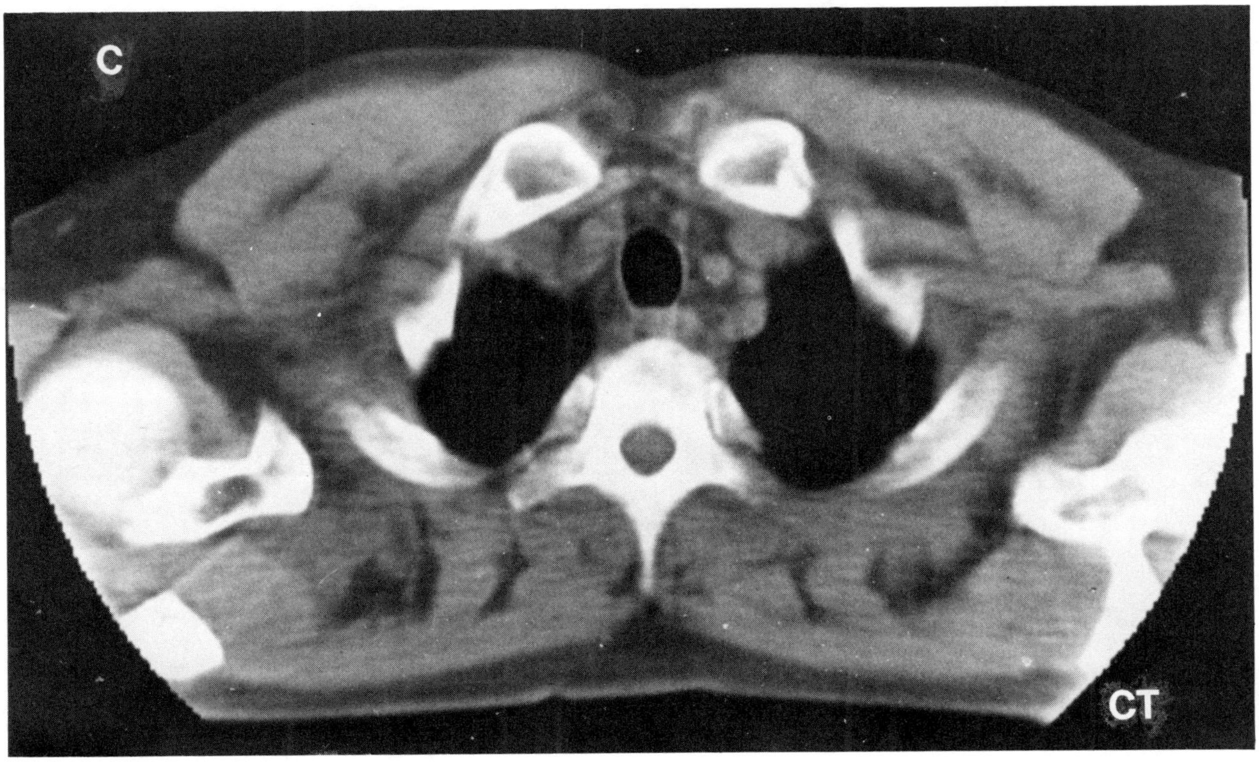
C
CT

The low signal intensity cortical bone can be seen surrounding bone marrow, the intensity of which is high and similar to fat, while the spinal cord is recognized by its intermediate signal intensity and surrounding it, the low-intensity cerebrospinal fluid is clearly visualized (Figure 3.1).

Within the sternal notch two small symmetrical structures represent the anterior branch of the jugular vein. Laterally on both sides, are the heads of the sterncleidomastoid muscles.

On the next lower level, at the sternoclavicular junction, five vessels can usually be identified on both sides of the trachea: the right brachiocephalic vein, the braciocephalic artery, the left carotid artery, the left subclavian artery, and the left brachiocephalic vein. The last one can be commonly seen at a lower level crossing the midline to join the right brachiocephalic vein and form the superior vena cava. Among these vessels, the largest one is usually the brachiocephalic artery and the smallest one, the left carotid artery (Figure 3.2).

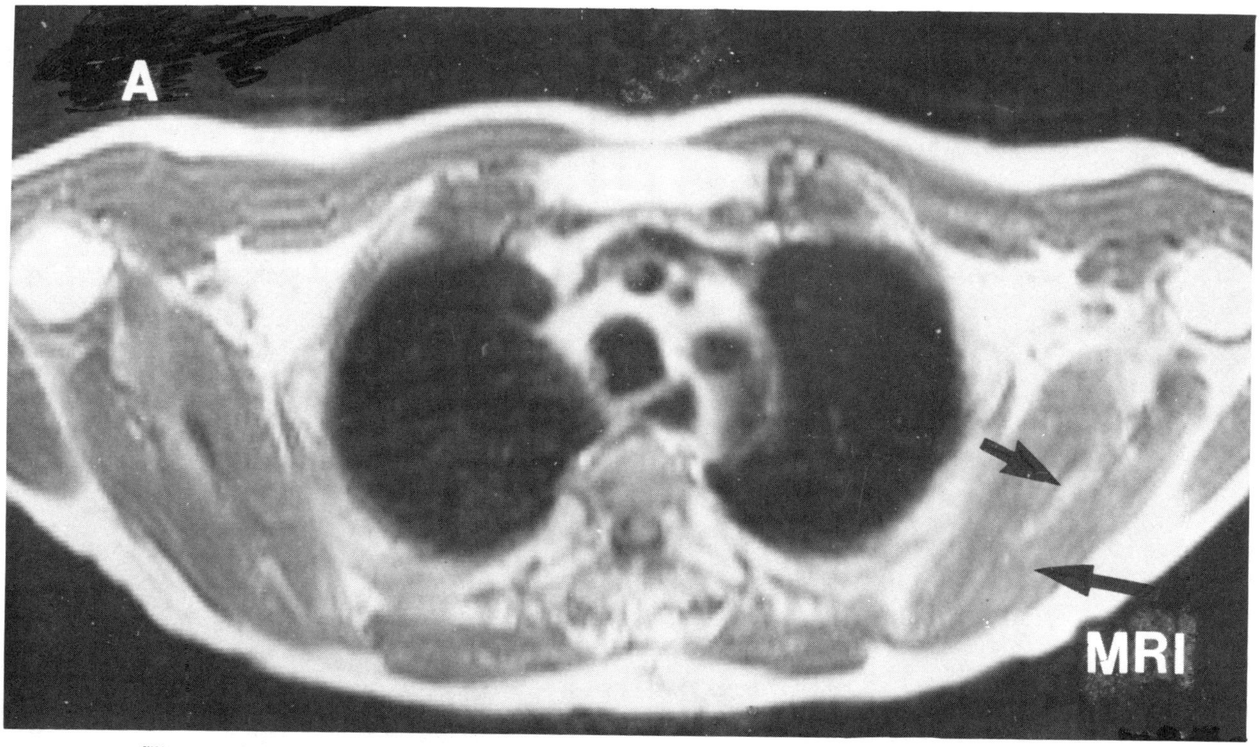

Figure 3.2 (A,B,C). At the level of the sternoclavicular junction, the left brachiocephalic vein (bcv) can be seen crossing the midline to join the right brachiocephalic vein (rb) and form the superior vena cava. Other vessels, clearly identified on CT and MRI sections are the small left carotid artery (c) and the larger brachiocephalic artery. The esophagus (e) is identified posteriorly to the trachea containing variable amounts of air. Muscle groups (large arrows) are recognized on MR images by their intermediate signal intensity separated by adipose tissue of high signal intensity.

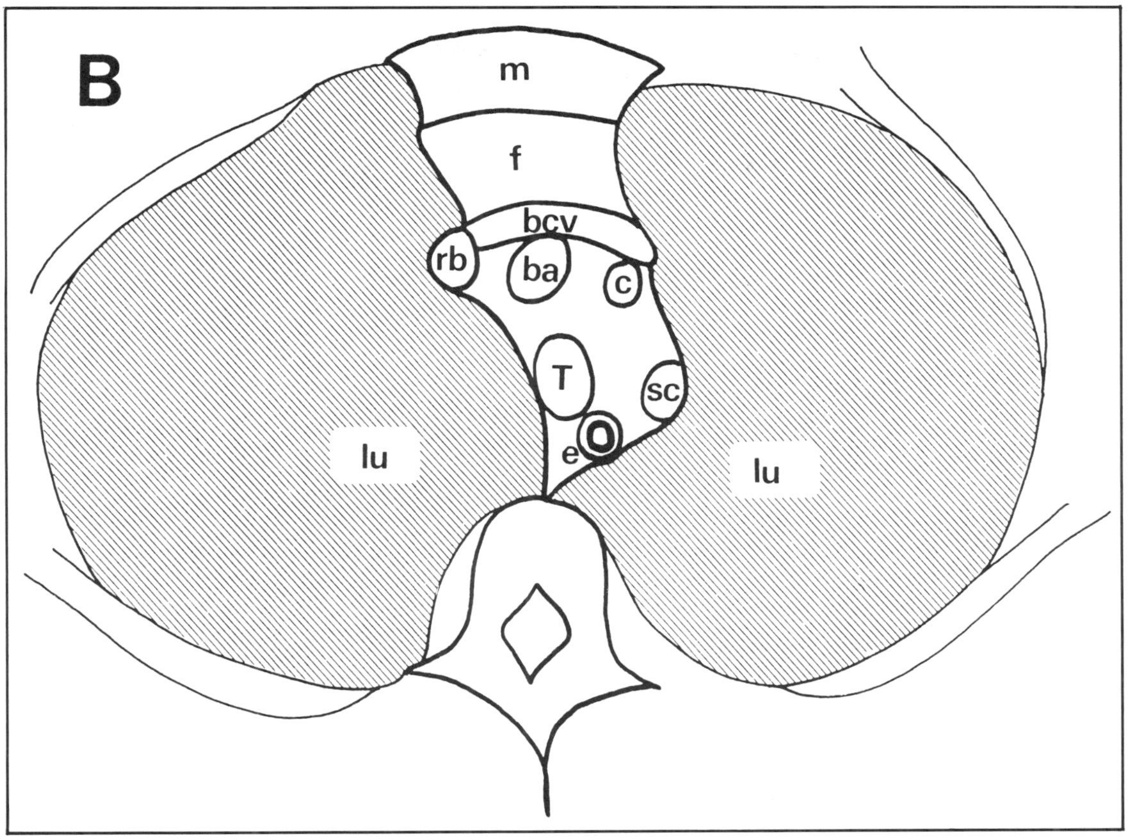
B
m
f
bcv
rb
ba
c
T
sc
e
O
lu
lu

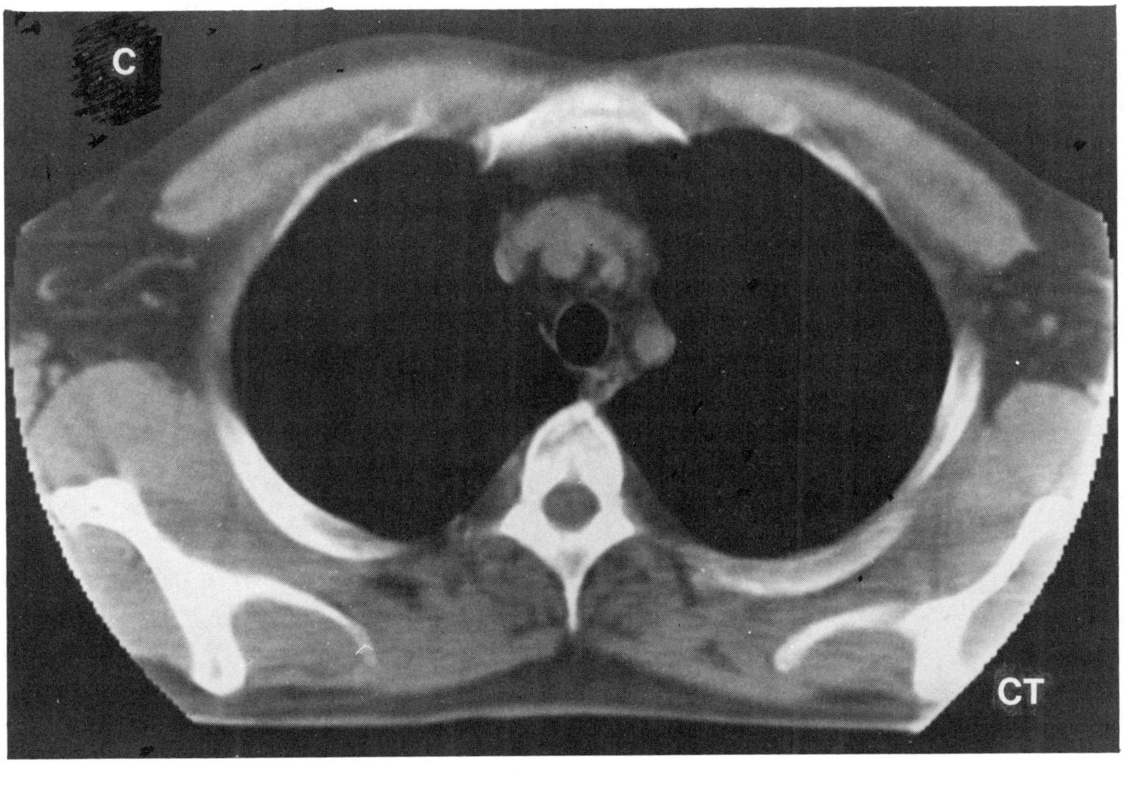
C
CT

At the level of the aortic arch,spin-echo images clearly depict the arch itself and the superior vena cava. In some cases, the azygos vein arch can be seen as high as this level laterally to the trachea and the esophagus. Usually, the lung will then be seen penetrating medially to the azygos vein adjacent to the postero-lateral tracheal wall and the posterior side of the superior vena cava (Figure 3.3).

Caudad to the level of the aortic arch, the ascending and descending aorta can be identified separately. The azygos vein advances at this level anteriorly to enter the superior vena cava in its posterior aspect. At the left of the large distal trachea is the aortic pulmonic window in which high signal intensity fat and moderate signal intensity lymph nodes can be identified.

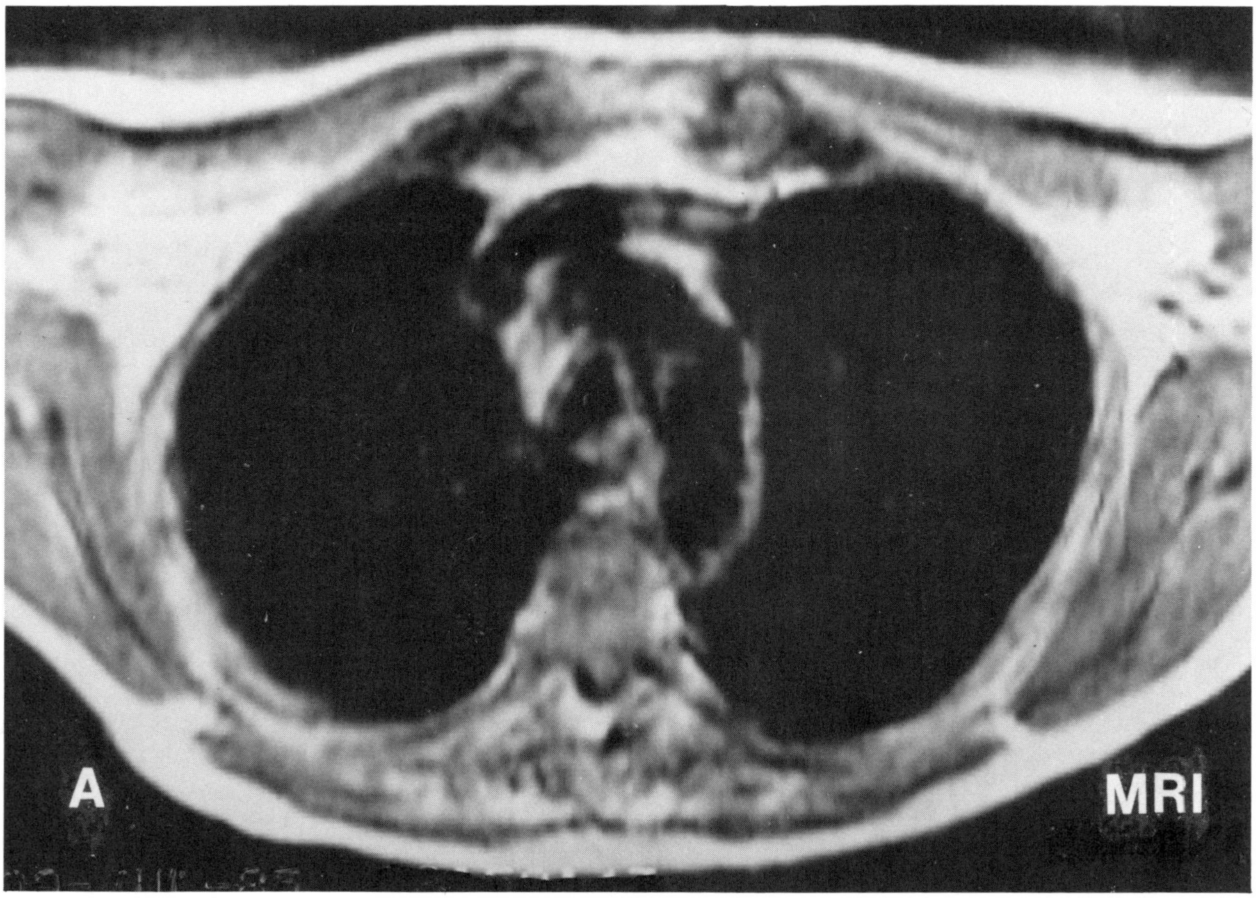

Figure 3.3 (A,B,C). At the level of the aortic arch, spin-echo images (3.3A) clearly depict the arch itself and the superior vena cava.

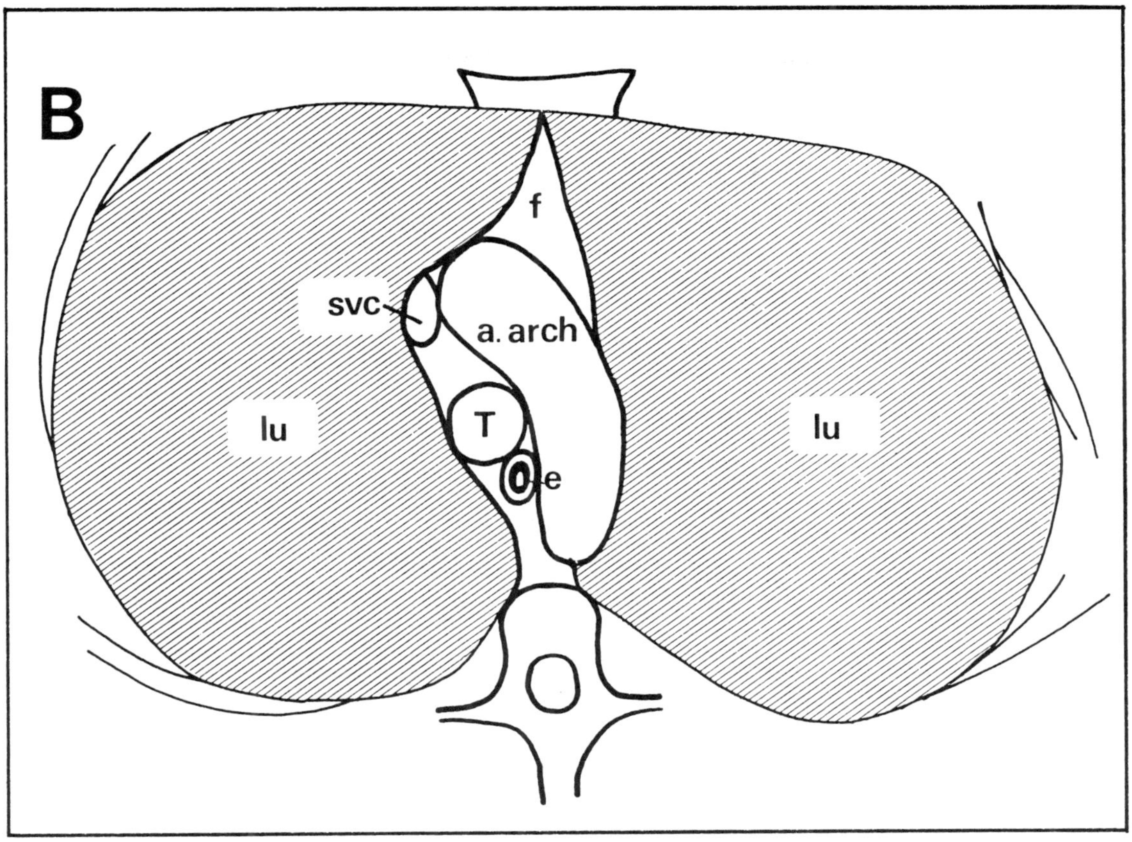
B
f
svc
a. arch
T
lu
lu
e

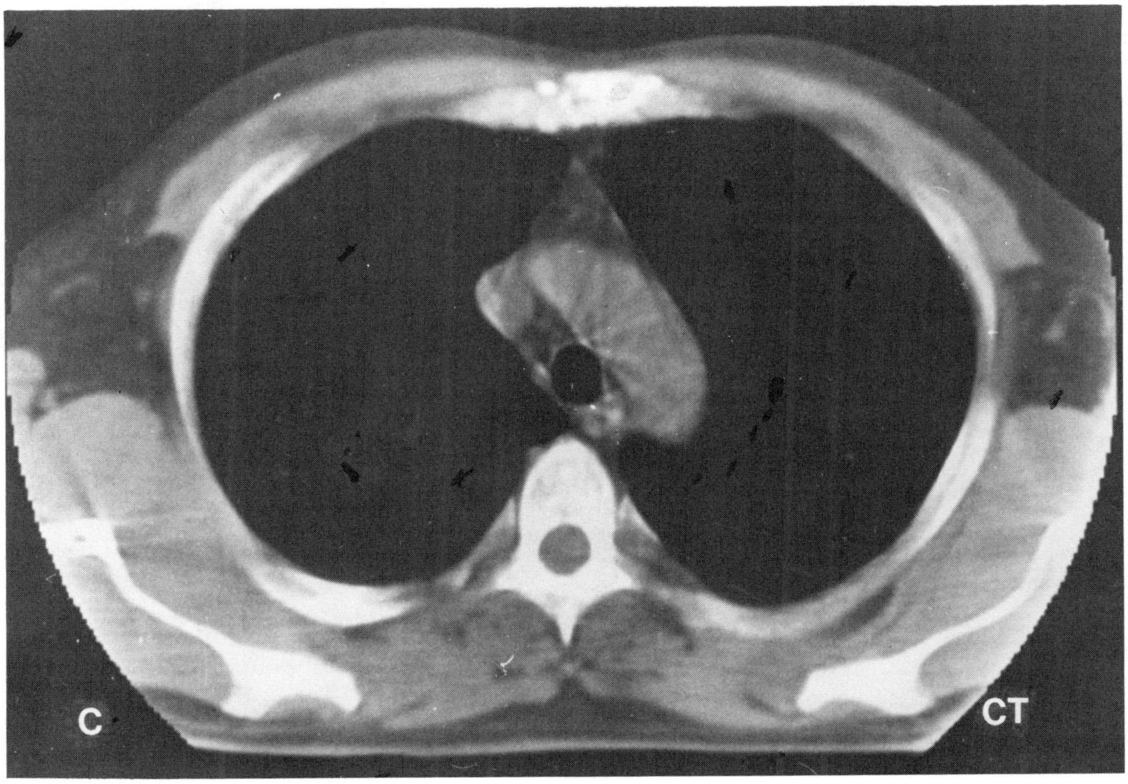
C
CT

The immediate lower level brings up the left pulmonary artery anteriorly to the left main stem bronchus, which is usually clearly seen on spin-echo images. At the same level, additional vascular structures can be recognized, such as the ascending and descending aorta, the superior vena cava, and the right upper lobe pulmonary artery or truncus anterior. In most of the cases, a moderate amount of high signal intensity mediastinal fat can be seen surrounding the vessels (Figure 3.4).

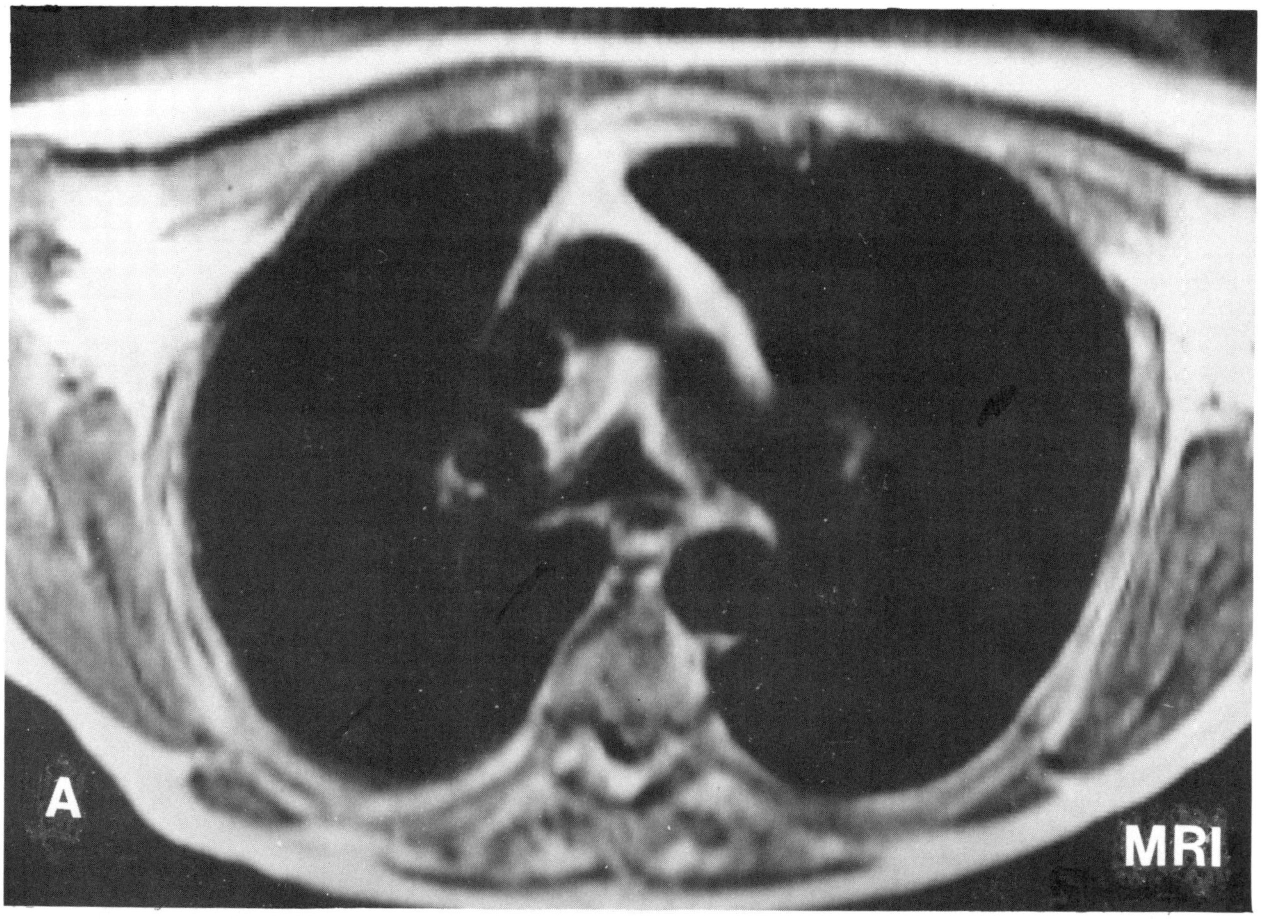

Figure 3.4 (A,B,C). Transaxial CT and MRI sections at the level of the left pulmonary artery (LPla) demonstrate also the ascending and descending aorta (AA, DA), the superior vena cava (svc) and the right upper lobe pulmonary artery or truncus anterior (ta). Notice the extremely well delineation of low signal vascular lumen on the MR image.

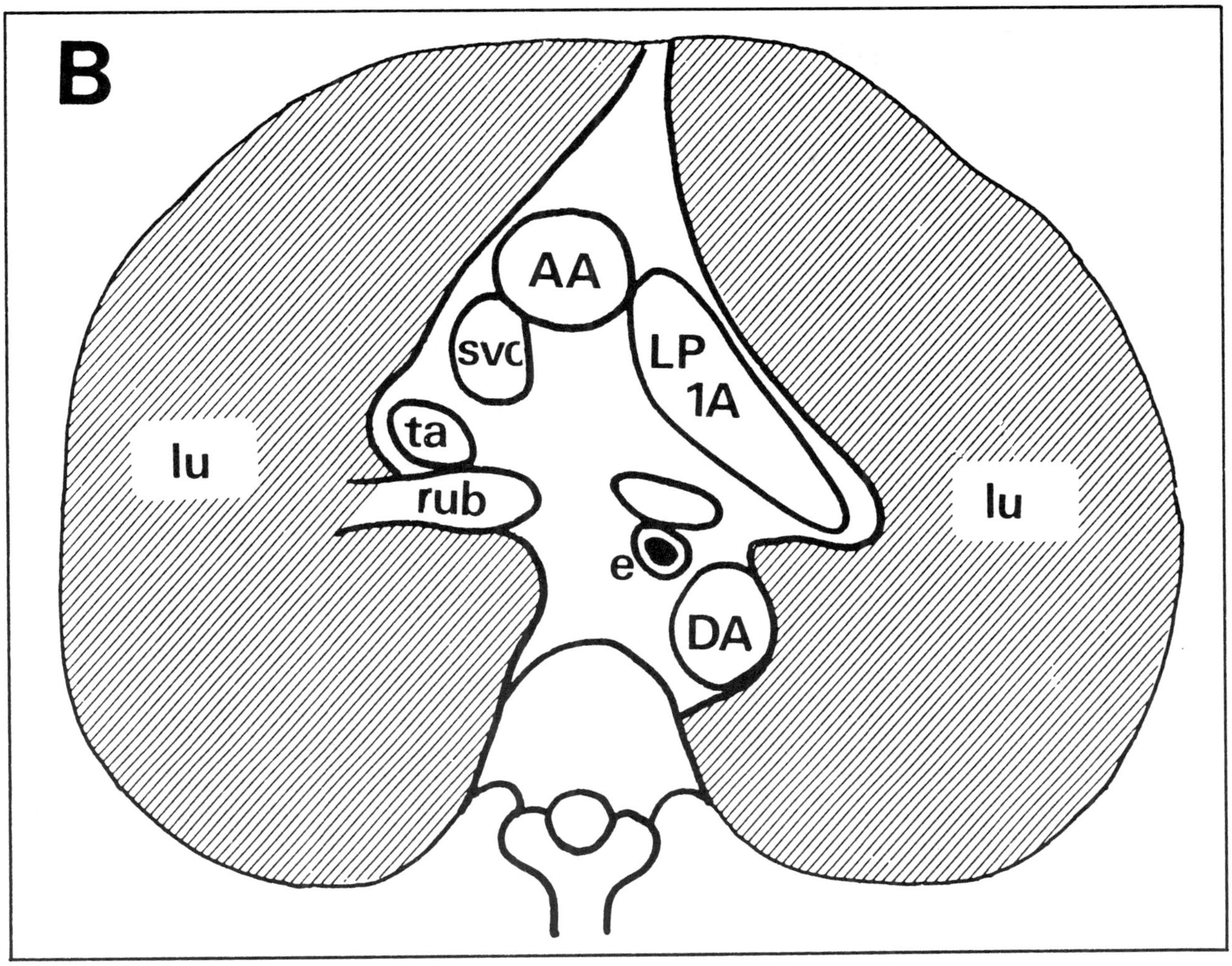
B
AA
svc
LP
1A
ta
lu
rub
lu
e
DA

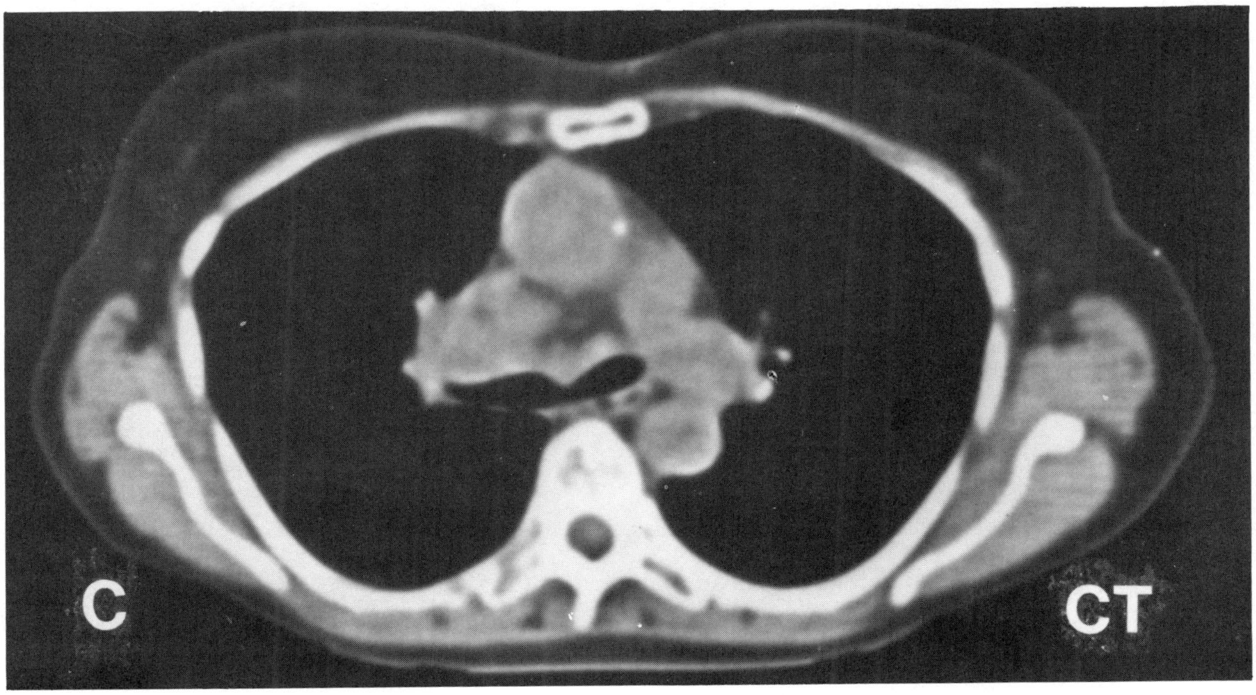
C
CT

On a more inferior MR section, the right pulmonary artery can be seen as it runs to the right, from the main pulmonary artery, anteriorly to the bronchus intermedius and behind the superior vena cava. Posteriorly to the bronchus intermedius, the lung forms the azygoesophageal recess (Figure 3.5).

While the distribution pattern of the pulmonary arteries is quite constant, a variable number of pulmonary veins are draining the upper and lower pulmonary lobes on each side converging into two large major veins that enter the mediastinum anteriorly and below the pulmonary arteries.

The right superior pulmonary vein can be identified as it runs laterally to the anterior segmental bronchus of the right upper lobe, more precisely, at the bifurcation of the right upper lobe bronchus into anterior and posterior segmental bronchi. In a section through the middle lobe bronchus, while it bifurcates into the lateral and medial segmental bronchi, the right superior pulmonary vein is commonly visualized just next to the medial segmental bronchus and the middle bronchus.

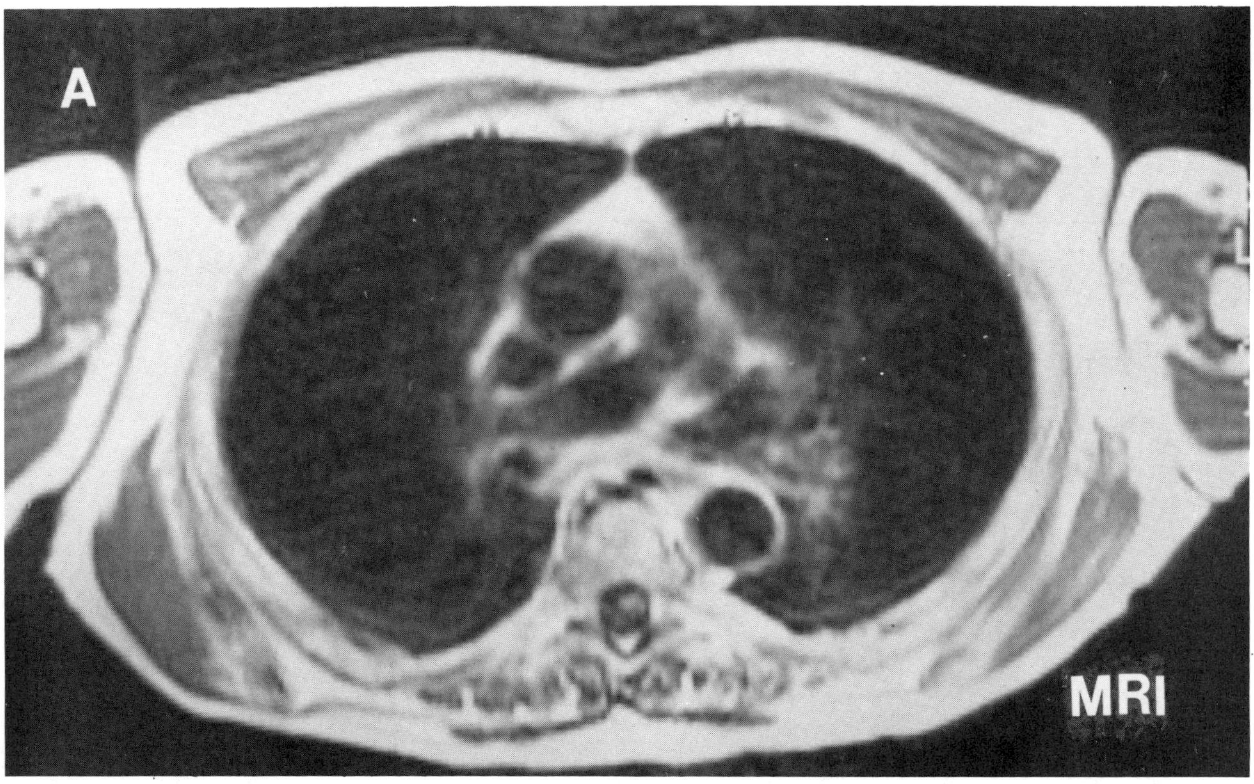

Figure 3.5 (A,B,C). At the level of the right pulmonary artery (RP1A), the vessel can be seen clearly on MR image, emerging from the main pulmonary artery (MPA) anteriorly to the bronchus intermedius (bi) and posteriorly to the superior vena cava.

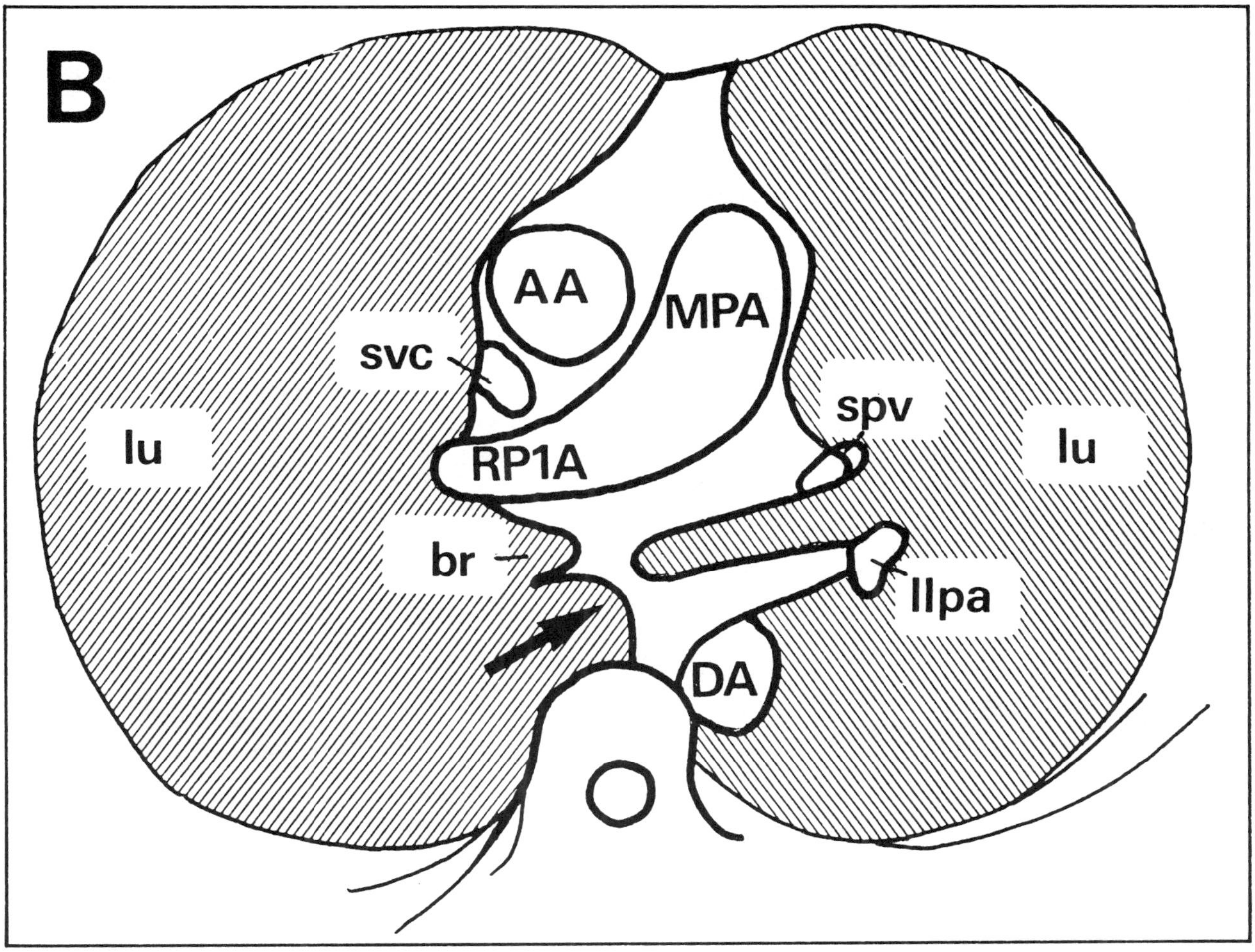
B
AA
MPA
svc
spv
lu
lu
RP1A
br
llpa
DA

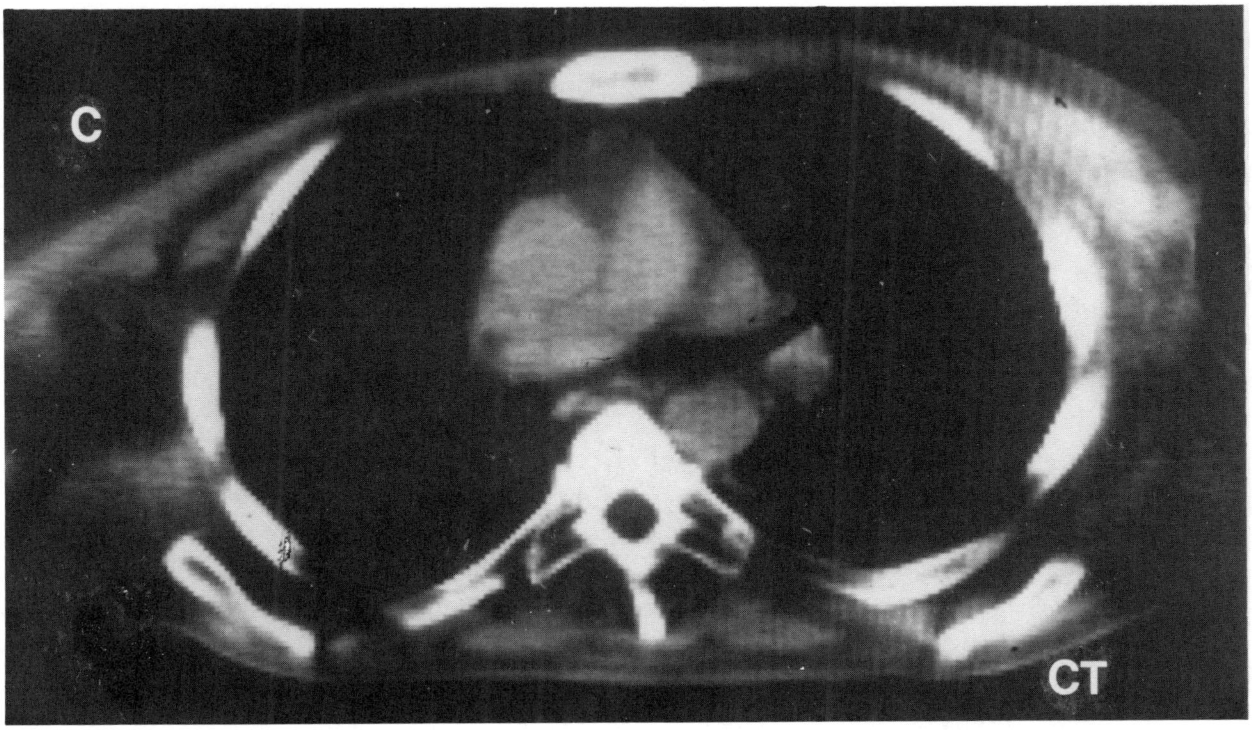
C
CT

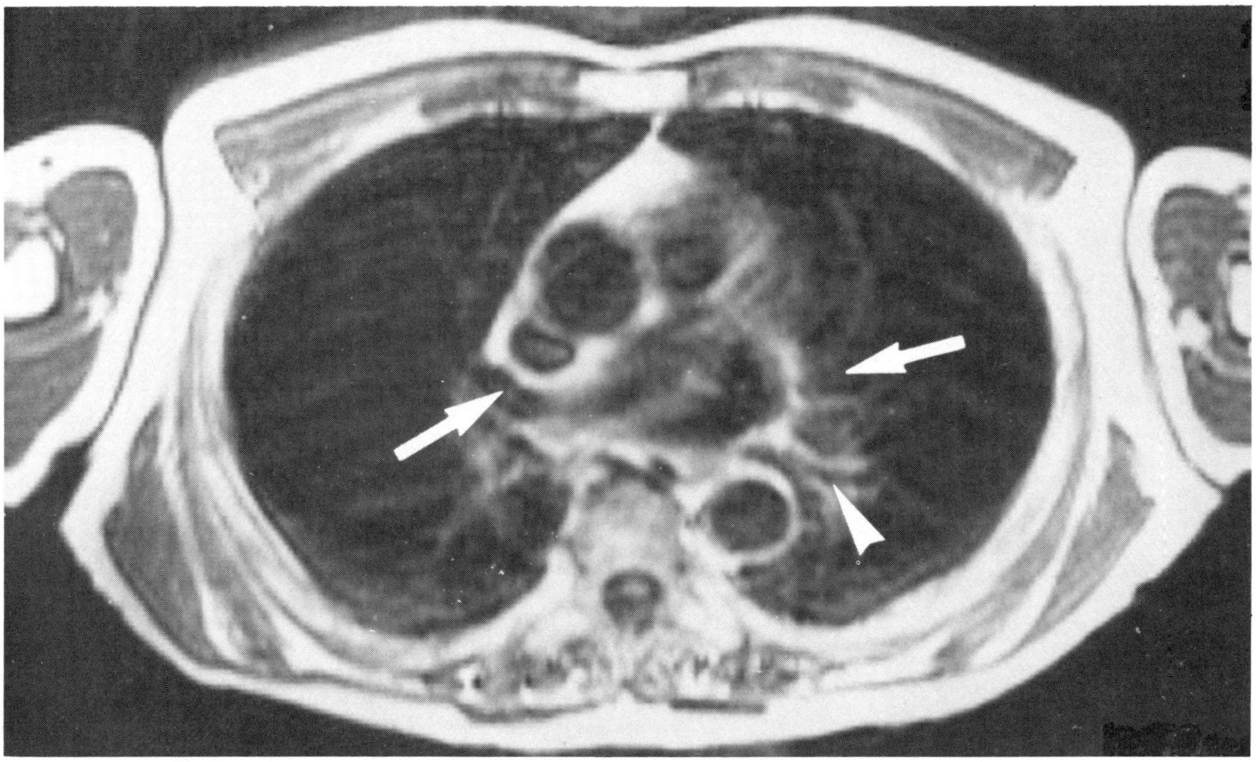

Figure 3.6. MR imaging through bronchus intermedius demonstrates the superior pulmonary vein on the right (large white arrow) and on the left, the pulmonary vein (large white arrow) is visible anterior to the descending pulmonary artery (arrowhead).

The right inferior pulmonary vein is also usually clearly identified on normal MR images, located medially to the basilar segmental bronchi and coursing horizontally towards the left atrium. At the level of the carina, on the left side, the superior pulmonary vein can be found as it lies medially to the left upper lobe pulmonary artery and borders anteriorly the left upper lobe bronchus. As a rule, only pulmonary veins close to the mediastinum and the left atrium seem to be routinely demonstrated on MR images (Figures 3.6 and 3.7).

The use of coronal and sagittal planes in MR imaging seems to bring an important addition to the anatomic display of the thorax, not only by their similarity to the conventional PA and lateral radiographic views of the chest, but mainly by their ability to visualize longer segments of major vessels and bronchi, allowing an accurate assessment of their very important and constant relationships (4, 7, 8, 9). With coronal and sagittal imaging, hilar and mediastinal structures are depicted while the cardiac chambers are accurately visualized and their relation to the surrounding mediastinal organs is clearly delineated (10) (Figure 3.8 and 3.9).

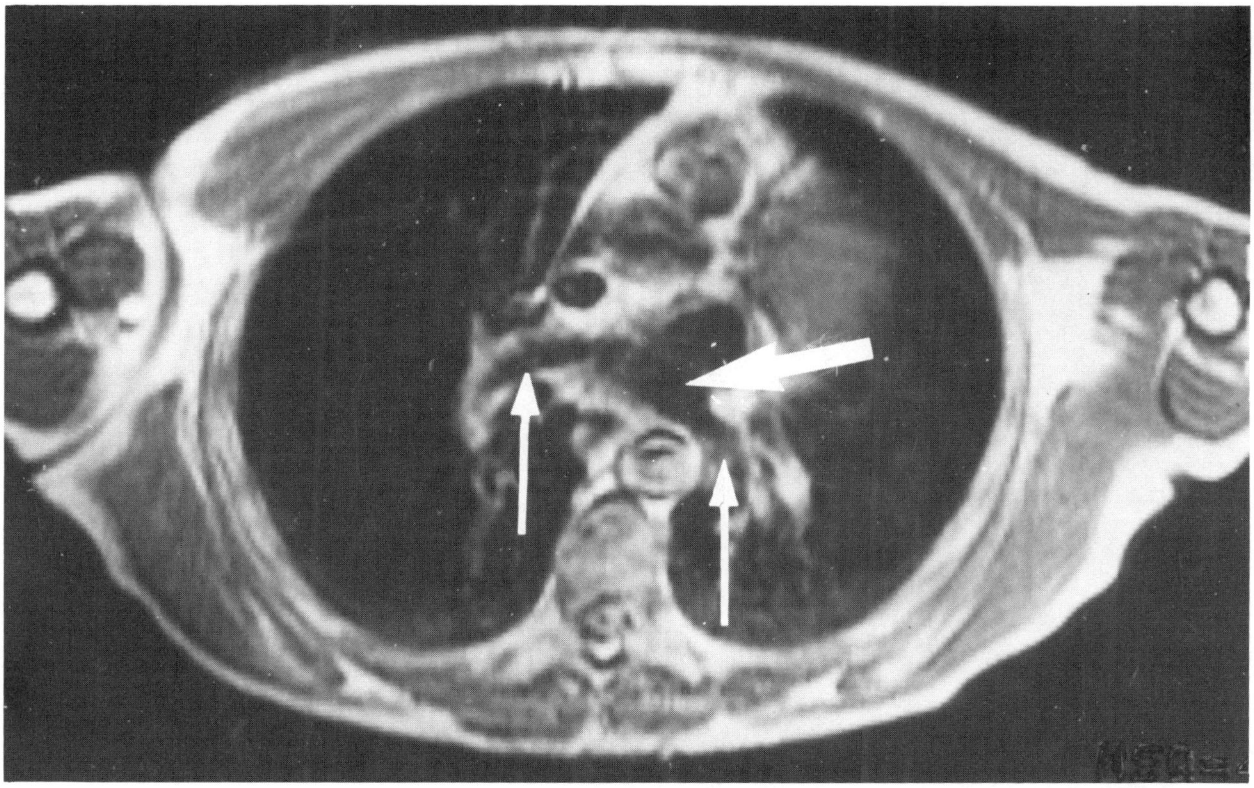

Figure 3.7. Normal MR image through the lower lobe bronchi. On the right, the bronchus intermedius is medial to the descending pulmonary artery. The left descending pulmonary artery is lateral to the lower lobe bronchus. The superior pulmonary veins (narrow arrows) enter the left atrium (large arrow) from both sides.

While MRI seems to be a reliable method in demonstrating enlarged lymph nodes at various sites in the mediastinum, easily separating them from the low signal intensity within the vascular lumen, normal-sized lymph glands are seldom identified on spin-echo images. In fact, the lack of signal from the flowing blood brings to the visualization of pulmonary hila which are composed of vascular and bronchial markings and some fat.

Normal pleura, located along the thoracic wall is not identifiable on routine MR images of the thorax. The identification of a zone of a relatively signal-free pulmonary parenchyma adjacent to the expected location of a pulmonary fissure has been described (4) and represents possibly the only manner to recognize this anatomical detail on MR images.

Good quality spin-echo images commonly allow the demonstration of the thymus gland which although appearing to be the largest in the neonate period, due to the small chest size, increases its proportions and reaches its maximum volume at puberty.

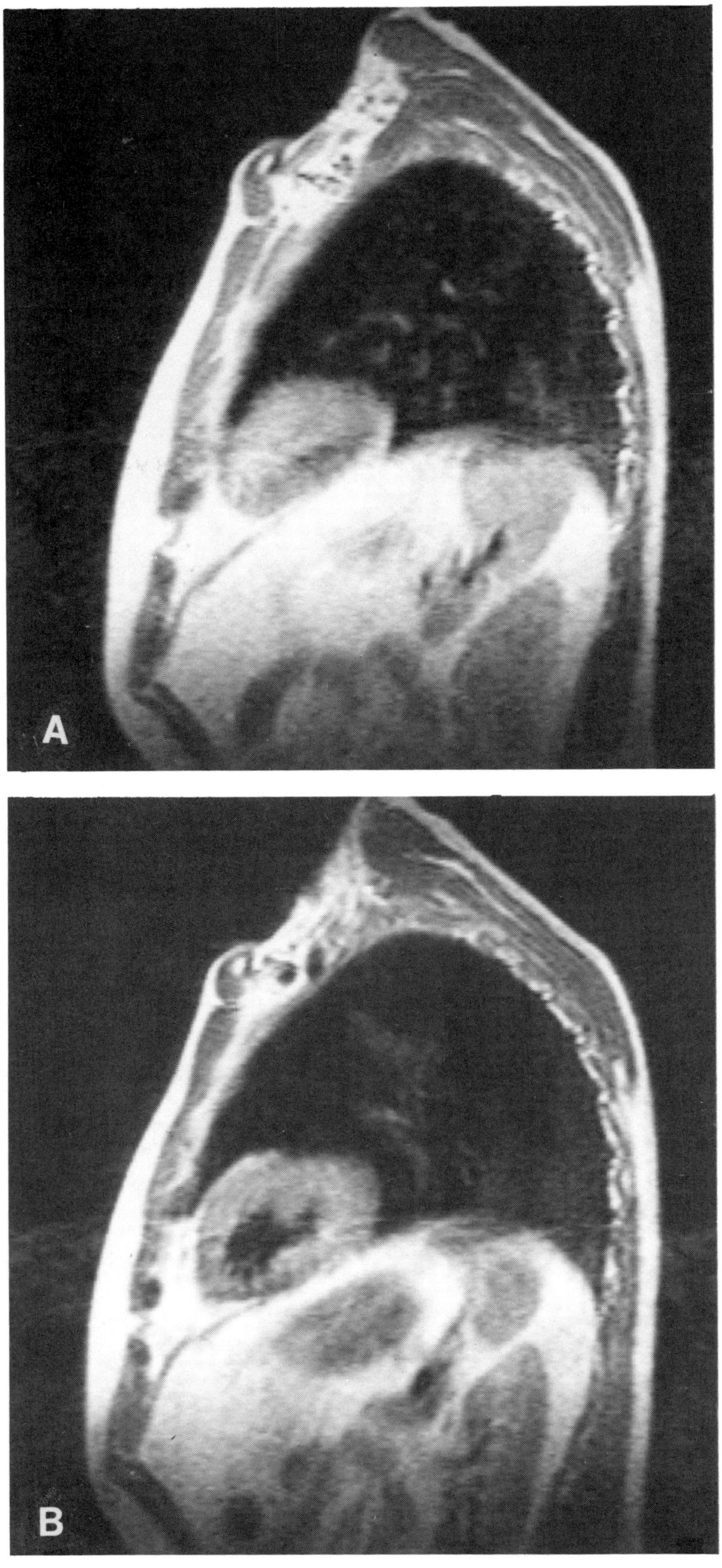

Figure 3.8 (A-K). Consecutive sagittal SE 3000/32 scans in a normal thorax from (A) to (K) accurately demonstrate normal hilar and mediastinal structures.

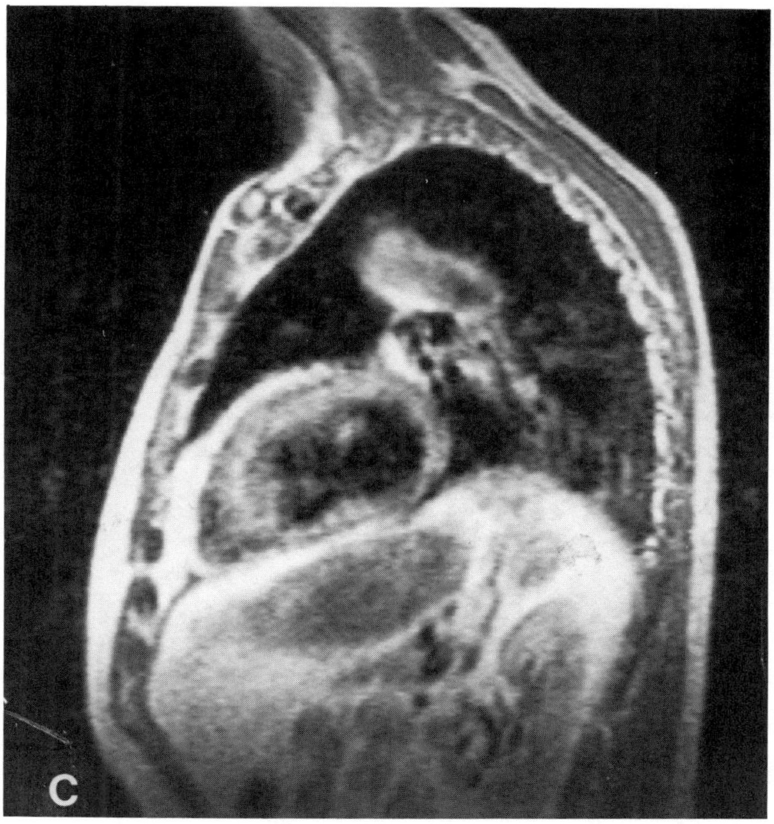

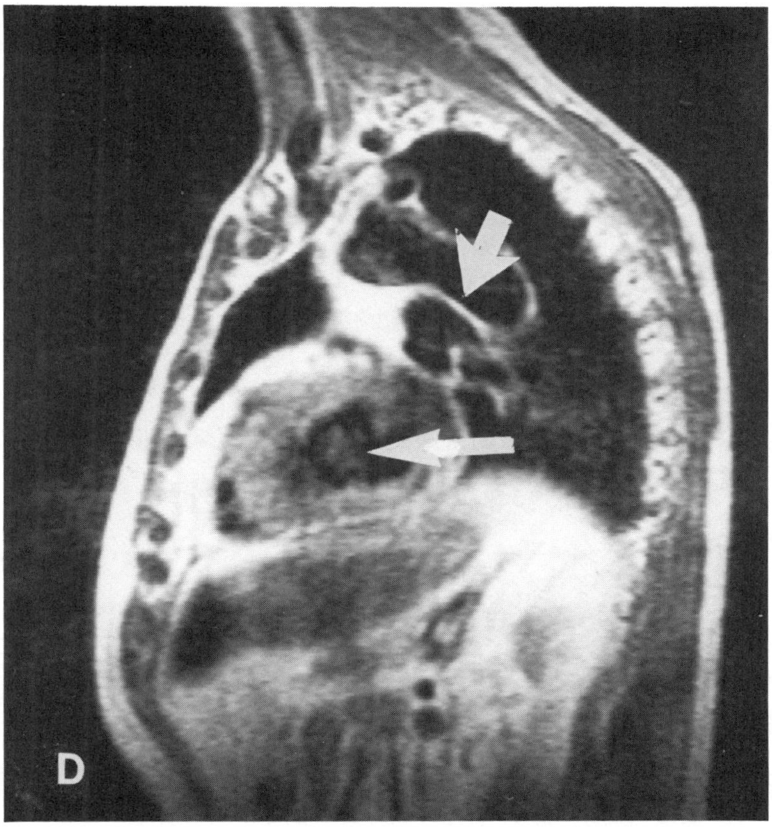

(D) left ventricle (narrow arrow), aorta (large arrow).

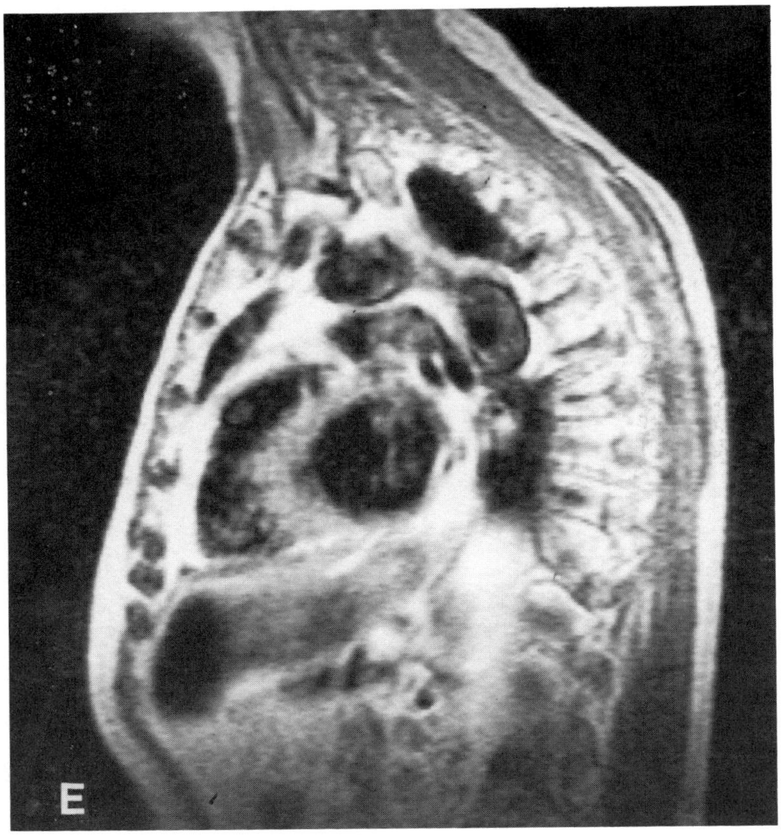

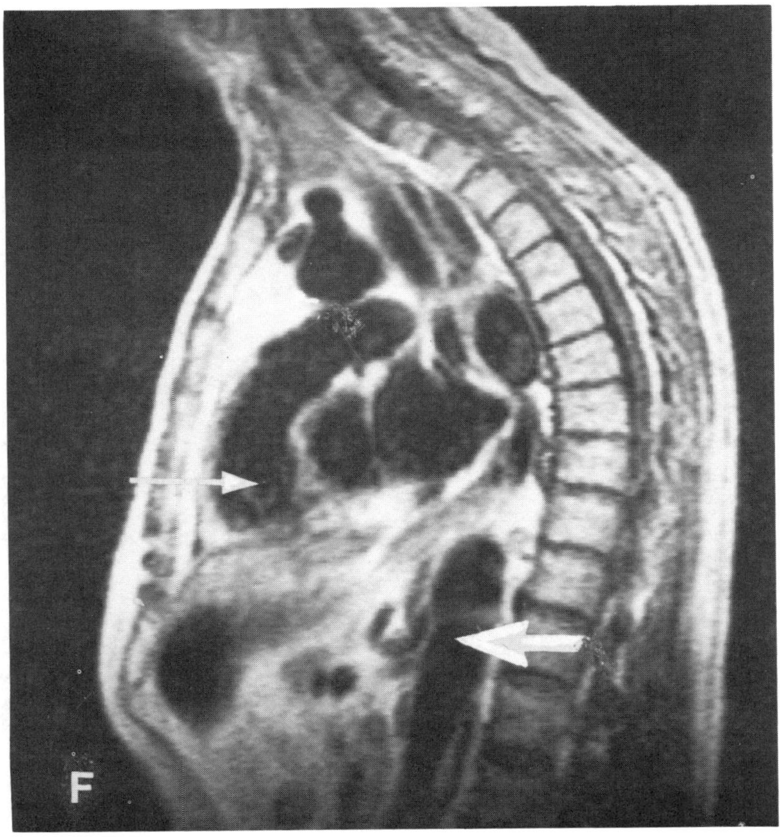

(F) right ventricle (small arrow), abdominal aorta (large arrow).

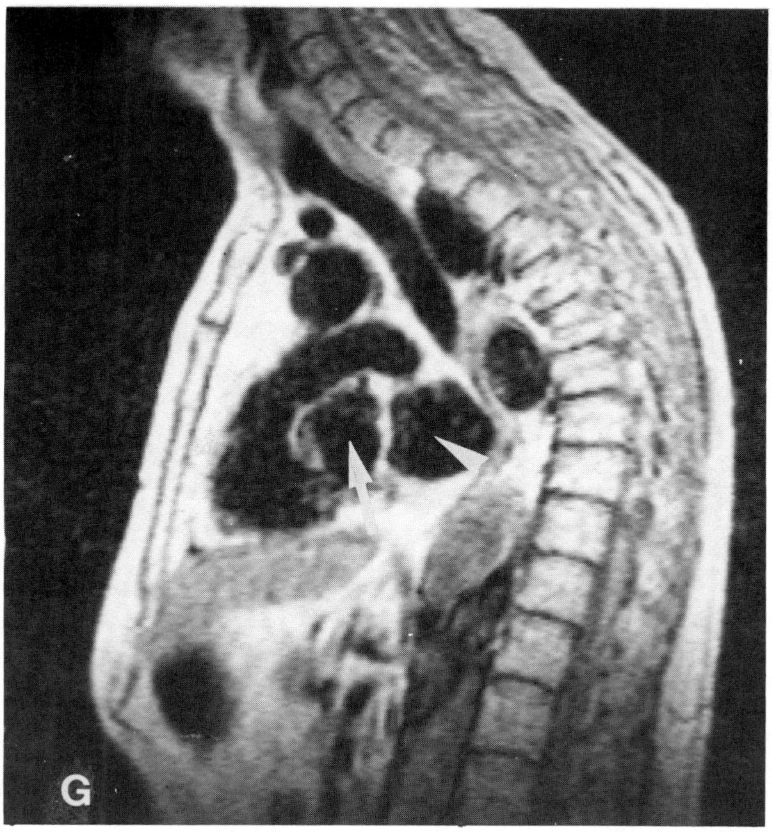

(G) left atrium (arrowhead), left ventricle (arrow).

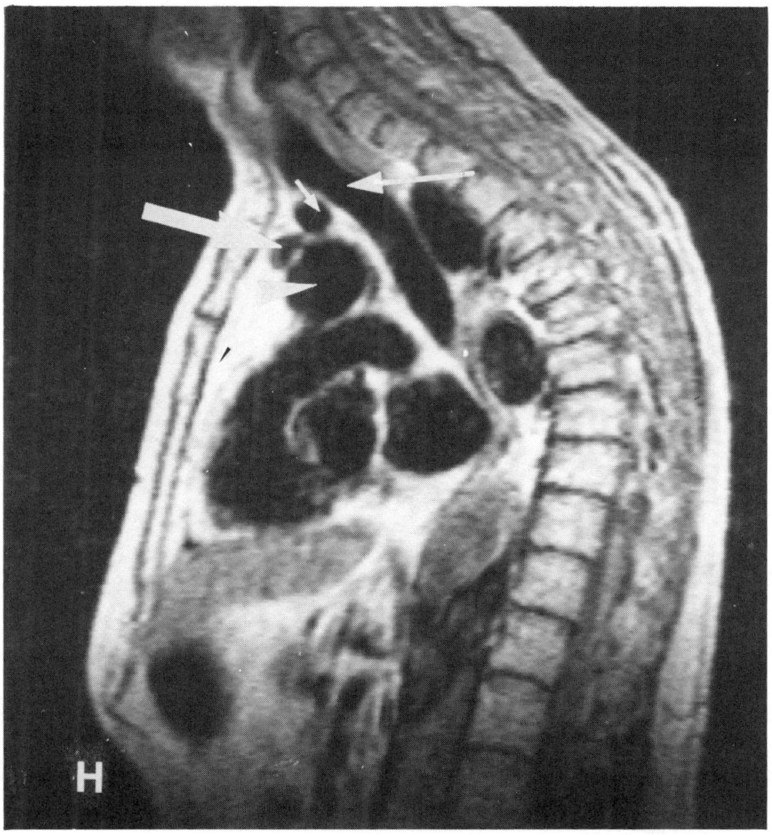

(H) trachea (long arrow), ascending aorta (arrowhead), innominate artery (small arrow), left brachiocephalic vein (wide arrow).

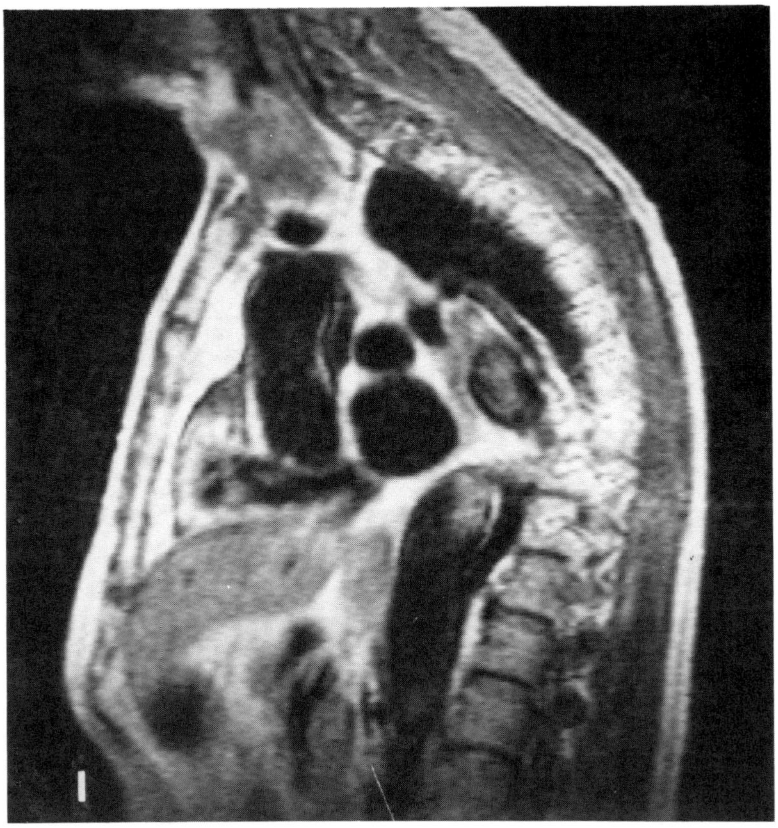
I

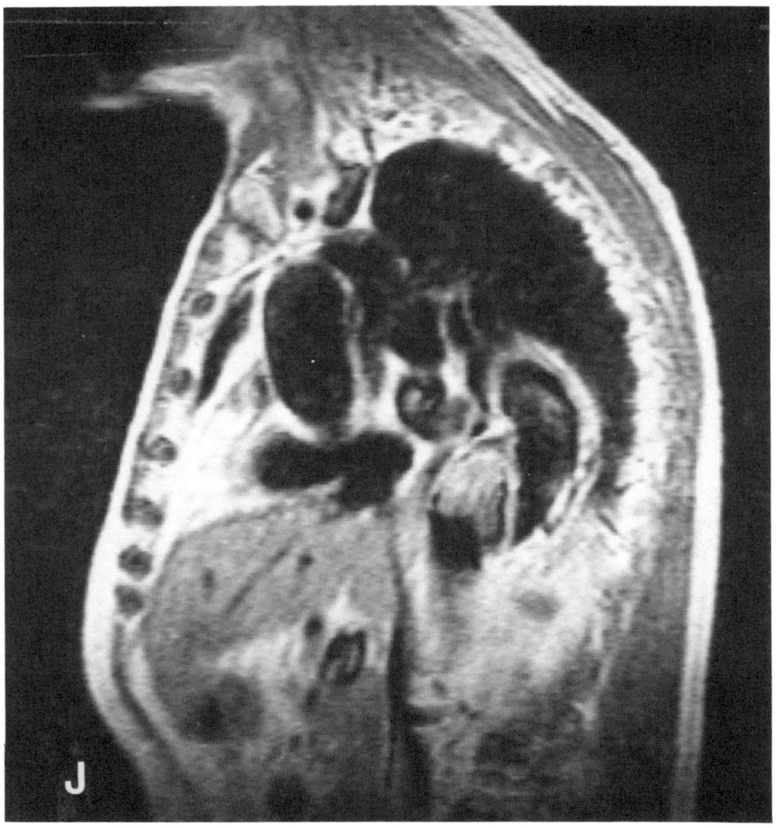
J

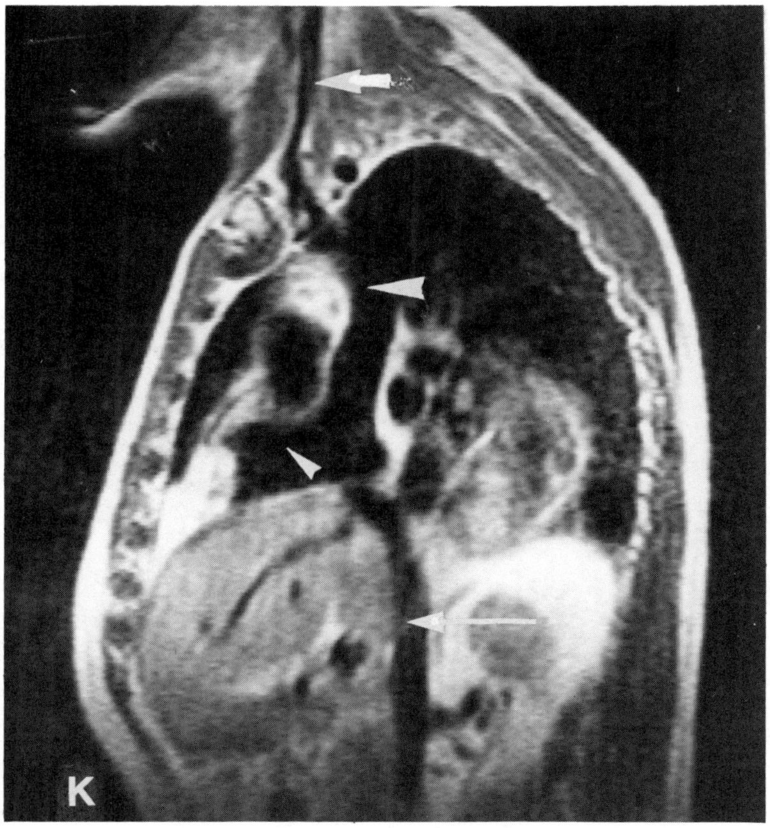

(K) inferior vena cava (narrow arrow), superior vena cava (arrowhead), brachiocephalic trunk (short arrow), right atrium (small arrowhead).

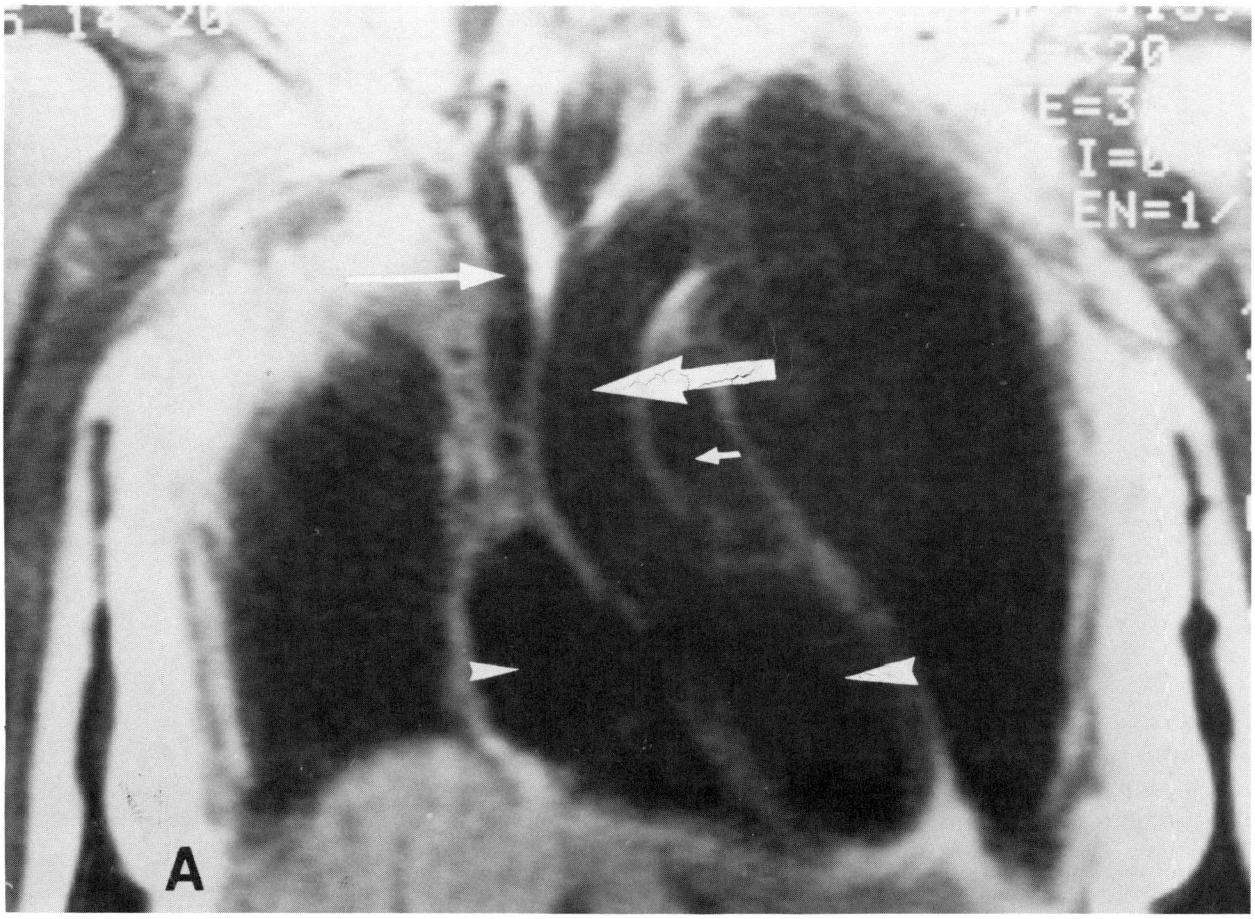

Figure 3.9 (A,B,C,D). Normal coronal SE images performed with TR/TE of 320/32 and 500/30 in various patients, from anterior (A) to posterior (D) demonstrate: (A) ascending aorta (large arrow), left ventricle (large arrowhead), right atrium (small arrowhead), superior vena cava (long arrow), pulmonary artery (short arrow); (B) left ventricle (large arrow) right atrium (large arrowhead) right pulmonary artery (long arrow) trachea (small arrow), aorts (small arrowhead); (C) left ventricle (large arrow), left and right common carotid arteries (small arrowheads); (D) aorta (long arrow).

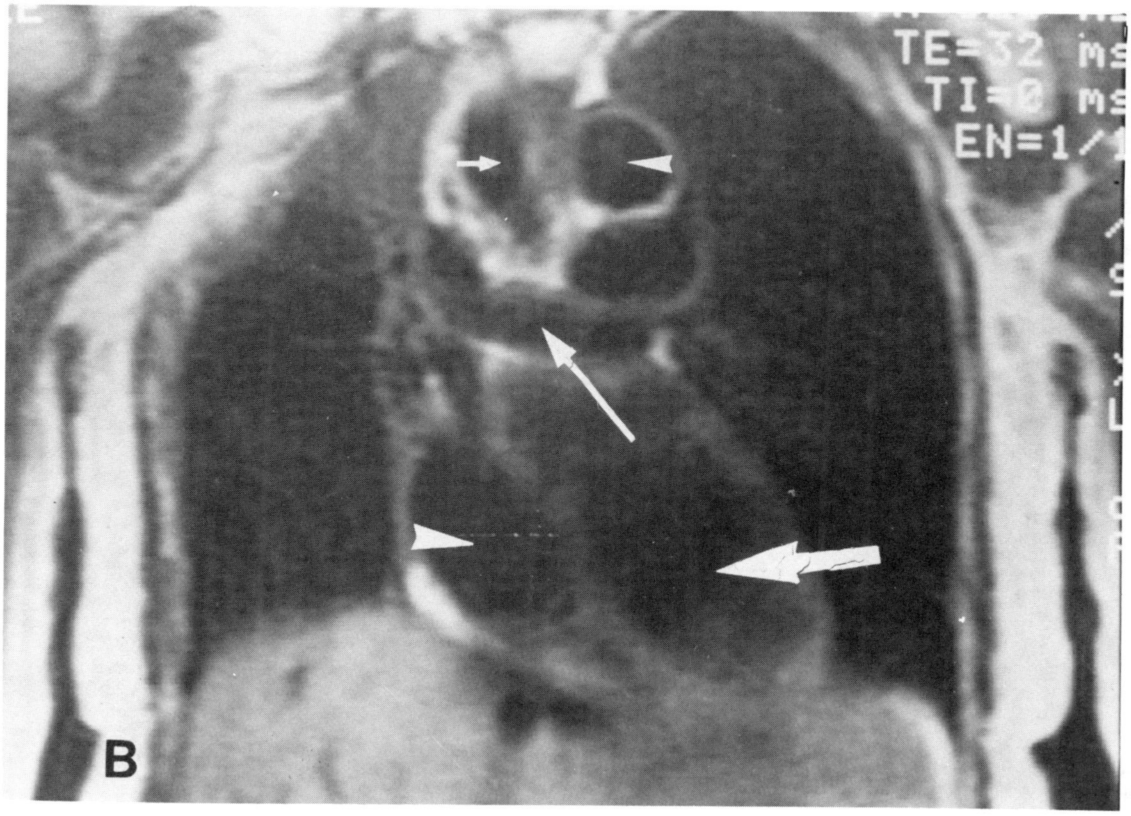
B

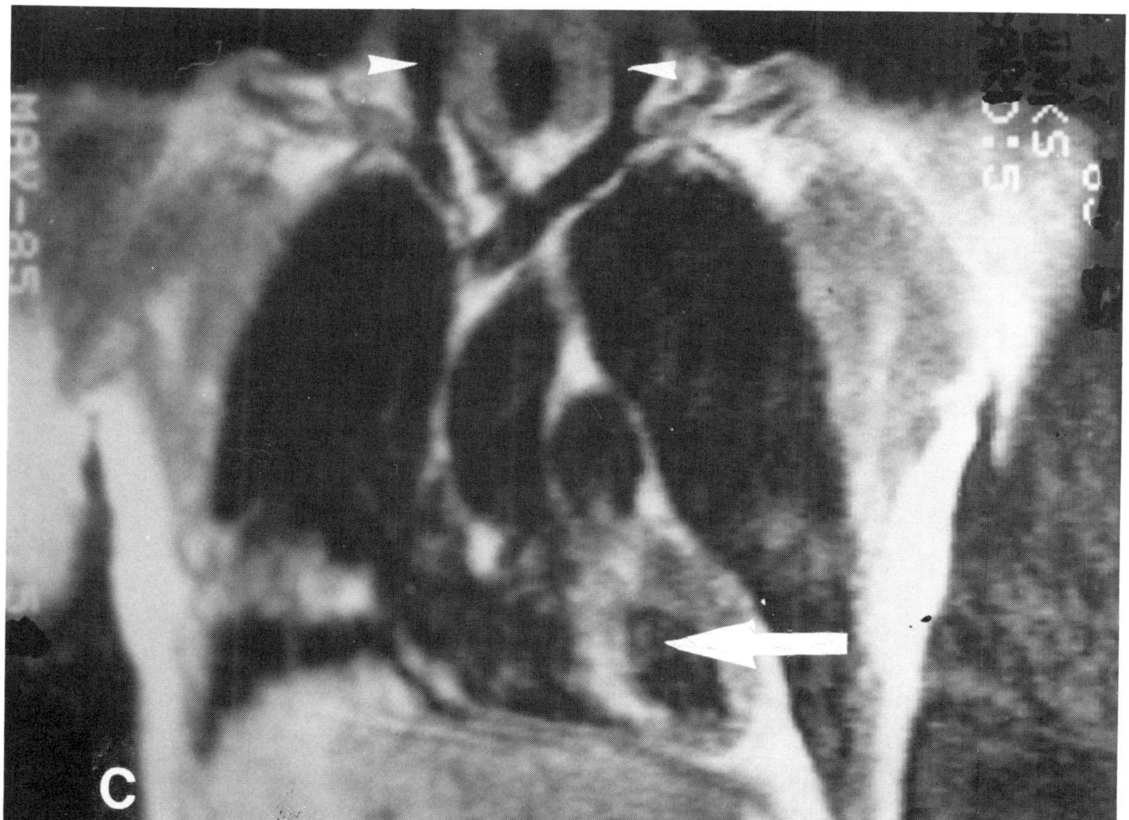
C

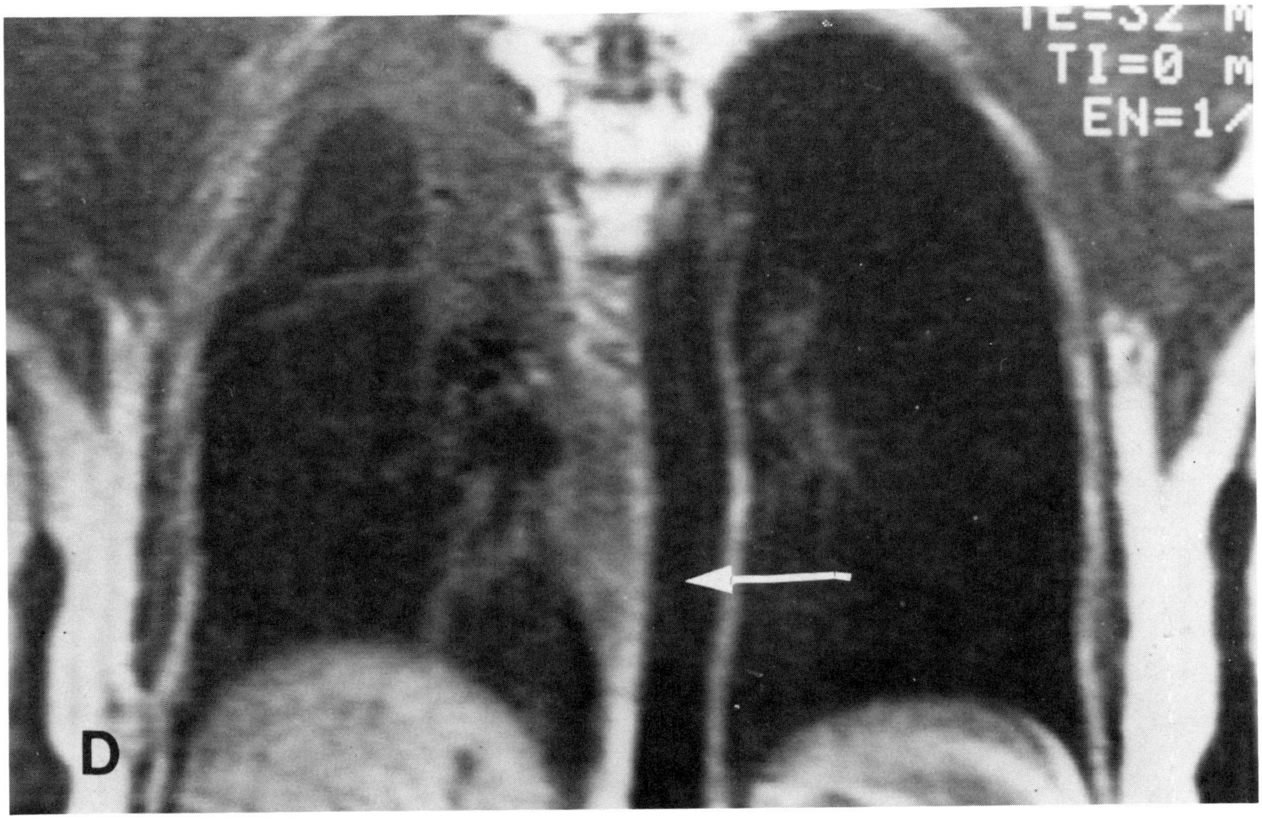

On MR images, the gland is usually intermediate in intensity being less intense than fat and more intense than the air-filled lung or mediastinal vessels. With advancing age, the thymus undergoes a progressive replacement of its parenchyma with fat and increases in size. When short TR values are used on spin-echo images, the intensity of such glands will be very close to the intensity of fat.

MRI seems to be also successful in delineating the diaphragmatic crura. The retrocrural space is limited by the diaphragmatic crura anteriorly and by the vertebral column posteriorly and contains important structures such as the descending aorta, the distal esophagus, the azygos and hemiazygos vein, lymph glands, and fat which surrounds the constituents of this space. By accurately imaging this area, MRI may prove to be an important adjuvant in the recognition of disease processes affecting the base of the lung and the upper abdomen, for example, in the differentiation between pleural and intraperitoneal fluid collections (Figure 3.10). Absence of signal from calcifications prevents the visualization of these pathological changes in the diaphragmatic pleura.

Normal anatomy of the heart as demonstrated with magnetic resonance imaging will be discussed as a separate topic (Chapter 4).

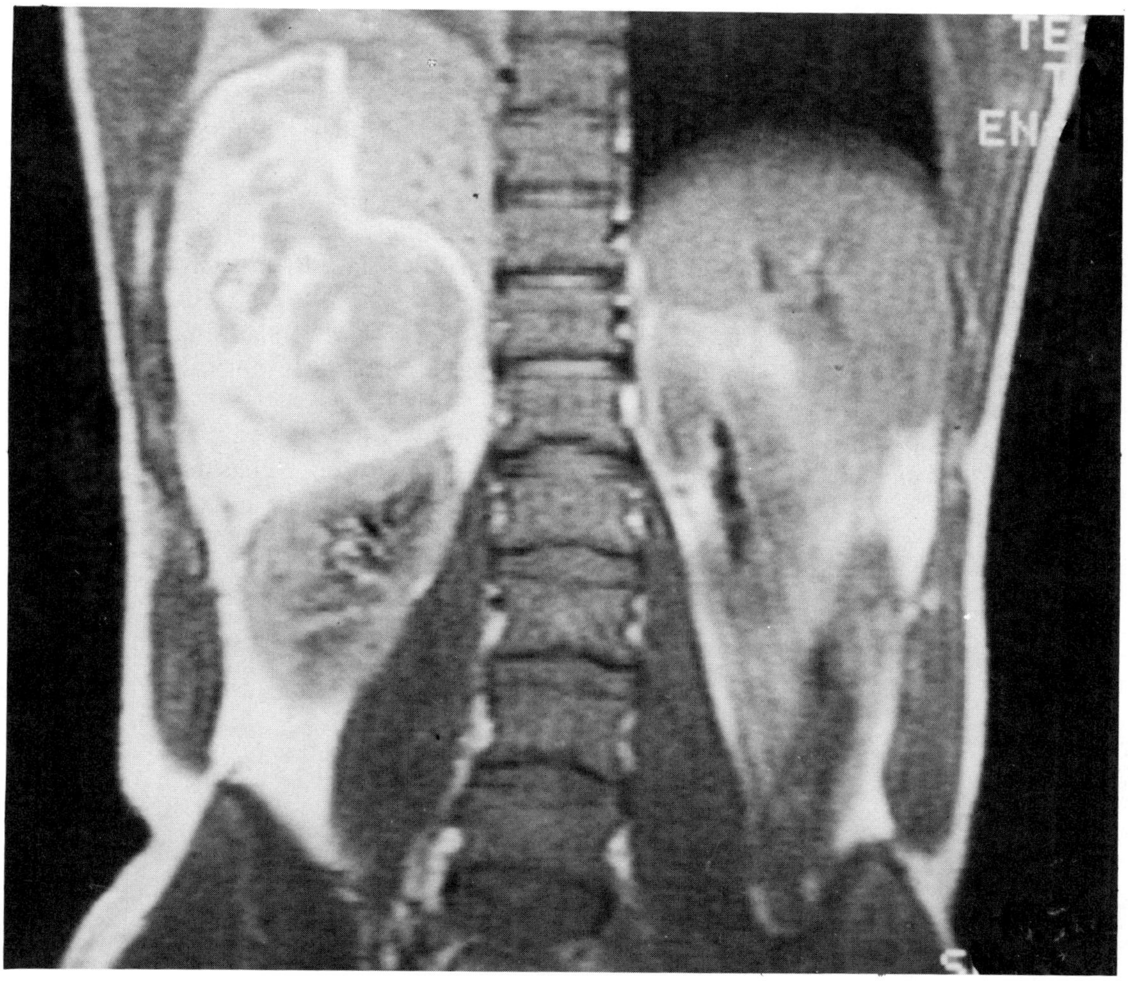

Figure 3.10. Coronal MR image performed with a TR of 500 and a TE of 32, demonstrates clearly the high position of the right hemidiaphragm secondary to the presence of a large post-traumatic subcapsular liver hematoma.

REFERENCES

1. Kundel HL, Kressel HY, Epstein D: The potential role of NMR in thoracic disease. *Rad Clin N Am, 21:* No. 4, 1983.

2. Gamsu G, Webb WR, Sheldon P, *et al.*: Nuclear magnetic resonance imaging of the thorax. *Radiology, 147:*473-480, 1983.

3. Axel L, Kressel HY, Thickman D, *et al.*: NMR imaging of the chest at 0,127: Initial clinical experience with a resistive magnet. *AJR, 141:*1157-1162, 1983.

4. O'Donovan PB, Ross JS, Sivak ED: Magnetic resonance imaging of the thorax: Advantages of coronal and sagittal planes. *AJR, 143:*1183-1188, 1984.

5. Ross JS, O'Donovan PB, Novoa R, *et al.*: Magnetic resonance of the chest: Initial experience with imaging and in vivo T_1 and T_2 calculations at 0.6T. *Radiology, 152:*95-101, 1984.

6. Cohen AM: Magnetic resonance imaging of the thorax. *Radiol Clin N Am, 22:*829-846, 1984.

7. Webb WR, Gamsu G, Crooks LE: Multisection sagittal and coronal magnetic resonance imaging of the mediastinum and hila. *Radiology, 150:* 475-478, 1984.

8. Webb WR, Jensen BG, Gamsu G, *et al.*: Coronal magnetic resonance imaging of the chest: Normal and abnormal. *Radiology, 153:*729-735, 1984.

9. Webb WR, Jensen BG, Gamsu G, *et al.*: Sagittal MR imaging of the chest: Normal and abnormal. *J Comp Assist Tomogr, 9:*471-479, 1985.

10. Higgins CB, Stark DD, McNamara M, *et al.*: Multiplane magnetic resonance imaging of the heart and major vessels: Studies in normal volunteers. *AJR 142:*661-667, 1984.

11. Sperber M: *Computerized Tomography of the Lung: Normal Anatomy and Most Common Disorders.* New York: Futura Publishing, Inc., 1984.

4

Cardiovascular System

Magnetic resonance allows high-resolution tomographic imaging in three planes without the use of ionizing irradiation. The technique can be used to assess cardiac function and to evaluate blood flow. In addition this new modality may allow tissue characterization and metabolic assessment.

MR IMAGING OF THE HEART

Cardiac Morphology

With the exception of the echo-planar related methods (1, 2), all MR imaging techniques rely upon the measurement of a large number of nuclear signals, which are acquired under different experimental conditions. The free induction decay and spin echoes, obtained in response to radio frequency pulses, arise from all tissues located within the sensitive volume of the RF antenna. Due to this inherent three-dimensional character of the experiment, the MR signals must be spatially encoded and images are derived from subsequent spatial decoding of a set of measurements. Spatial encoding of the nuclear signal is applied through the use of a set of three orthogonal linear gradients of magnetic field which spatially vary the resonance frequency of the nuclei. The gradients, some of which are varied stepwise from one measurement to the next, introduce the spatial encoding either into the frequency of the nuclear signal, or into its phase or amplitude. Decoding of the spatial information is usually performed by multidirectional Fourier transform of the raw data set.

Under the assumption that the signal-to-noise ratio is such that only a single measurement per spatial encoding step is required, a full 3D set, with a resolution of 256 x 256 x 12 points for instance (i.e., 12 planes imaged on a 256 x 256 matrix each), would require 256 x 12 different measurements with Fourier Zeugmatography related techniques (3, 4). Total imaging time would then amount to 51 minutes, under the further assumption that the time interval between successive measurements would be set to 1 second. The choice of this time interval is usually free, and it determines to what extent the longitudinal relaxation times (T_1) will affect image contrast.

To reduce total imaging time and size of the data set, selective excitations can be applied. Nuclear signals can selectively be obtained from planar areas by applying radio frequency pulses of limited bandwidth in the presence of a linear gradient of magnetic field. Thus, the total number of measurements needed (for single plane imaging) can be reduced to 256, and total imaging time to 4.3 minutes, under similar assumptions as above.

When imaging the heart, the total number of measurements required for a single plane, for instance 256 measurements, fixes the total minimal acquisition time to 4.3 minutes, assuming that the RR interval is of one second. It is essential, indeed, that the heart configuration be identical while performing the different measurements related to different spatial encodings. Thus, triggering of the RF pulses with respect to heart cycle is paramount, and this constraint fixes the repetition time (i.e., the delay between successive excitations) to multiples of the RR interval. Consequently, with cardiac MR imaging, image contrast cannot as freely be modulated as when imaging non-moving tissues. Usually, measurements are triggered every QRS peak, leading to repetition times ranging between 600 and 1000 msec depending upon the patient's heart rate. Thus, appreciable T_1 weighting is present with spin echo sequences, particularly when measurements are performed with high field systems (T_1 of heart muscle is around 300 msec at .08 Tesla[5] and around 870 msec at .6 Tesla [6]). T_2 contrast can be superimposed by appropriately choosing the echo time (TE). Optimal cardiac morphology is depicted in short (TE) images, due to the short transverse relaxation time (T_2) of the normal myocardium (about 35 msec) (7).

Inversion recovery sequences, as usually implemented, do not seem to be extremely well suited for cardiac imaging. The long delay between the inversion pulse (triggered by the QRS peak) and the read pulse increases the sensitivity of the sequence to irregularities of the heart rhythm. If these are present, the position of the read pulse will cover a range of different heart phases during the acquisitions related to a particular image, so that blurring and movement artifacts will adversely affect image quality. But optimal results might be reached in favorable conditions. Furthermore, different triggered IR imaging schemes are conceivable which would reduce the sensitivity of the sequence to heart rhythm fluctuations.

The high contrast between cardiac muscle and blood derives from a large variety of phenomena affecting blood signal, and it underlies the vast amount of cardiovascular applications of MRI.

The discussion of the often very complex flow related features can not be done within the scope of this chapter. They are related to the relative directions of flow and image plane (8–10) and of flow and imaging gradients (11, 12), to the echo number (13, 14), to image type (15), to voxel size (16), and to many other flow and pulse sequence related parameters (17).

The effectiveness of cardiac MR imaging has greatly been enhanced through the introduction of multiple slice techniques. As mentioned earlier, total imaging time of a heart slice is fixed, and related to image matrix size and heart rate. When performing single slice cardiac imaging considerable acquisition time is consequently being wasted between successive measurements triggered at every QRS peak. In multiple slice imaging, one takes advantage of the delay time between successive excitations of a particular slice to perform measurements on nearby slices. The total number of different slices which can be measured during the delay time depends on instrumental parameters and on the pulse sequence used (for instance the total number of echoes and the echo time in a spin echo pulse sequence will affect this number).

The different slices measured between successive QRS peaks will obviously reflect different phases of the heart cycle. If one is interested in depicting different anatomical levels at a particular heart phase, then necessarily a penalty in total number of measurements will have to be paid.

Cardiac Function

Cardiac function may be assessed by imaging a particular level at regularly spaced time intervals during the heart cycle. The time resolution which can be achieved with standard spin echo sequences is rather poor, due to the relatively long values of the minimal repetition times. The latter are determined by a combination of pulse sequence and instrumental parameters, and by the recovery times (longitudinal relaxation times) of the tissue water protons. A considerable improvement in the time resolution of cardiac functional imaging has recently been obtained by the combined use of gradient recalled echoes and small flip angle excitations (18). Small RF pulses (i.e., small with respect to the usual 90 degree pulse) tip into the transverse plane only a fraction of the longitudinal magnetization, so that most of the longitudinal component is kept unaffected by the pulses. As a consequence, the stationary state established by excitation with a series of equally spaced small flip angle pulses, will be characterized by the existence of an appreciable amount of longitudinal magnetization prior to each excitation. This remains the case even when the repetition times are set to values which are very short with respect to the longitudinal relaxation times of the tissues. The presence of 180 degree refocusing pulses, needed in the usual spin echo experiments, would have a deleterious effect upon this scheme, in that these pulses also would invert the longitudinal magnetization. Consequently, with short repetition time, small flip angle sequences, spin echoes are generated by inversal of the sign of the readout gradient, rather than by the application of a refocusing pulse. An additional advantage of this approach is the short echo time which can be achieved, as no delay is introduced by a selective 180 degree pulse.

The minimal repetition time which can be achieved with this type of technique is determined by a variety of parameters, such as field of view, matrix size, maximum gradient strength and other instrumental factors. A TR of about 20 msec seems within the possibilities of most imagers, assuming a 40 mm field of view and a 256 points resolution in the readout direction. Thus, assuming a one second RR interval, about 50 measurements can in principle be performed during one heart cycle. In other terms, within a time span of 4.3 minutes, a particular slice through the heart can be imaged on a 256 square matrix at nearly 50 different equally spaced heart phases. Given this excellent time resolution, the heart function can be viewed in "cine" mode, by rapid and repetitive scanning through the set of appropriately ordered images (19).

Image contrast obtained with these fast imaging techniques (20) obviously depends on the repetition (TR) and spin echo times (TE). In addition, the pulse angle plays a determinant role. When the latter is varied from very low (e.g., around 5 degrees) to high values (e.g., 45 degrees), the dominating image contrast mechanism shifts from transverse to longitudinal relaxation. Furthermore, as the repetition times used are very often comparable to or even shorter than the T_2 values of the tissues, some inherent T_2 weighting is usually present, unless spoil gradients are used to cancel phase coherence in the transverse plane prior to each excitation. Contrast between blood pool and cardiac muscle depends on a large variety of parameters as is the case with standard spin echo sequences. But, in contrast with the latter techniques, fast imaging methods very often provide highlighted signal intensity in the blood pool.

The ultimate goal of cardiac MR would be high resolution, high contrast real-time imaging of the heart. One should realize that the fast imaging techniques mentioned until now provide what may be called "pseudo" real-time imaging, in that any of the images obtained is reconstructed on the basis of many data acquired during different heart cycles. "True" real-time cardiac imaging, in contrast, requires that the images be reconstructed on the basis of a single nuclear signal, measured during a time lapse which is small with respect to the cardiac period.

The "true" real-time requirement has been met by echo-planar related methods (1). These methods acquire the total amount of information needed for subsequent image production during a single measurement, lasting a few tens of milliseconds. Thus "true" real-time cardiac functional imaging is in principle possible, by combination of this type of acquisition technique with small flip angle excitations. This approach has recently been followed, and image acquisition at a rate of 20 images per cardiac cycle has been reported (21). The method has appropriately been named "BEST" (Blipped Echo-planar Single-pulse Technique).

A basic principle of physics, however, relates the attainable signal-to-noise ratio to the total measurement time. With real time imaging, as a consequence, an inherent penalty in signal-to-noise is necessarily paid with respect to standard MR imaging. With the former techniques the spatial resolution is consequently decreased (the voxel size is increased), in order to transform the signal-to-noise into a spatial resolution penalty. Until now, no echo-planar related methods have been made available on commercial imagers, presumably due to the stringent technical requirements.

CLINICAL APPLICATIONS*

Normal Cardiac Anatomy

The cross-sectional imaging displays cardiac anatomy similar to Computed Tomography, but a major advantage of Magnetic Resonance is its ability to provide images in sagittal, coronal and oblique planes as well as in the axial plane (Figures 4.1 and 4.2). The intrinsic contrast between the blood pool and cardiovascular structures results in clear discrimination of cardiac chambers, myocardium, papillary muscles, valves and pericardium (Figures 4.3, 4.4, 4.5). Cusps of the aortic and pulmonary arteries are sometimes visible. Pulmonary veins entering into the left atrium are always identified (Figure 4.6). Coronal sections show the tracheal bifurcation and its relationship with the pulmonary arteries (Figure 4.7). Sagittal sections optimally demonstrate the aorta (Figure 4.8).

---

* All examinations displayed in this chapter were performed on a 1.5 Tesla superconductive Gyroscan system operating at 0.5 Tesla.

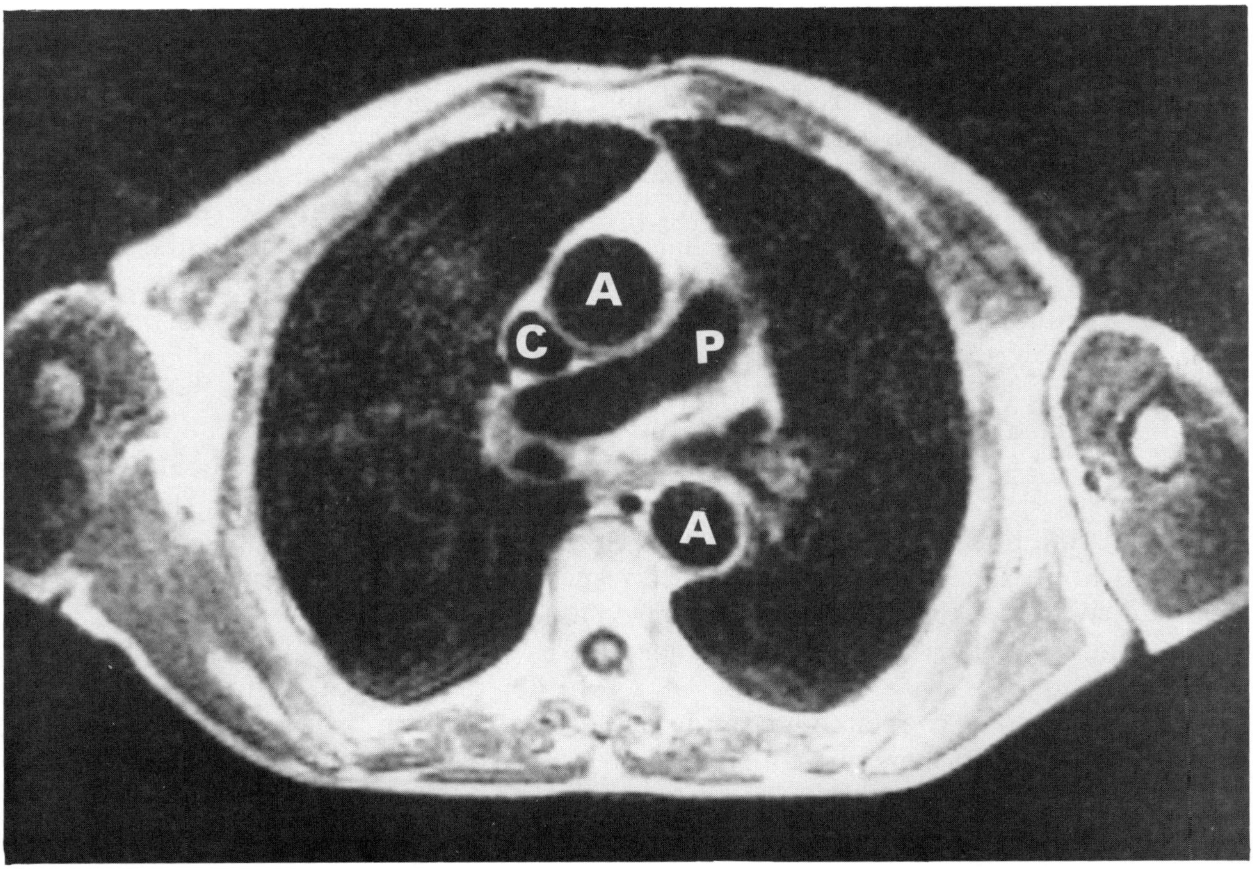

Figure 4.1. Normal anatomy. Transverse section. The right pulmonary artery extends posteriorly and to the right from the main pulmonary artery (P) to course posterior to the superior vena cava (C). Ascending and descending aorta (a).

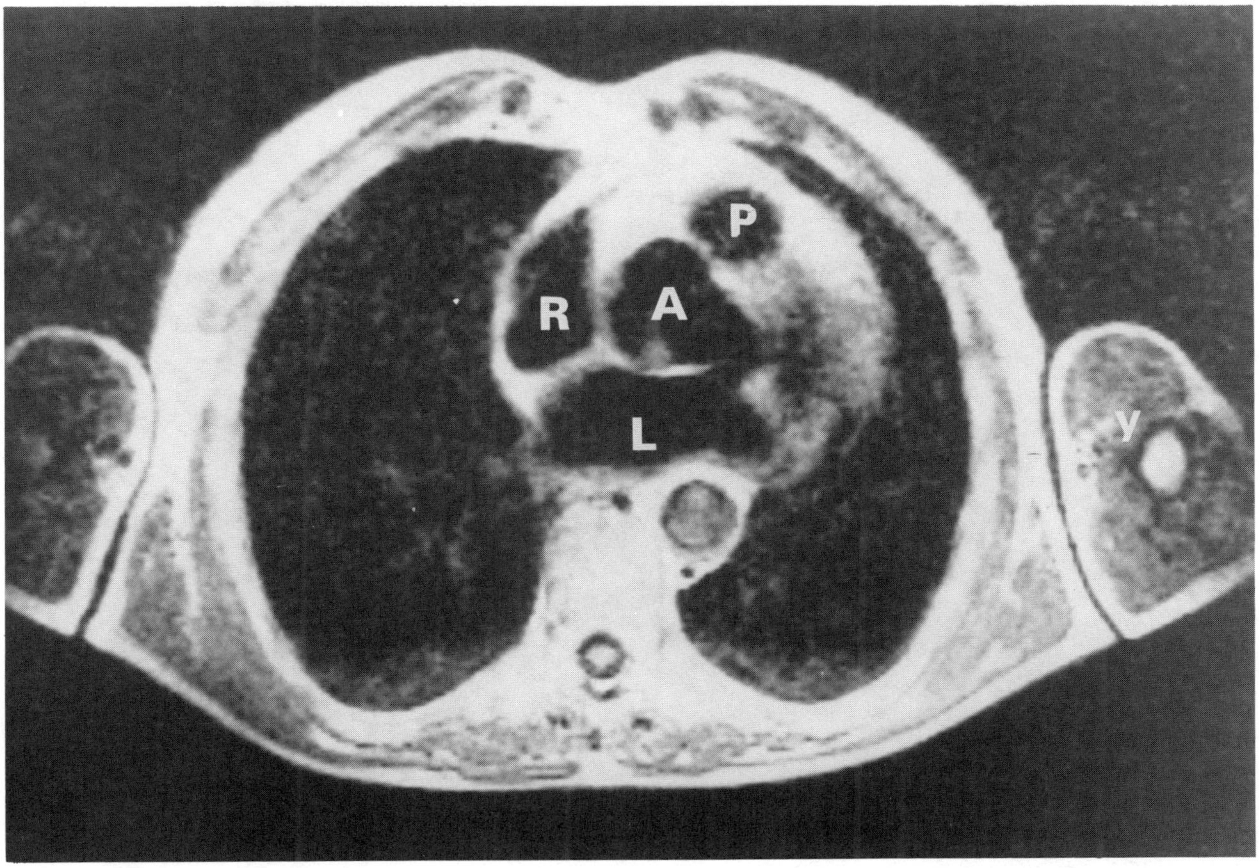

Figure 4.2. Normal anatomy. Transverse section, centered at the base of the heart, shows the right atrium (R), the left atrium (L), the main pulmonary artery (P) and the aorta (A).

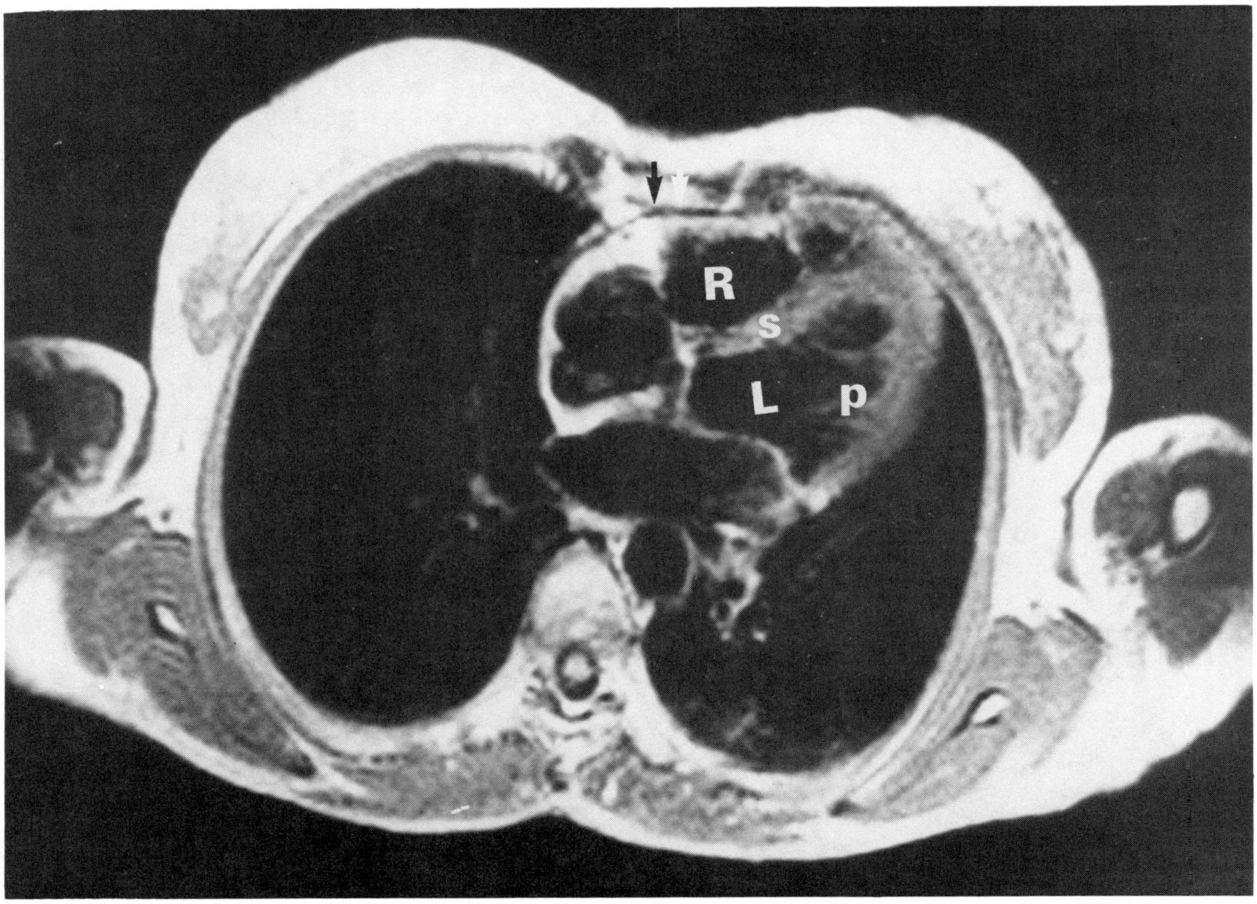

Figure 4.3. Normal anatomy. At the ventricular level, the pericardium (arrow) is seen as a rim of low signal intensity. The papillary muscles (p) are clearly visible. s = septum, L = left ventricle, R = right ventricle.

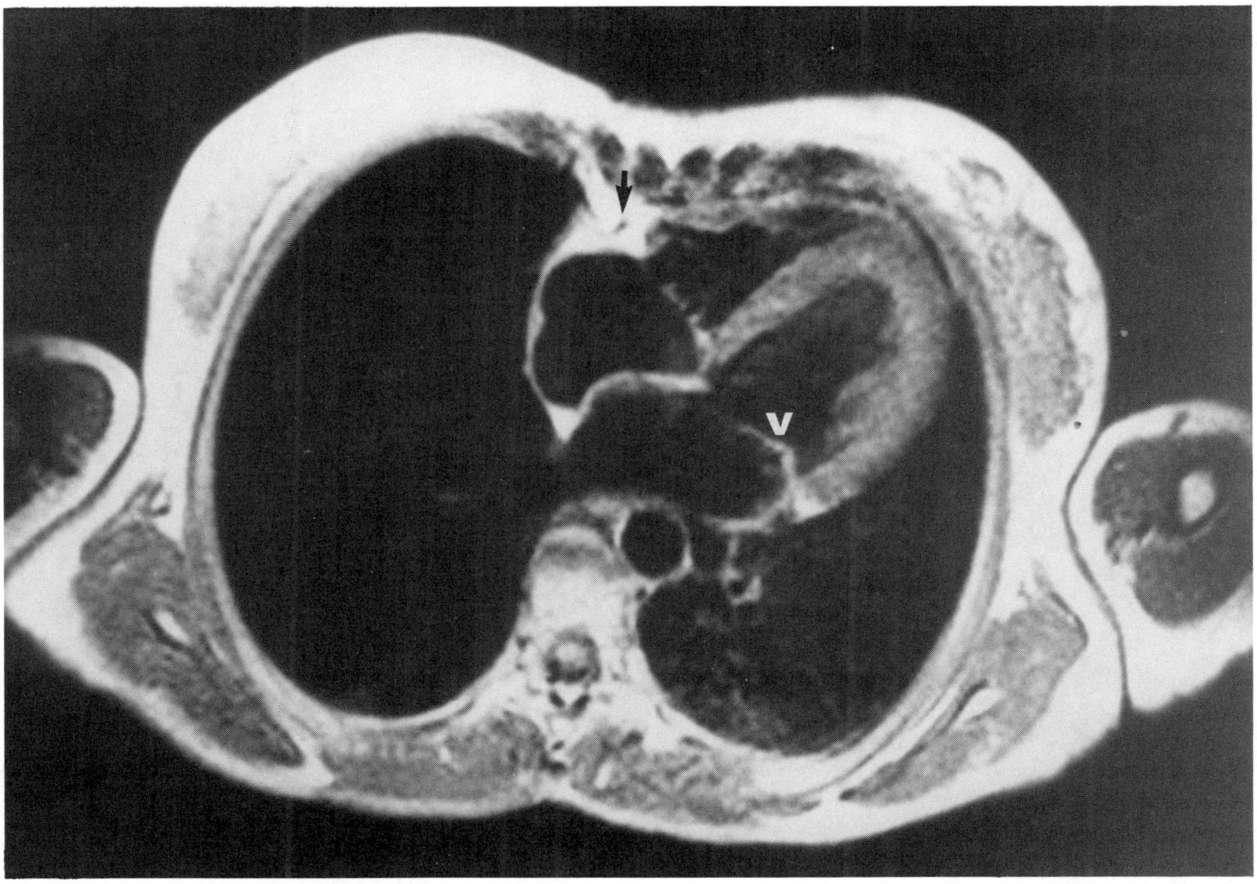

Figure 4.4. Normal Anatomy. Transverse section in the middle of the left ventricle. The mitral valve (v) is visible. The right coronary artery (arrow) is visible in fat tissue.

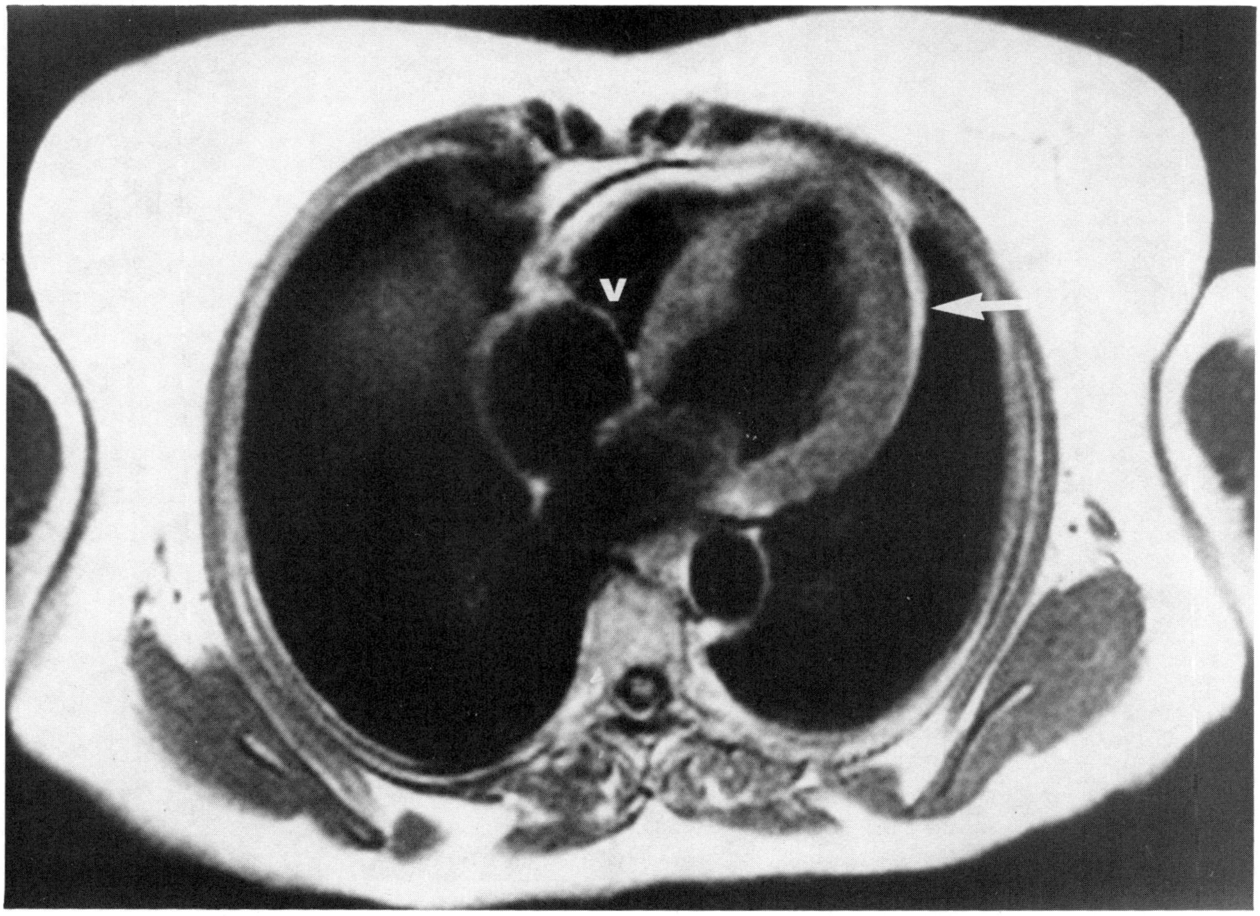

Figure 4.5. Normal anatomy. This transverse section is performed below the level of Figure 4.4. This section shows clear discrimination between pericardial fat (arrow) and myocardium; (v) is the tricuspid valve.

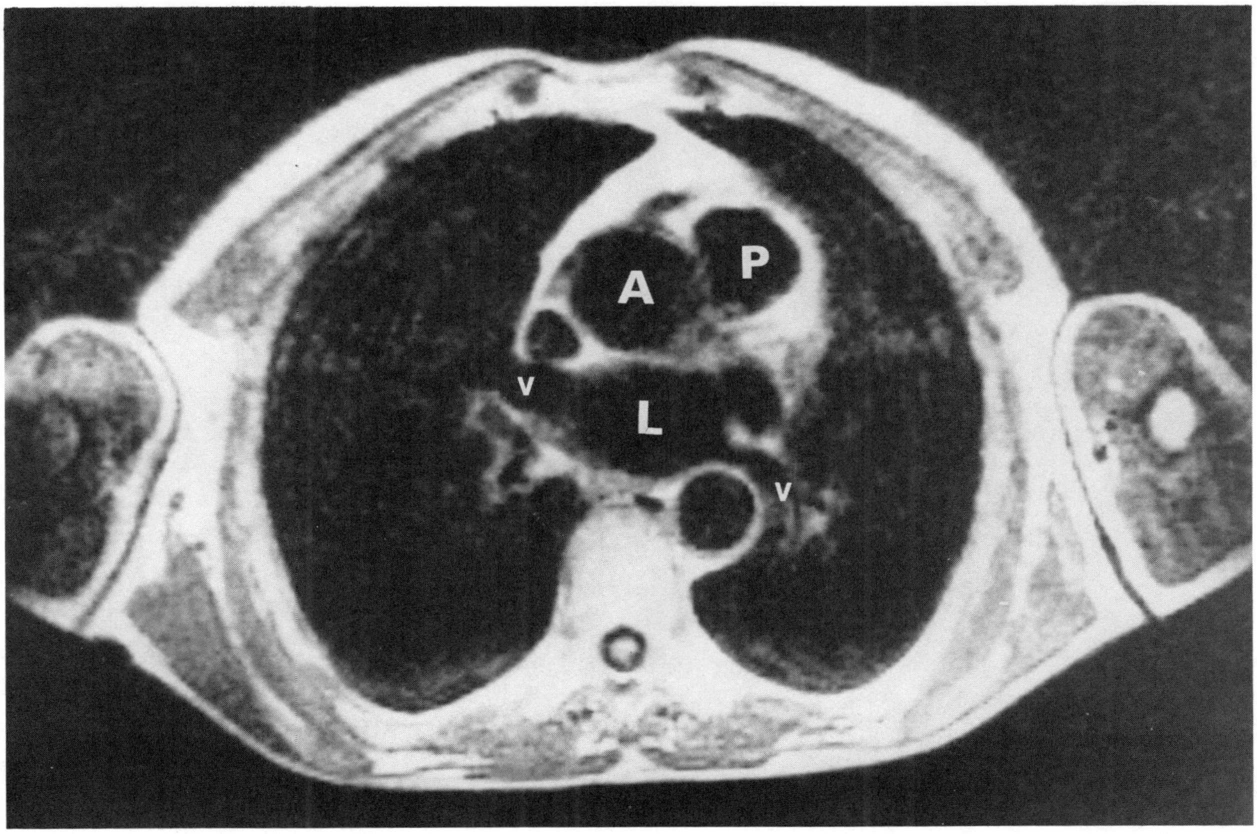

Figure 4.6. Normal anatomy. Transverse section centered at the level of the left atrium (L). The main pulmonary artery (P) is somewhat anterior to the aorta (A). The main pulmonary veins (v) are seen coursing into the left atrium.

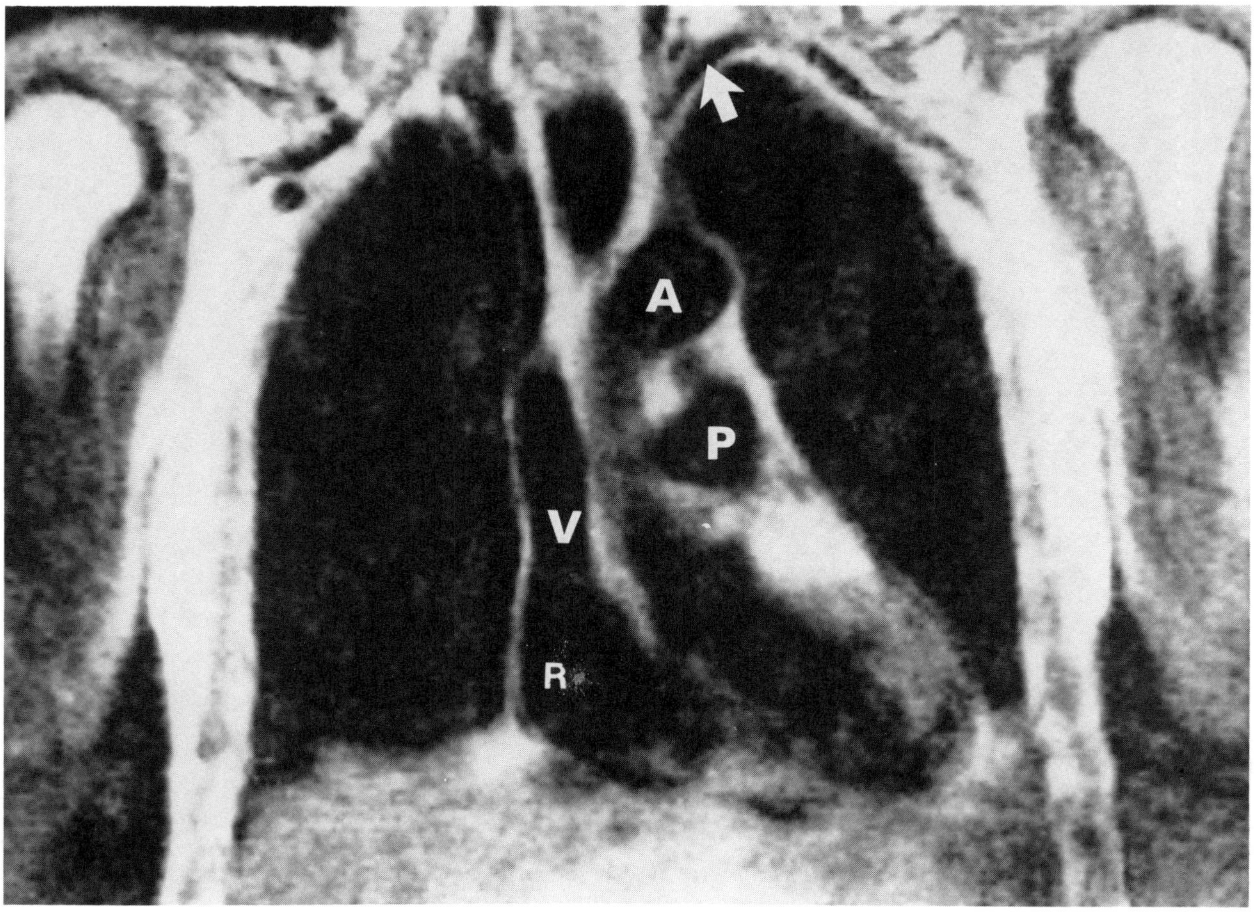

Figure 4.7. Normal anatomy. This coronal section shows the pulmonary artery bifurcation (P), the aorta (A), the left subclavian artery (arrow), the superior vena cava (V) and the right atrium (R).

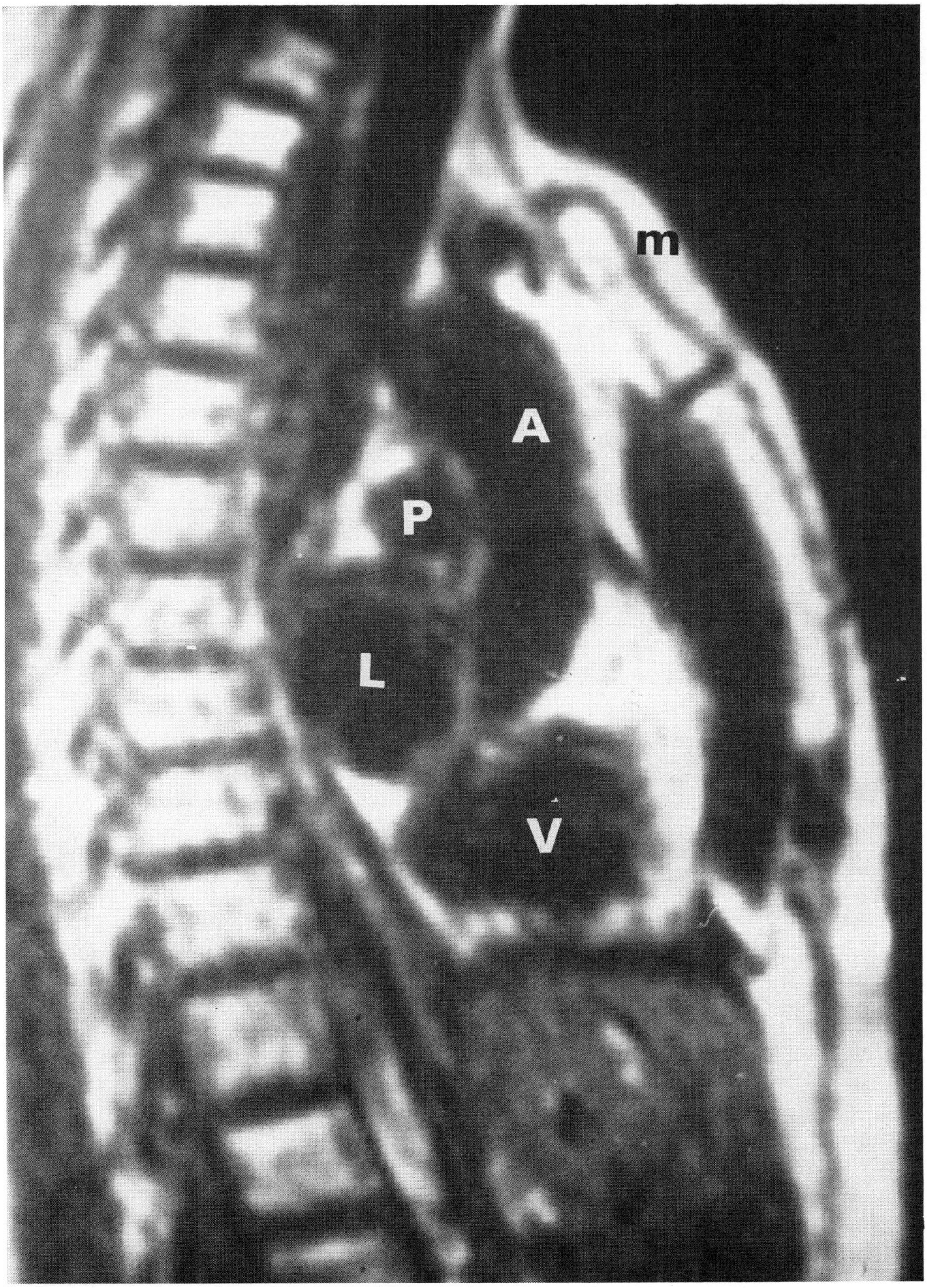

Figure 4.8. Normal anatomy. This sagittal section demonstrates the aorta (A), the left pulmonary artery (P) the left atrium (L), the left ventricle (V) and the left internal mammary artery (m).

The proximal portions of the native right and left coronary arteries are often identified on axial SE images as longitudinal tubular structures with a low signal intensity, but their tortuous course makes them difficult to follow (Figure 4.4).

The pericardium seen by MRI is usually described as a dark line between epi- and pericardial fat layers which are seen as high signal intensity structures. On axial SE images the pericardium is well seen over the anterior and right aspect of the heart. CT scans of the pericardium are acquired over several cardiac cycles, thereby inducing some uncertainty about the actual pericardial thickness (80). The minimal thickness of the pericardium reported by CT measurements is more than twice the thickness observed on cadaveric specimens. CT studies also show variations in the regional distribution of the pericardial thickness. MR, in contrast, acquires data at particular phases of the cardiac cycle, thus allowing the pericardial thickness to be measured. In a MR study of U. Sechtem, *et al.* (78, 79), in the mid ventricular section, in front of the right ventricle the pericardial thickness was 1.2 +/— 0.5 mm in diastole and 1.7 +/— 0.5 mm in systole, both values exceeding the thickness of 0.4 to 1.0 mm reported for anatomic measurements of pericardial thickness. The authors suggest that the pericardial fluid normally present in the pericardial spaces, which also has low signal intensity, likely contributes to the overall pericardial thickness as visualized. The sensitivity of MR to detect a small amount of pericardial fluid should be an argument to use this technique for detection and quantification of even small pericardial effusions. In children, the fat layers are absent. Therefore, the detection of the pericardium is only possible in the anterior part of the heart. As there is less epi- and pericardial fat behind the posterior and lateral walls of the left ventricle and right auricle, demonstration of the pericardium in these regions is more difficult also in normal adults. In addition we have observed that the pericardium is better visualized in systole than in diastole. According to the literature and our own experience, pathological conditions raise the pericardial signal intensity (78, 79, 80).

Ischemic Heart Disease

MRI allows direct visualization of the myocardium and excellent delineation of endocardial and epicardial interfaces. Consequently, the technique can easily identify segmental wall thinning resulting from a previous myocardial infarction (Figure 4.9). Left ventricular aneurysms can also easily be identified. Cine mode imaging allows the study of wall motion and consequently permits demonstration of akinetic or hypokinetic myocardial areas. M.T. McNamara and C.B. Higgins evaluated signal intensities and T_2

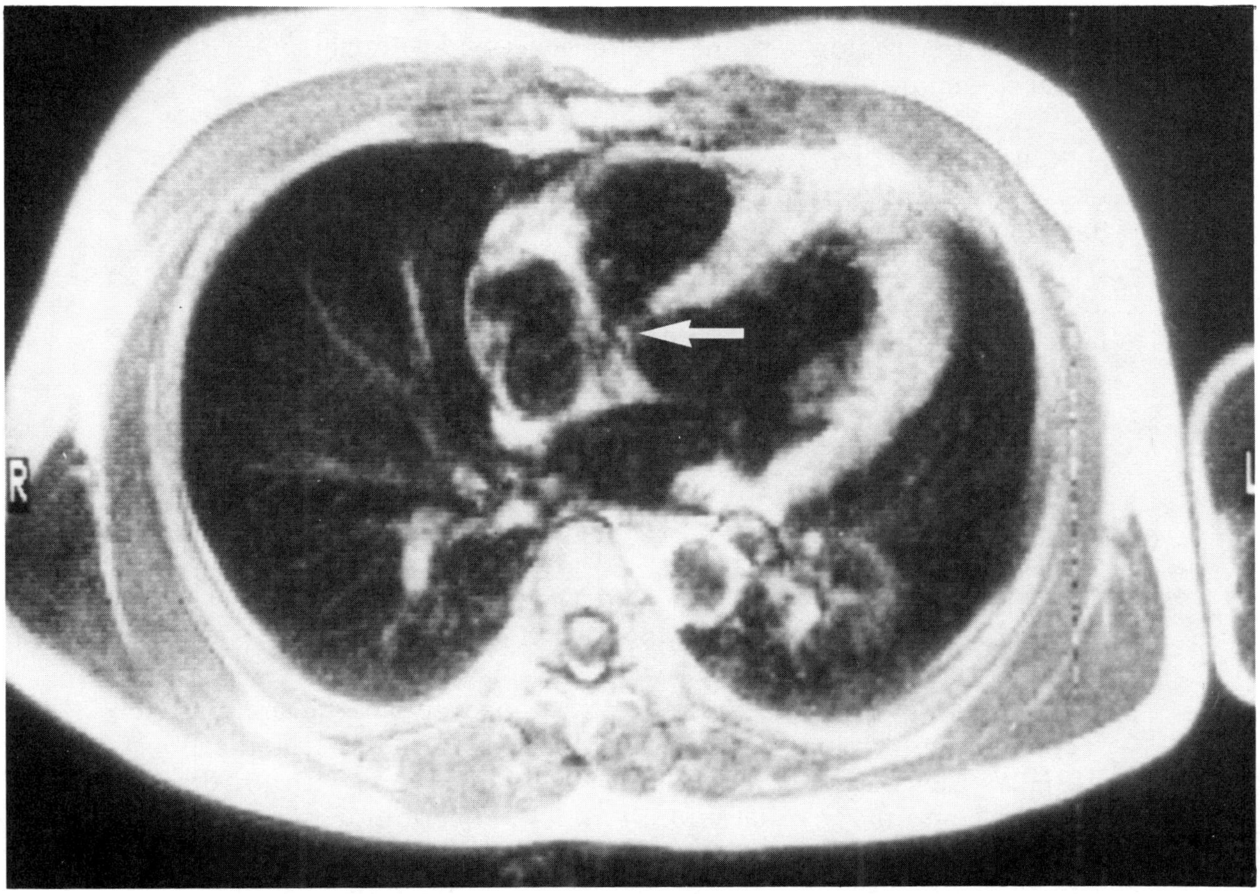

Figure 4.9. Transverse section through the left ventricle in a patient with a recent septal myocardial infarction complicated with septal defect (arrow). The MRI examination was performed one week after surgical repair of the septal perforation. The prosthetic (Teflon) material gives no signal.

relaxation times in normal patients and in a population of patients with evolved myocardial infarction. The study was performed with a superconductive system operating a 0.35 Tesla. Region-of-interest analysis demonstrated a significantly greater signal intensity of normal myocardium versus infarction in most patients. The difference in T_2 between normal and infarcted myocardium was also significant. The mean T_2 of thinned evolved infarction was shorter than the mean value for myocardium of the normal volunteers. On the contrary, acute myocardial infarcts have been shown to have increased signal intensity compared with adjacent normal myocardium in both experimental animals and in humans (64, 65).

J.J. Brown, *et al.* (93) have demonstrated that ischemic myocardial injury aged between three hours and four days results in a prolongation of T_1 relaxation times, whereas 56-day-old infarcts show a decrease in T_1 values. Increased T_1 values in early stages of myocardial ischemia are closely related to increase in myocardial water content. In the early stages of ischemic injury, the increase in myocardial water is primarily intracellular although some interstitial edema occurs as well.

Another group (92) evaluated the capability of MRI to detect acutely injured myocardium in the first five hours period after a one hour period of occlusion followed by reperfusion. Also to determine if relaxation times could be used to differentiate injured from normal myocardium. This study shows that ECG-gated MRI detects acute reperfused infarcts in vivo, as early as 30 minutes following reperfusion, as high signal intensity areas caused by prolonged T_2 relaxation times. The T_2 relaxation times of the reperfused infarcts remains significantly higher compared to normal myocardium at any time from 30 minutes on up to 5 hours postreperfusion. Multiple factors appear to play a role in the rise of relaxation times after coronary occlusion and reperfusion: increase of total water content, loss of myocardial integrity and blood accumulation into the damaged myocardium. Areas of hemorrhage, frequently encountered in autopsy series, tend to increase signal intensity by T_2 weighted images.

Uptake of paramagnetic contrast medium in the area of a myocardial infarction is a potentially interesting adjunct in diagnosis. H.W. Eichstaedt, *et al.* (66) investigated patients with the diagnosis of acute myocardial infarction. I.V. injection of a 0.1 mmol/kg body weight Gadolinium-DTPA was followed by an average 70% increase in signal intensity within zones of acute infarction, as compared to a 20% increase in normal myocardium. In case of subacute or chronic infarction there was no significant signal enhancement. Uptake of Gadolinium-DTPA in the area of acute myocardial infarction may be used as a positive marker of acute myocardial necrosis. Intraventricular thrombi are often associated with infarction and usually located in the apical region (Figure 4.10). Usually cardiac thrombi have higher signal intensity than the normal myocardium on the first echo and the contrast is further accentuated on the second echo (86). In our experience, a homogeneous or heterogeneous character of an intracavitary lesion is not sufficiently diagnostic to allow the discrimination between thrombi from other intracardiac structures. Differentiation of thrombi from slowly flowing blood is not easy, however as blood signal intensity might vary during the cardiac cycle in contrast to the thrombus signal intensity, there is potential for differentiation. Various degrees of organization and fibrotic reactions within the thrombus also limit discrimination.

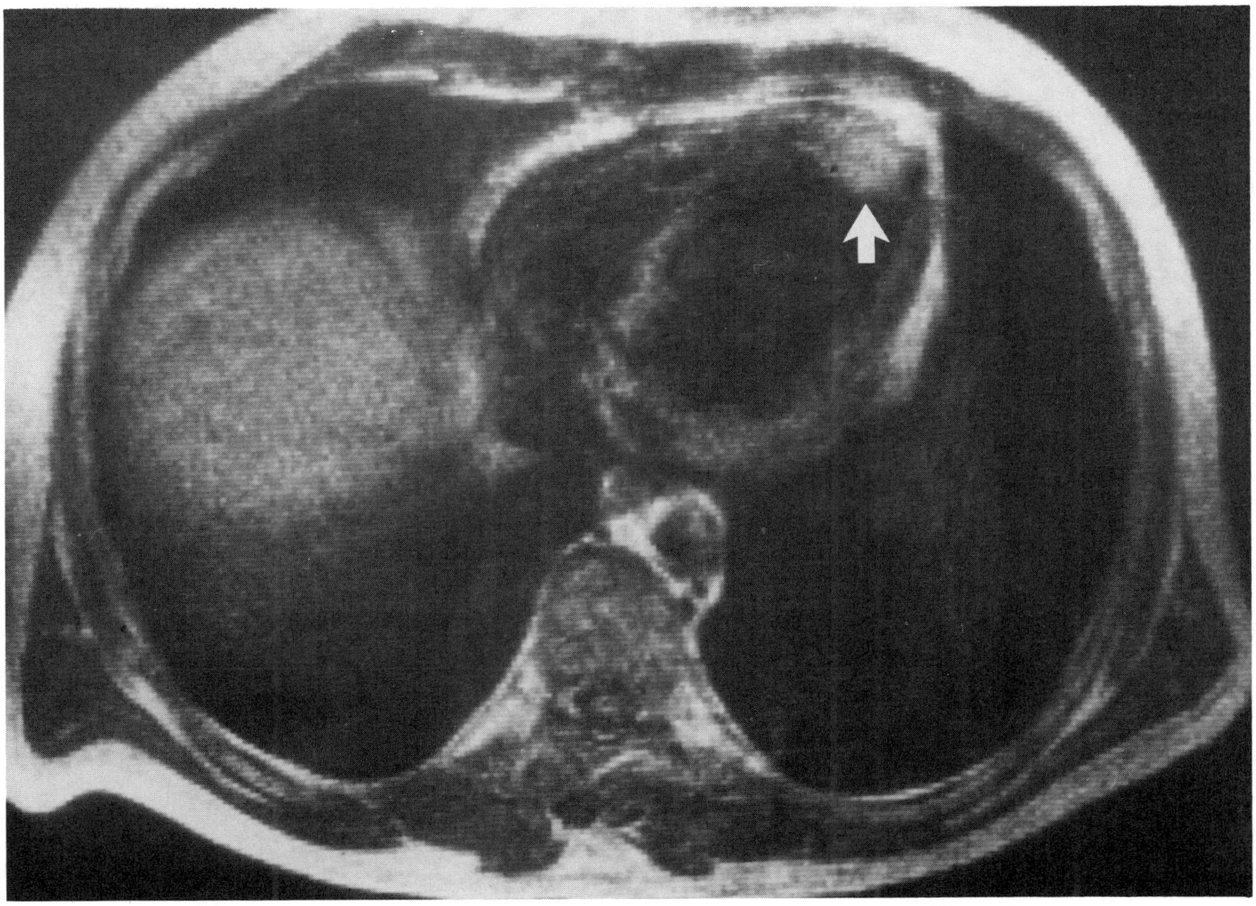

Figure 4.10. Second spin-echo transverse section through the left ventricle in a patient with a previous myocardial infarction. The apical thrombus (arrow) is identified as a high signal image. Note myocardial thinning.

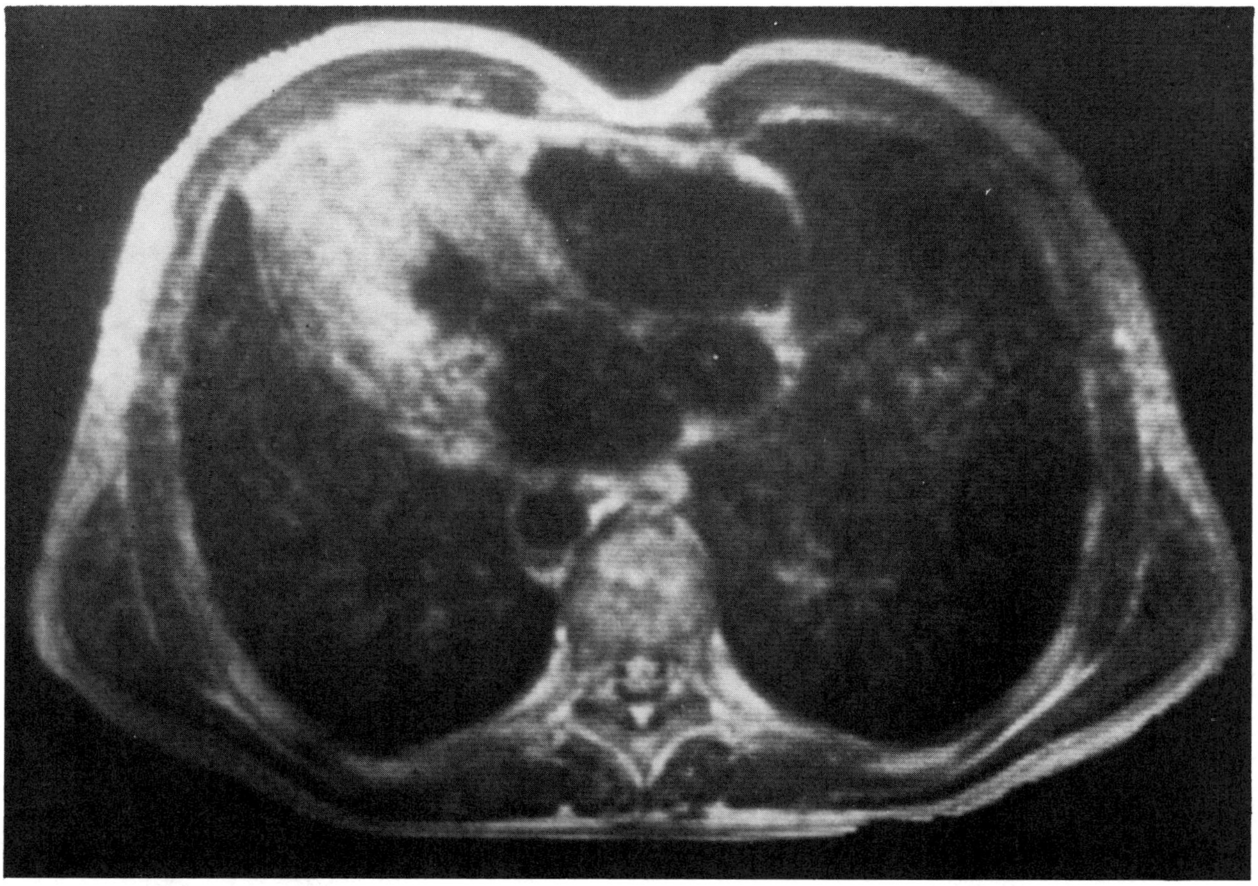

Figure 4.11. Transverse image through the left ventricle obtained in a patient with hypertrophic cardiomyopathy shows diffuse hypertrophy of the myocardial muscle.

Cardiomyopathies

Cardiomyopathies are heart muscle diseases of unknown cause. Primary or idiopathic, they are classified into dilated, hypertrophic and restrictive types. Until now, two-dimensional echocardiography has been used to identify the disease and to evaluate the effects of therapy. MRI can be used in addition to echocardiography to evaluate myocardial wall thickness and cardiac chamber volume in cardiomyopathies (Figures 4.11 and 4.12).

M.S. Florentine, *et al.* (67) tested the ability of ECG triggered MRI to determine the left ventricular mass in living animals. The left ventricle was imaged in the transaxial plane and multiple adjacent 10 mm thick slices were obtained. The ventricular wall area and volume were calculated by computer. The calculated left ventricular mass was compared with its real postmortem mass using linear regression analysis. An excellent relation between calculated and real mass was found (r = 0.95). Intraobserver and

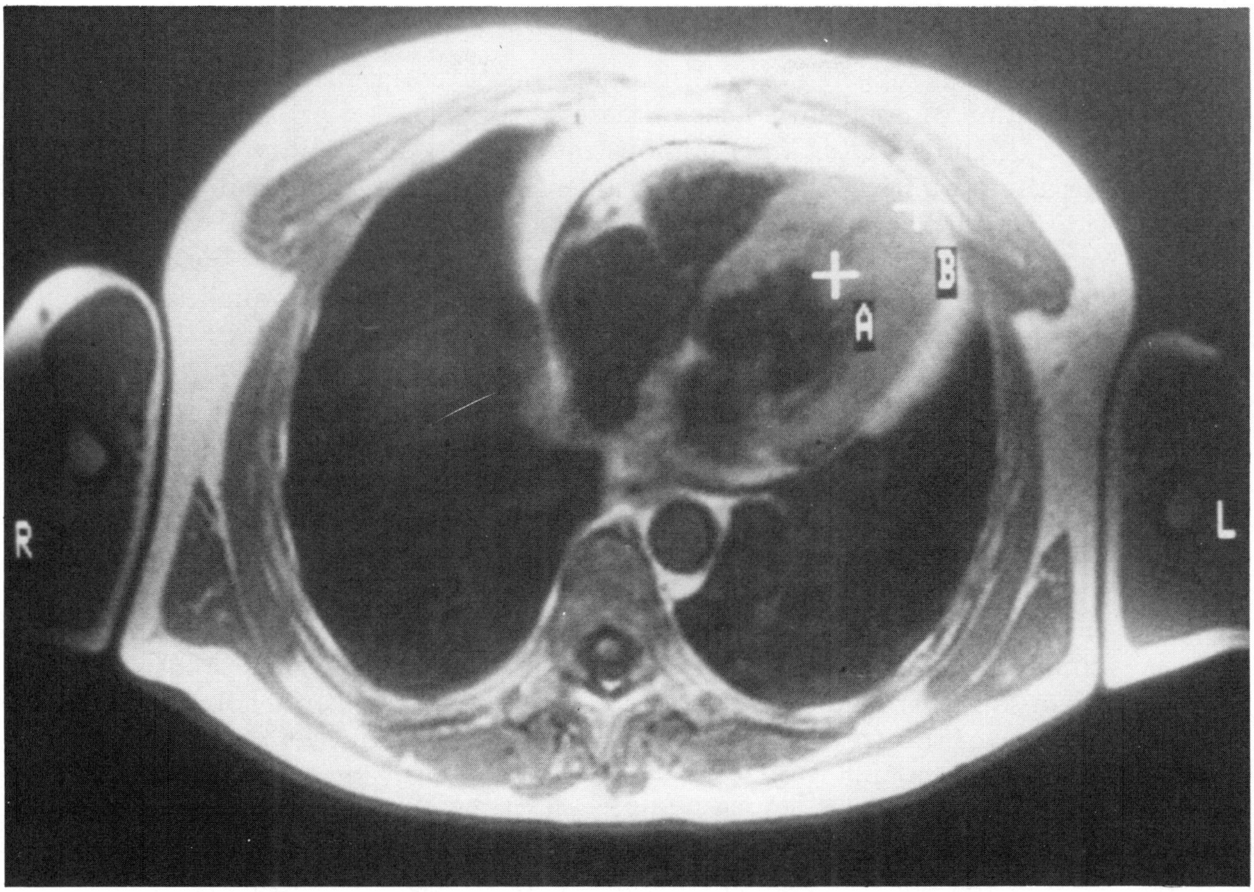

Figure 4.12. Transverse image in a patient with hypertrophic cardiomyopathy depicts apical location of muscle enlargement.

interobserver reproducibility was also excellent (r = 0.99). The ability of MRI to provide quantitative cardiac morphologic informations makes it particularly appealing for humans, although some problems such as partial volume effects or respiratory motion artifacts should be solved.

MRI, in our experience, has proven valuable in assessing various types of hypertrophic cardiomyopathy such as midventricular, generalized or localized forms. In some cases morphologic evaluation by MRI is superior to that of echocardiography and angiography because of anatomical limitations of the latter techniques.

Congenital Heart Disorders.

Several reports (71-74) indicate the potential of MRI in the evaluation of congenital heart diseases.

D. Didier, *et al.* (74) demonstrated the clinical utility of MR for the definitive diagnosis of segmental anatomy and the detection of cardiac abnormalities in a series of 72 patients aged two months to 75 years. MR findings were corroborated by angiography and echocardiography. Forty-four out of 47 abnormalities of the great vessels were outlined by MRI. In transposition of the great vessels, the aorta and the pulmonary artery with its bifurcation are easily identified on MR images. On sagittal sections the typical pathological changes of this condition are clearly visualized. Imaging of the pulmonary arteries and their main branches is mandatory for surgical planning in patients with diminished pulmonary blood flow due to a variety of cyanotic congenital diseases. In such situations, opacification by antegrade catheterization may be difficult or impossible and MRI can provide the most complete delineation of these structures. B.D. Fletcher and M.D. Jacobson (84) studied 19 children for suspected congenital abnormalities of the great vessels. MRI demonstrated lesions where echography either failed to visualize or was inconclusive in 11 patients. MRI complemented echographic diagnosis in 4 patients. All cases were angiographically documented.

Atrial and ventricular septal defects are usually diagnosed by MRI, however thin membranous septa giving poor signal can be misdiagnosed as defects. The latter are usually best demonstrated on long-axis views. Dilatation of the left atrium and the pulmonary veins can be demonstrated in left-to-right shunts. Although evaluation of most congenital heart diseases is possible, the visualization of cardiac valves is often difficult. Moreover, MRI is currently unable to provide accurate haemodynamic data.

Pericardial Diseases

Until recently, pericardial diseases were diagnosed by angiocardiography and echocardiography. Lately, CT has proven to be able to delineate the pericardium. However, all these techniques have major shortcomings in the evaluation of pericardial abnormalities. Therefore, MRI seems to be a promising modality for the study of this area (78-81).

Pericardial effusions due to congestive heart failure generally show low signal intensity (Figure 4.13). Inflammatory pericardial effusions such as due to uremia or tuberculous pericarditis present

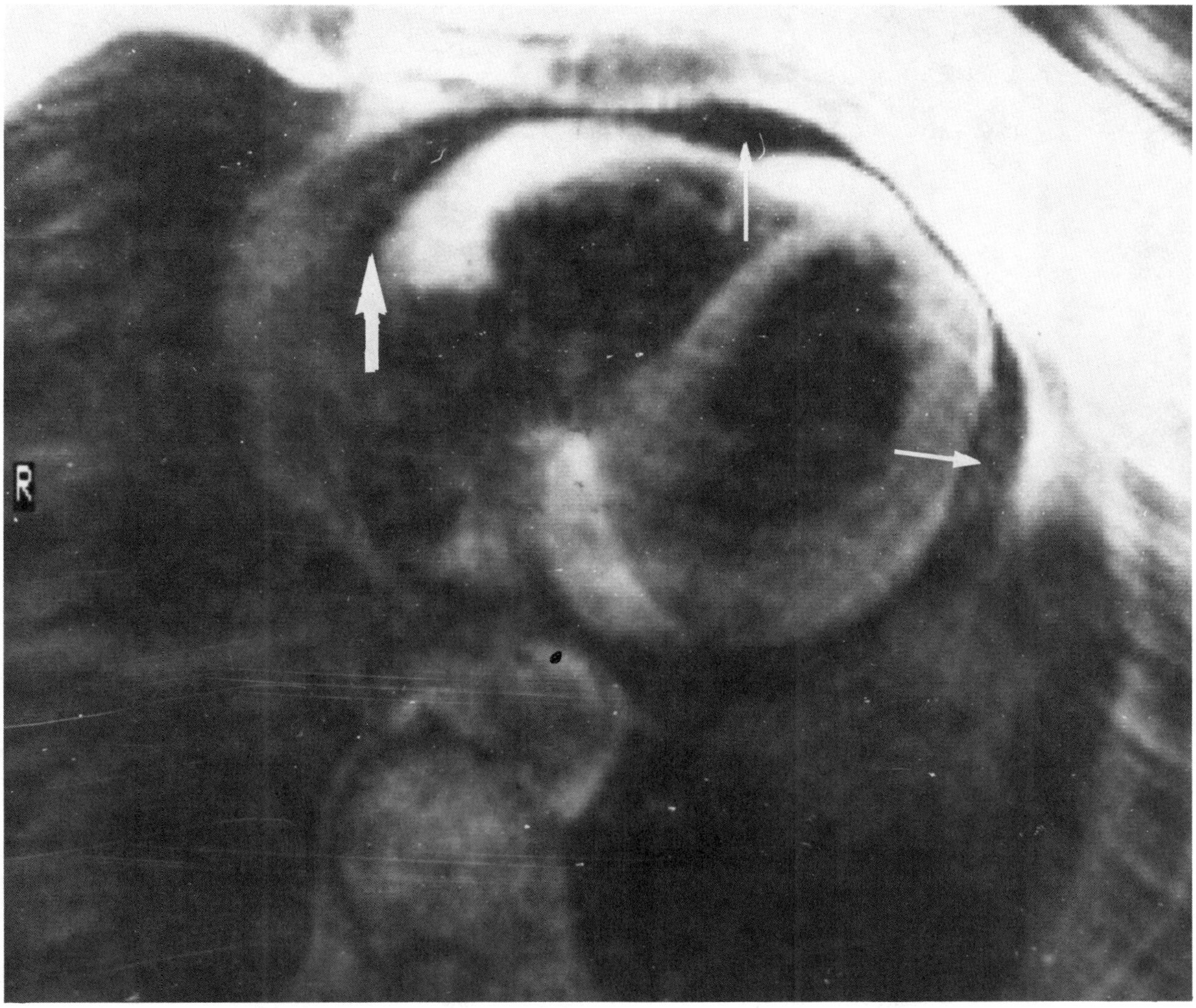

Figure 4.13. Pericardial thickening associated with chronic polyarthritis. The pericardium (arrows) is well recognized as a structure having similar signal intensity to the myocardium.

an increased signal intensity. In these cases, pericardial thickening and adhesions between the parietal and the visceral pericardium can be identified and differentiated from the pericardial fluid. This is particularly well seen when the TR is lengthened by skipping one or more heart cycles. A case of pericarditis due to lupus erythematosus has been published (49). The fluid was reported to have low signal intensity while the thickened parietal pericardium had intermediate signal strength. We observed one patient with pericardial manifestations of chronic polyarthritis and made

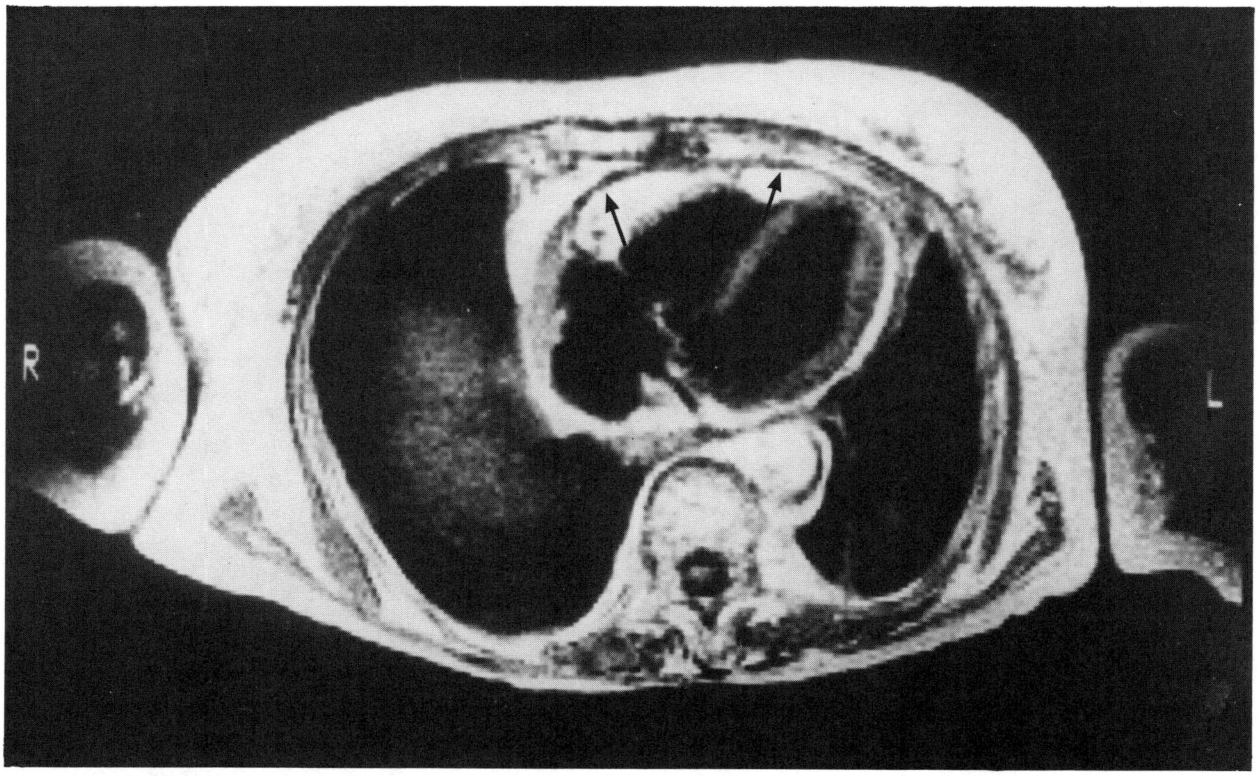

Figure 4.14. MRI study demonstrates fatty pericardial infiltration with high signal intensity. The pericardium itself is represented as a rim of low signal intensity (arrows).

similar observations (Figure 4.14). Pericardial fluid is not distributed evenly in the pericardial space, it is generally collected mainly dorsolaterally to the left ventricle. Sometimes the fluid is collected near the right atrium. The anterior pericardial recess situated between the aorta and pulmonary artery was enlarged in 11 out of 15 patients with pericardial effusion in Sechtem's study. Volume evaluation remained relatively unprecise owing to the uneven distribution of the effusion around the heart. In small effusions (less than 30 ml), however, MR detection was better than by echocardiography. Stark, *et al.* (81) stated that MR is able to differentiate and characterize pericardial fluid with different compositions. Proteinaceous or cellular impurities reportedly would increase the signal intensity of pericardial fluid when imaged with a technique using a long TR and TE. Therefore, blood would have intermediate or high signal intensity according to whether there are clotted or serous components. On the contrary, we personally observed two cases where purulent or hemorrhagic effusion had low signal intensity.

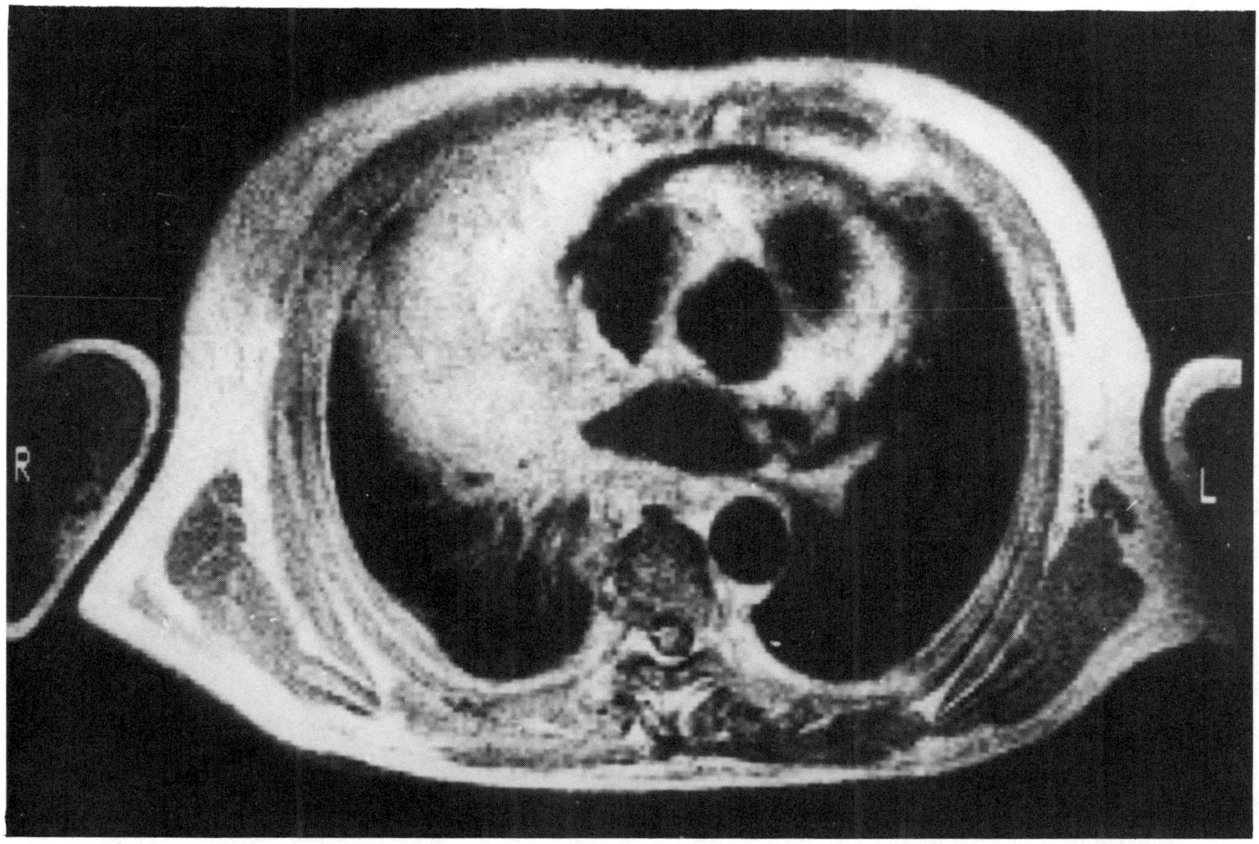

Figure 4.15. Neoplastic pericardial effusion in a patient with lung cancer. The neoplasm infiltrates the wall of the left atrium.

In chronic constrictive pericarditis the pericardium has low signal intensity due to thick fibrous tissue or calcification. With post operative patients, the signal of the pericardium is often of intermediate intensity representing an inflammatory reaction. MRI contributes to the diagnosis of restrictive cardiomyopathy by excluding pericardial thickening. In these cases, MRI is a useful tool for differential diagnosis between constrictive pericarditis and fibrous cardiomyopathy.

The inflamed pericardium is thickened and edematous, which results in an increase of its signal intensity. This can be seen in infectious pericarditis as well as in inflammatory processes of metabolic or systemic origin (uremia, connective tissue diseases, etc.). Pericardial cysts have long T_1 and T_2 values indicative of fluid-filled structures. Usually, there is a line of lower signal intensity surrounding the cyst, corresponding to the parietal pericardium. MRI distinguishes very well the paracardiac mass from the myocardium, showing the low intensity signal of the pericardium between the mass and the heart. Pericardial and myocardial invasion by adjacent masses is also well demonstrated (Figure 4.15).

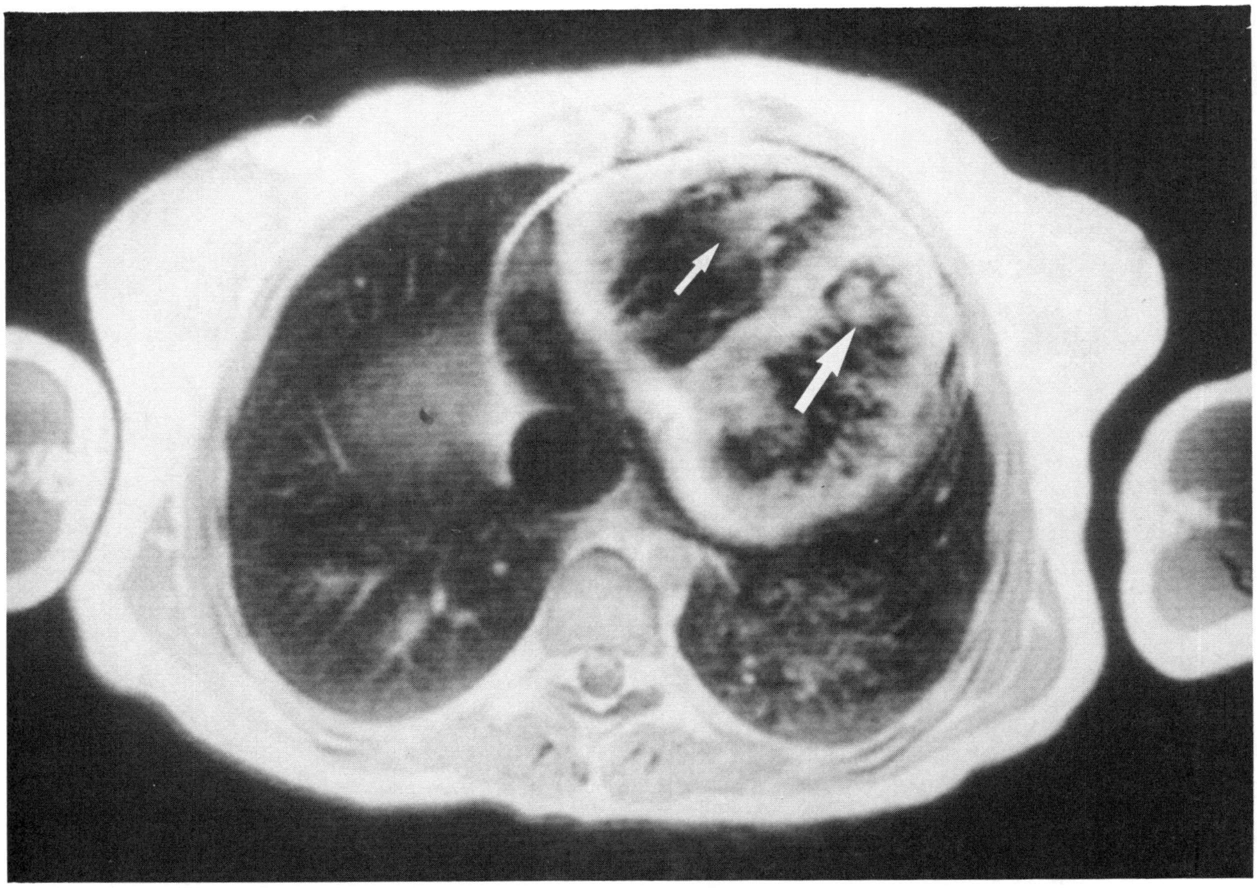

Figure 4.16. In this 12-year-old boy, echocardiography depicted intracavitary echogenic lesions in both ventricles. The MRI study confirmed intracavitary tumors in both right and left ventricles. The signal intensity was similar to that of the myocardium. Final diagnosis was myxomas of the right and left ventricles (arrows).

Neoplastic Diseases

MRI is likely to become the optimal imaging modality for the demonstration of intracardiac tumors. It has increasingly been used for refinement of the diagnosis of intracardiac masses suggested by other techniques.

Thrombi are identified on MR images as structures of intermediate signal intensity projecting into a cardiac chamber. The relative signal intensity of a thrombus increases with the echo number compared to the first echo leading to increased contrast with the myocardial wall.

It has been stated that MRI is a reliable method for detecting left atrial myxomas (87). In our experience and in accordance with the literature, the signal intensity of myxomas is similar to that of the myocardium (Figure 4.16). We also diagnosed left ventricular metastasis originating from a breast tumor which pre-

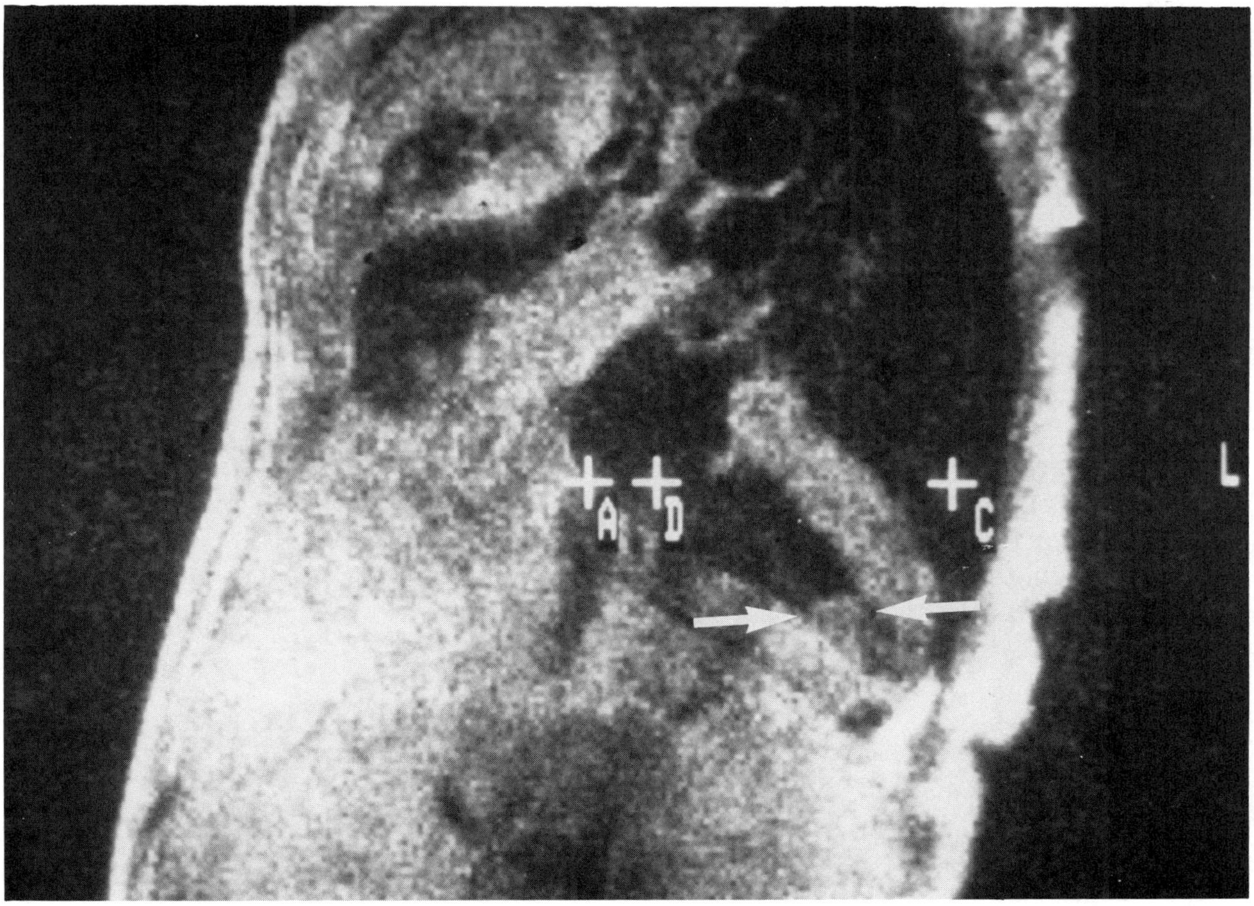

Figure 4.17. This proven metastasis (arrows) of a breast cancer in a 47-year-old woman shows a signal intensity similar to that of the myocardium.

sented similar signal behavior (Figure 4.17). The location of the lesion is the most important criterion for diagnosis. Myxomas usually are located in the left atrium and arise from the septum, while thombi usually occur on the posterior and lateral wall.

Because of the precise delineation of the pericardium, of the myocardial walls and of the great vessels, MRI appears to be more accurate than CT for assessing the extent of tumors adjacent to cardiovascular structures. Several reports (62, 63, 88) have documented the clinical utility of triggered MR for demonstrating invasion of the pericardium, cardiac chambers and pulmonary arteries. Great intrinsic contrast resolution is not only provided by the low signal from vessels but also by the high intensity of mediastinal fat. Coronal, sagittal and oblique projections are of great utility for evaluation of tumor extent. The fatty outline of an examined structure represents an excellent indicator for its integrity. In our experience, 11 patients with proven pulmonary neoplasm were referred for possible invasion of the pericardium, pulmonary veins or pulmonary arteries as suspected on CT. The patients subsequently underwent MRI. Whereas CT scans were equivocal, MR predicted resectability which was confirmed by surgery in 9 patients (Figures 4.18, 4.19 and 4.20).

➡

Figure 4.18. Sagittal section in a patient with an esophageal cancer. Echocardiographic findings suggested an intraatrial tumor. MRI diagnosis, confirmed by surgery, was atrial compression without invasion. This latter statement was based on the visible posterior fat plane suggesting pericardial integrity (arrow).

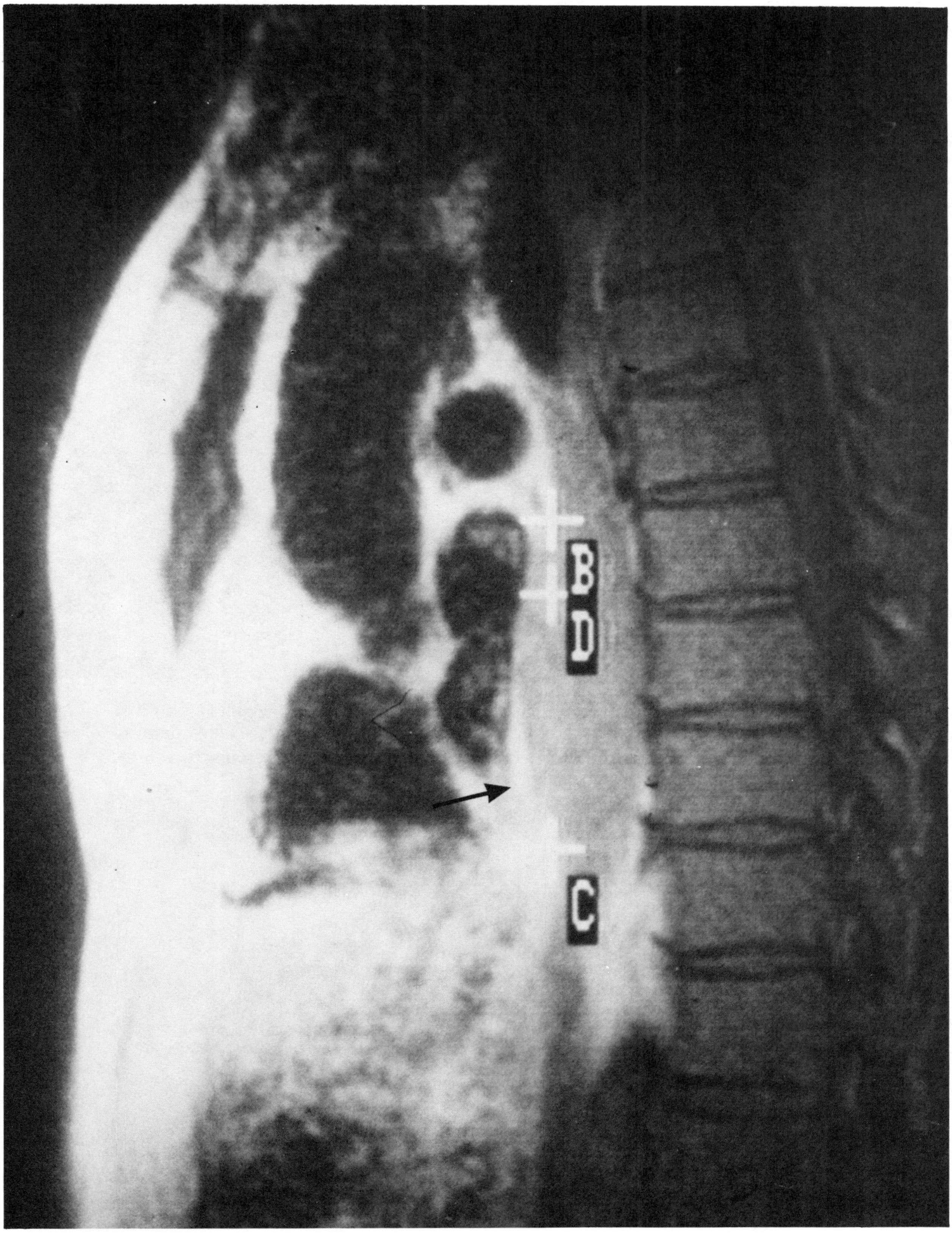
B
D
C

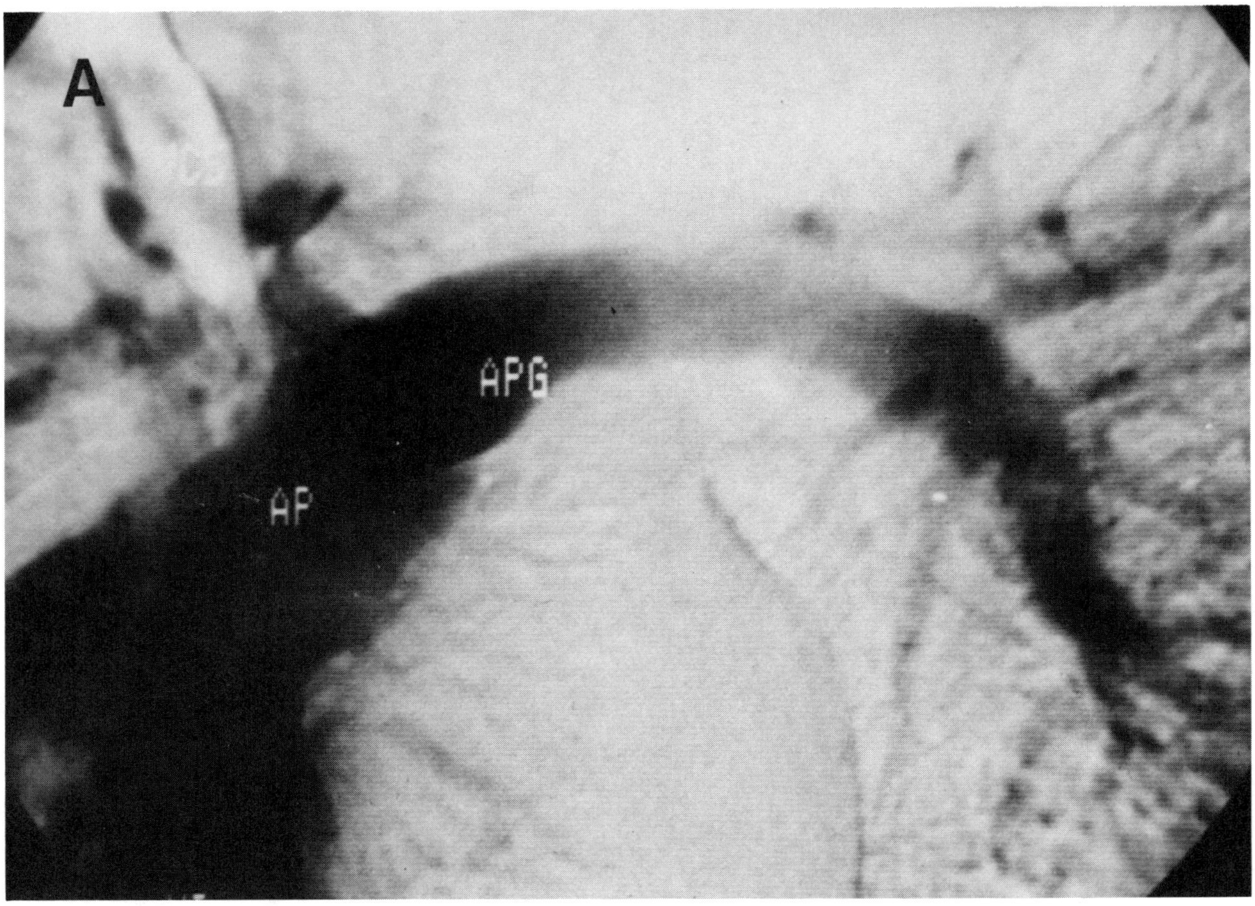

Figure 4.19. Patient with a left lung cancer. MRI oblique sagittal section (B) performed in the same projection as a DSA study (A). Both studies demonstrate similarly a carcinomatous involvement of the left pulmonary artery.

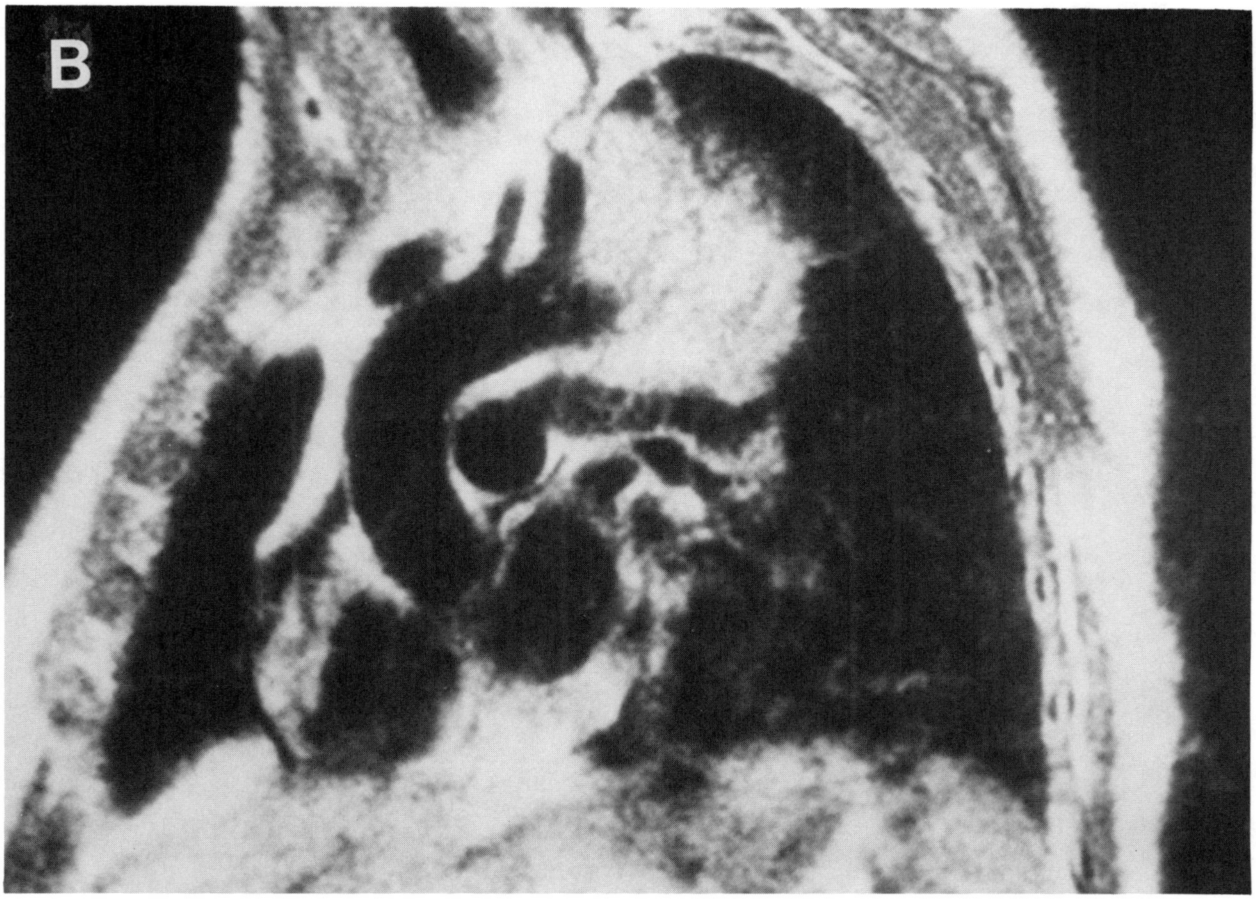
B

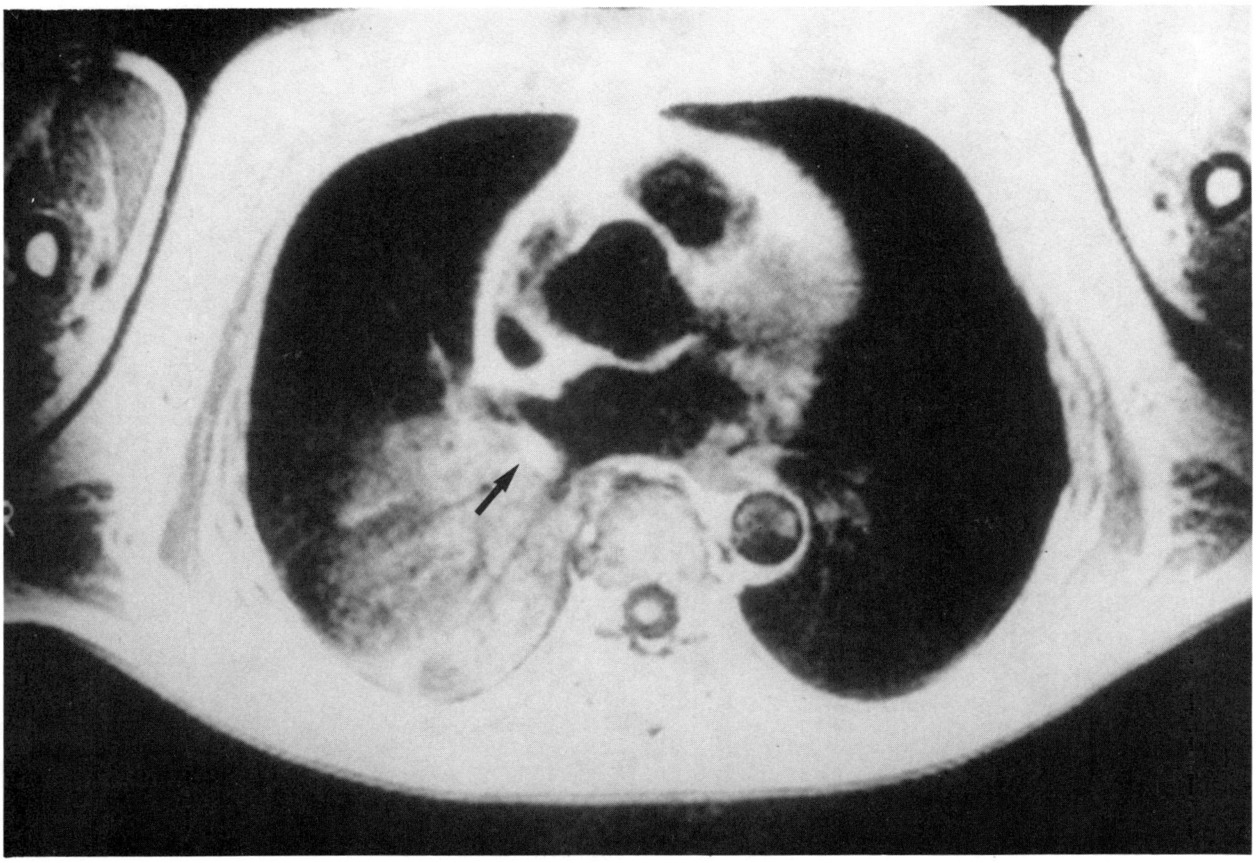

Figure 4.20. Transverse section on the level of the left atrium in a patient with lung cancer. Resectability was evaluated by ECG triggered MRI. The right pulmonary veins were involved, but pericardial invasion could be excluded on basis of fat plane integrity (arrow). Operative findings confirmed this conclusion.

Acquired Diseases of the Thoracic Aorta

MRI has several characteristics which are particularly well suited to study the aorta: high intrinsic contrast betweel flowing blood and stationary structures without the need for contrast injection, multidirectional imaging capabilities and measurement facilities. Therefore, the technique is able to provide visualization of the cephalic branches of the aorta.

Several methods for magnetic resonance angiography have been described (16, 94). As with conventional DSA, most of these techniques rely upon the acquisition of two projective images which differ only in the high signal intensities of the vascular structures. By substracting these images, stationary tissue signal intensities cancel out, thus highlighting the vascular tree (Figure 4.21).

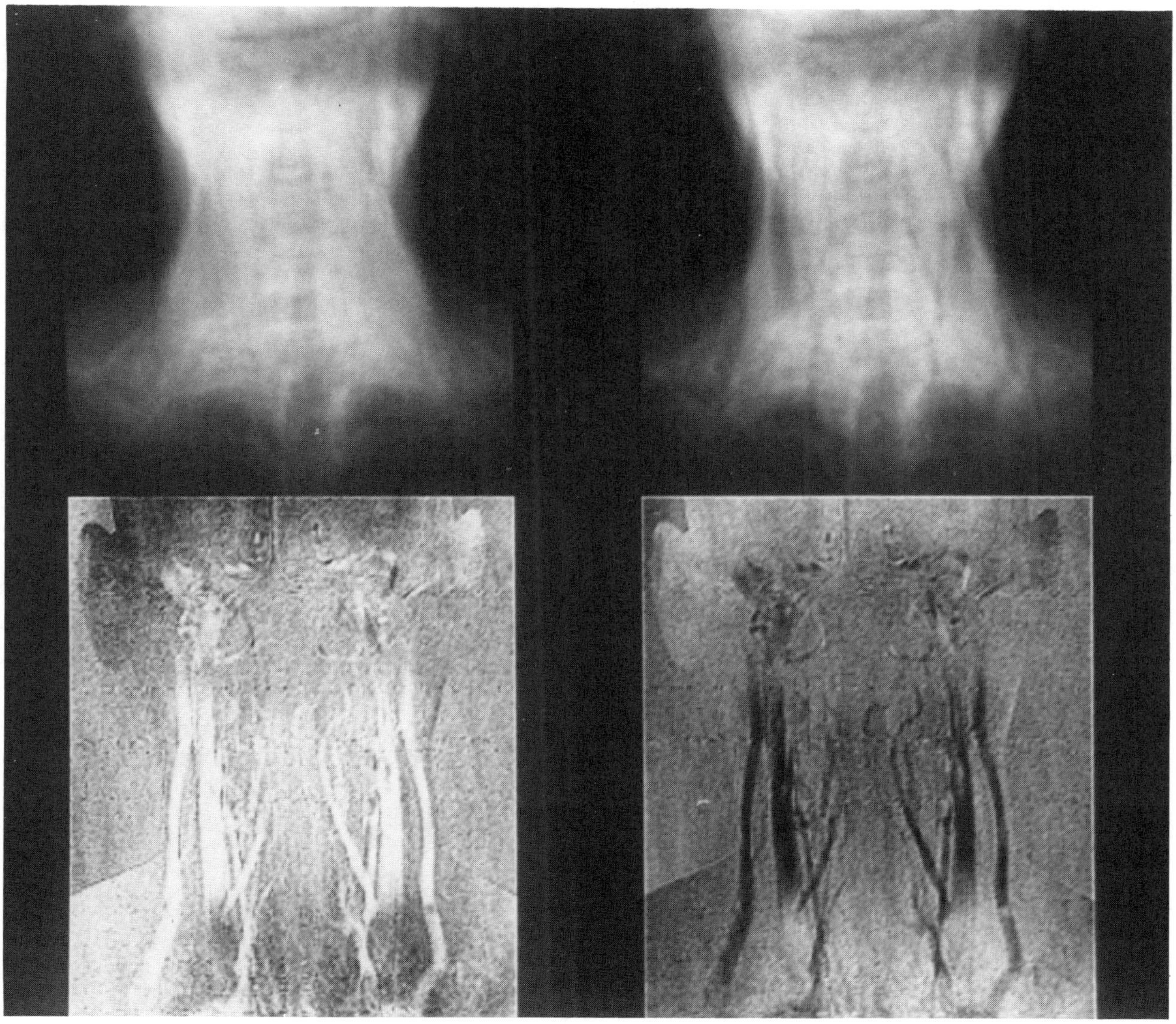

Figure 4.21. This figure shows coronal images of the cephalic vessels obtained in a volunteer. The upper projective images have been acquired respectively at diastole and at systole. The lower images result from the substraction of the two upper ones. By courtesy B. Poncelet.

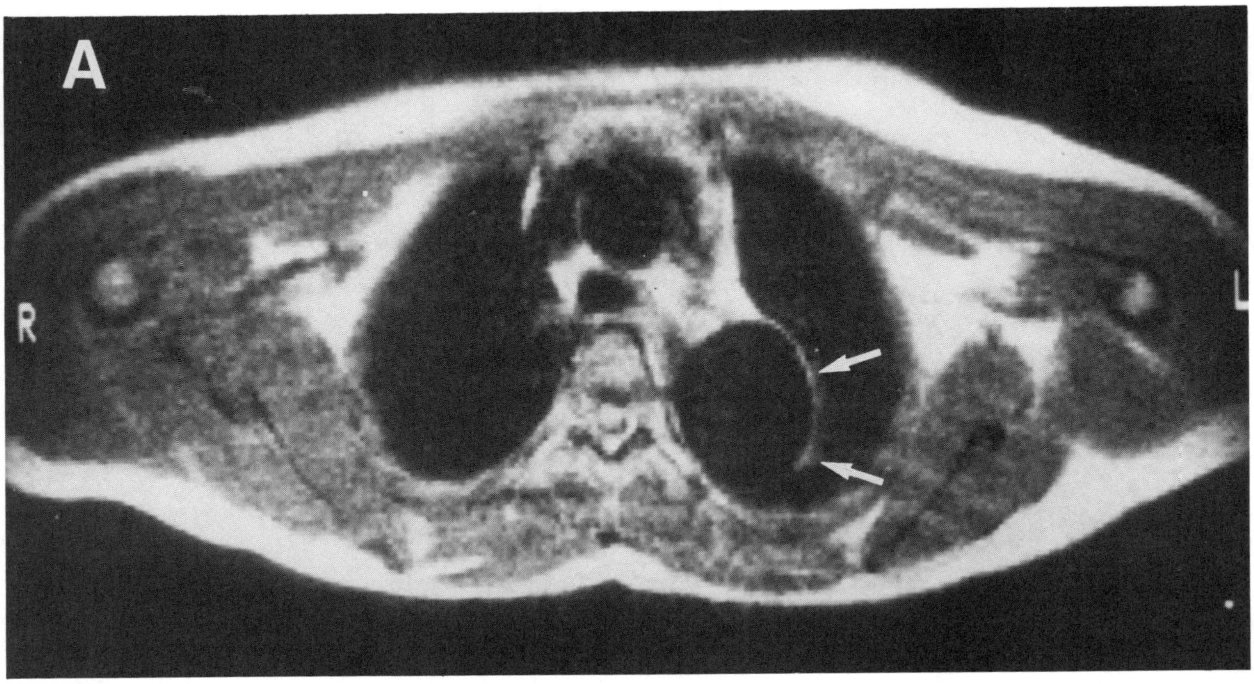

Figure 4.22, Transverse (A) and sagittal (B) magnetic resonance imaging in a 26-year-old woman. A widening of the left upper mediastinum was noticed on a check-up chest x-ray. MR study demonstrates a large saccular aneurysm of the proximal descending aorta. Surgery confirmed the diagnosis (arrows).

MRI studies have been reported (89-91) to provide reliable diagnosis in a variety of pathological conditions including dissecting, fusiform, saccular and post-traumatic aneurysms. Morphology, location and size of aneurysms could be adequately evaluated on either long or short-axis images. However, most information is provided by oblique long-axis images. Aortic wall thickness was well shown with pathological changes such as wall thickening secondary to giant cell aortitis (89). The use of MRI for recognition of aortic dissection has also been described (91) including identification of the true and false channels and eventual involvement of aortic branches. R.E. Dinsmore, *et al.* (89, 90) described additional features: the identification of the intimal tear in the ascending aorta and the enhancement of true and false channels by the use of phase-shift technique for the display of differential rates of flow. However, presently the evaluation of aortic regurgitation still requires conventional angiography (Figures 4.22, 4.23).

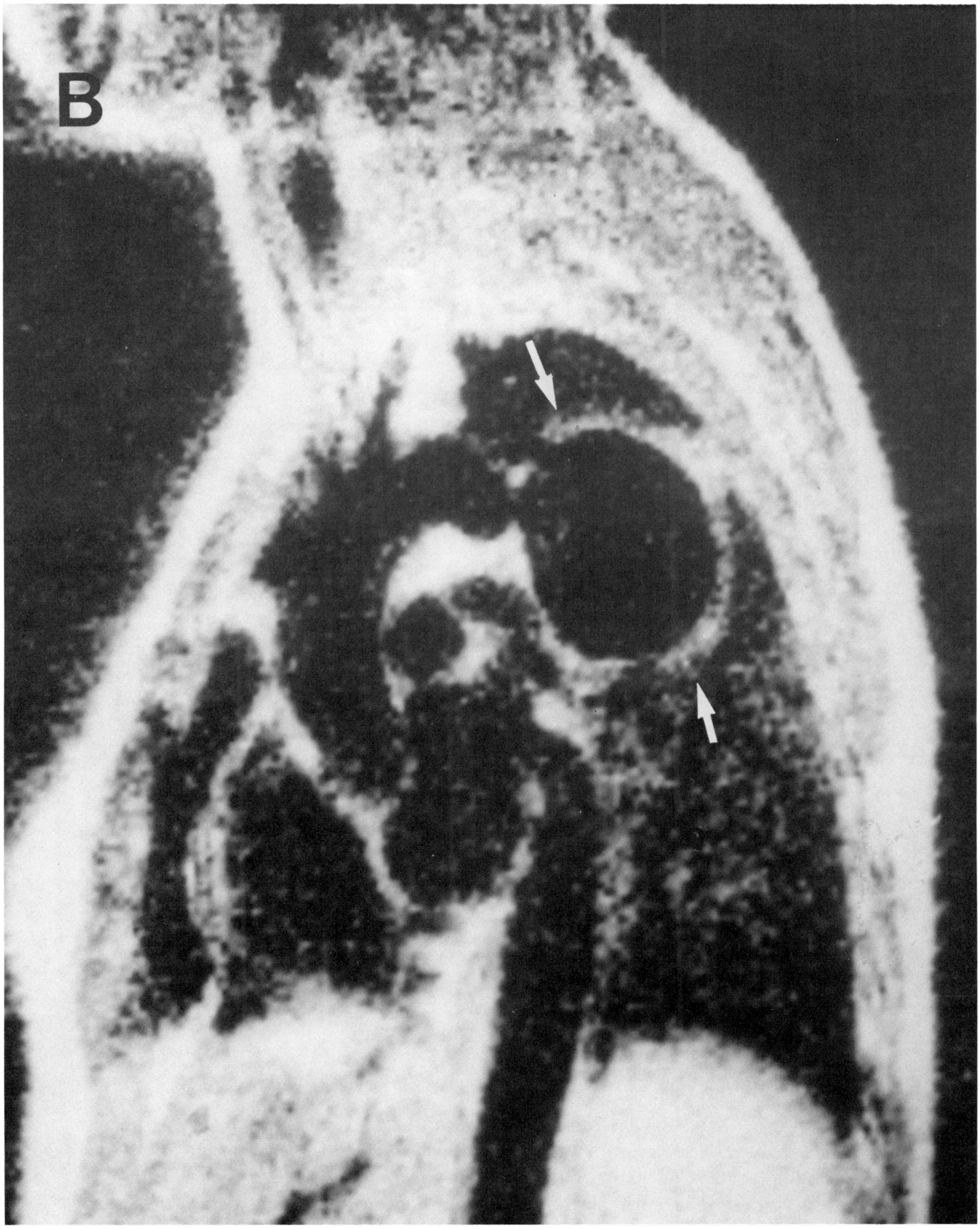
B

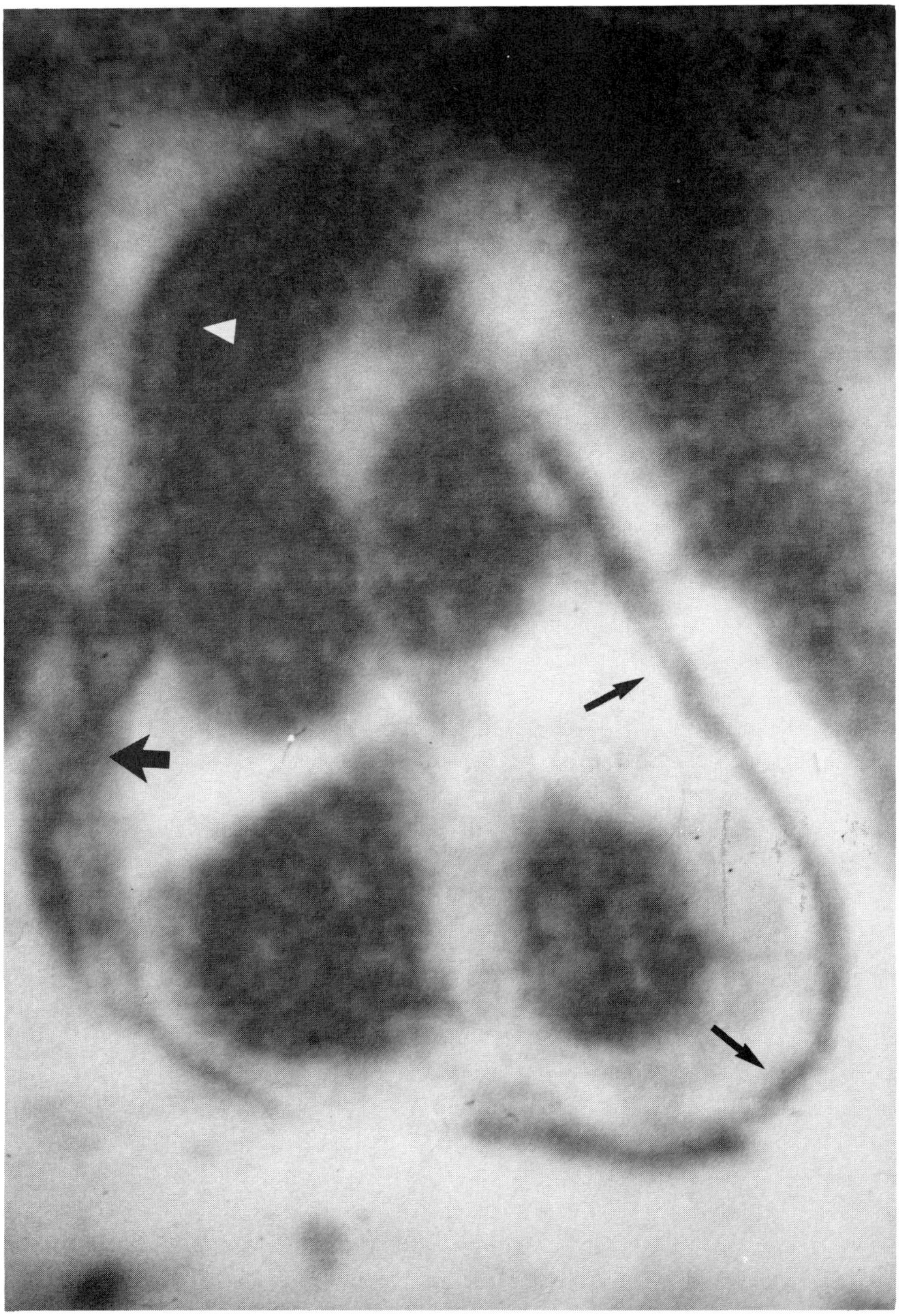

Figure 4.23. This 62-year-old man was admitted to the hospital having acute, severe pain in the anterior chest and neck. CT showed dissection of the ascending aorta. The patient was in stable condition and MRI was performed in emergency. The coronal oblique section demonstrates a dissection of the ascending aorta starting above the ostium of the right coronary artery (large arrow) and a pericardial hemorrhagic effusion (small arrows). The intimal tear is visible (arrowhead). These statements were confirmed by the surgical findings.

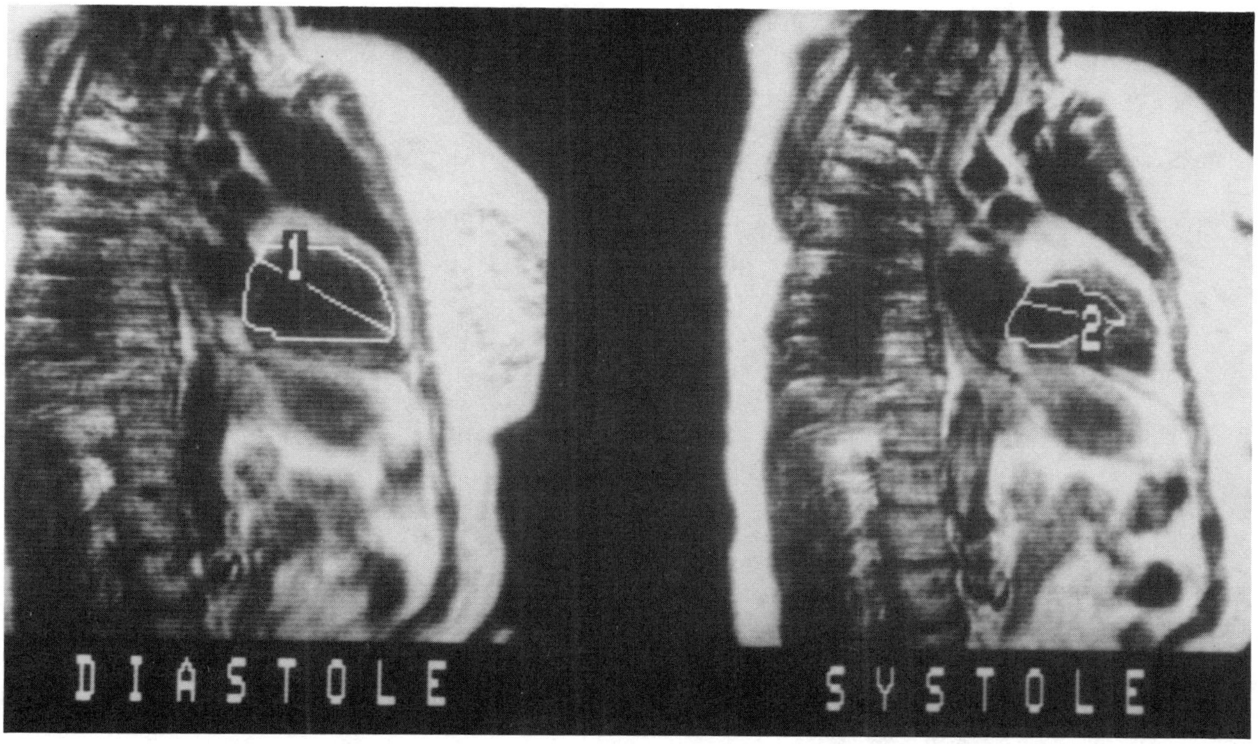

Figure 4.24. Area and length measurements on the left ventricle obtained by MR during diastole and systole.

CARDIOVASCULAR FUNCTION

Ventricular Function

Aside from its ability to visualize pathology in a RAO coronal plane parallel to the interventricular septum, it seems that a reasonable correlation exists between ejection fractions determined by MR imaging and those obtained from angiographic images (85). The ability of MR to determine regional left ventricular function was investigated by S.R. Underwood, *et al.* (83). Muscle thickness was measured in selected segments. Wall motion was analyzed. The technique depicts not only wall motion, but also permits quantitation of ventricular mass. Diminished wall thickening has been depicted in patients with chronic and acute myocardial infarctions. Volume and mass quantitation can be evaluated for both left and right ventricles (Figure 4.24, 4.25). In addition, it seems that reliable quantitation of blood flow will enhance our understanding of the physiology and pathological changes in various cardiac and vascular disorders.

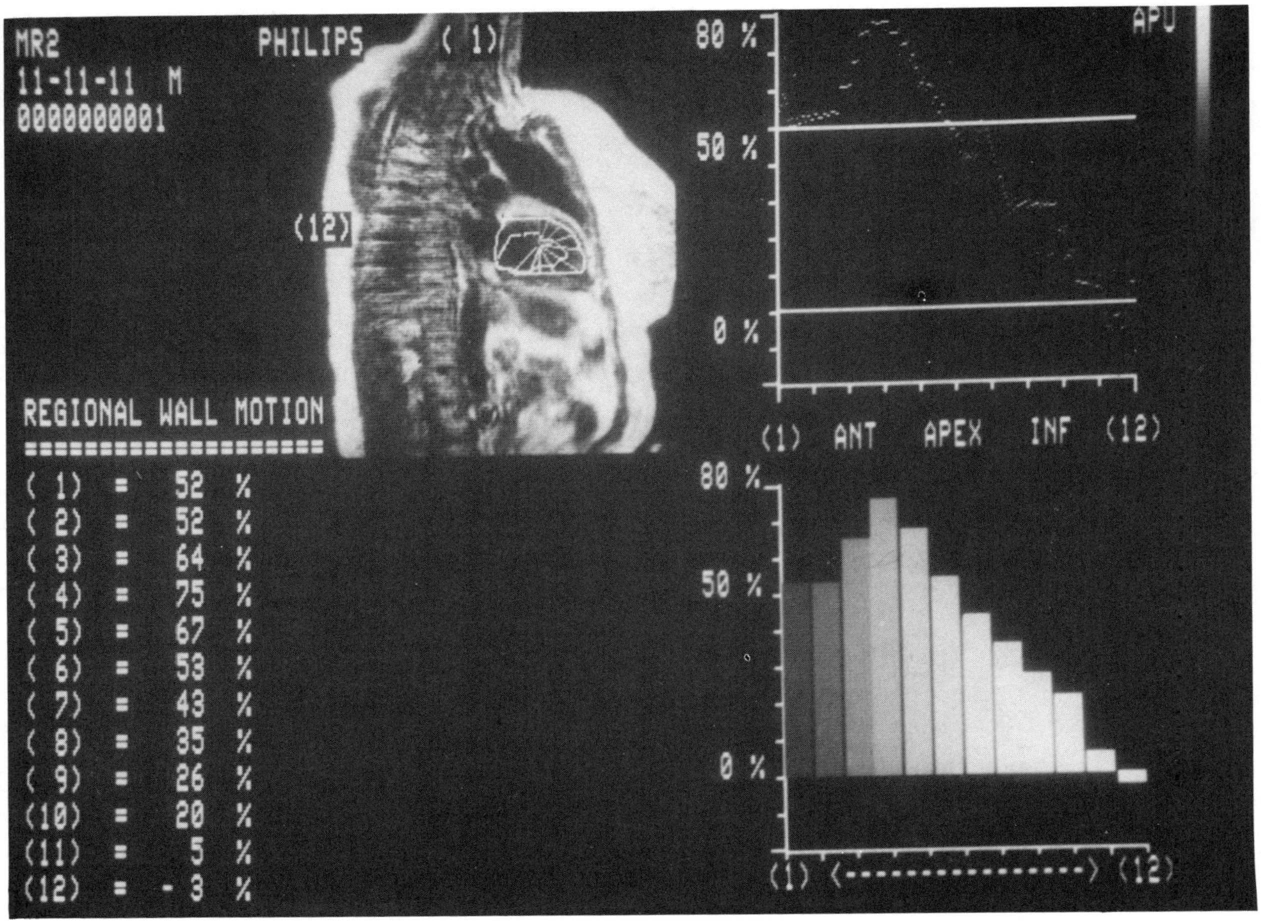

Figure 4.25. Segmentation of the sagittal oblique magnetic resonance images for the analysis of wall motion. This display indicates an inferior akinesia.

MR SPECTROSCOPY (MRS) OF THE HEART: A VIEW TO CARDIAC METABOLISM

The MRI investigation of cardiac morphology and function requires optimal spatial resolution in the images. Therefore, the instrumental frequency is set to the resonance frequency of the protons. The signal intensities of these nuclei outrange by far the intensities of other nuclei in biological tissues. The major contribution to the proton signal arises from the water molecules. In fatty tissues, mobile lipid molecules also generate observable signals. Image contrast is dominated by the differences between tissues in the densities of the water and lipid molecules and by the differences in the water proton relaxation times. The water proton relaxation rates vary with the molecular environment of the water molecules, and consequently are tissue dependent. With gradient recalled echoes, image contrast is furthermore modulated by phase differences between water and lipid signals (22).

With MRS, the signals generated by a particular nucleus are separated into different components, each arising ideally from nuclei embedded in a particular chemical substructure. For instance, the separation of the proton signals of biological tissue into the two dominating components, respectively arising from water and mobile lipid molecules, is a straightforward example of proton MR spectroscopy. In this particular case, the sensitivity of the experiment is such that this separation can be performed with the spatial resolution of standard proton imaging. Pulse schemes have been developed which generate separate water and lipid images ("proton chemical shift imaging" [23]), and which seem applicable to cardiac imaging. Proton chemical shift imaging of the heart might have some potential in the detection of increased myocardial lipids in post-ischemic myocardium (24).

With MRS of biological tissues, however, one is usually interested in the detection of metabolites which are present at considerably lower concentrations than the water molecules. As a consequence, one is led to sacrifice spatial resolution in favor of signal-to-noise, and to acquire signal from a single volume in most MRS applications. Hence these types of experiments have been called "localized MR spectroscopy experiments." Various techniques have been developed with the aim of extracting spectroscopic information out of a single volume. The least sophisticated of these techniques acquire signal from the sensitive volume of a surface coil (25), and do provide imperfect depth selection. Other methods rely on complex pulse schemes, and isolate signal from more or less well delineated volumes (26).

Within the realm of in vivo MRS, the isotopes which are likely to offer the greatest clinical potential are phosphorous-31, hydrogen-1 and carbon--13. Depending upon which of these nuclei is being focused on, different sets of metabolites will become visible.

Phosphorous-31 MRS

Phosphorous-31 MR spectroscopy of the heart has the potential of providing information on myocardial energy metabolism (27). The phosphorous-31 spectrum of heart muscle is composed of lines which may be assigned to the phosphate groups of the adenosine-triphosphate (ATP), of the phosphocreatine (PCr) and of the inorganic phosphate (Pi) molecules present. In addition, observable signal is present in the phosphomonoester and phosphodiester regions of the spectrum. Signal intensities are such that usable 31P spectra of the human heart can be obtained within 5 to 10 minutes acquisition time (28). The spectral position of the inorganic phosphate line is pH dependent, due to the rapid chemical exchange process between different inorganic phosphate groups. As a consequence, the tissue pH can be derived from the 31P spectrum, and this constitutes the only non-invasive way to obtain this information. In addition to the relative concentrations of the MR observable phosphate metabolites and to the pH, the phosphorous-31 spectra can provide information about the fluxes of intracellular enzyme catalyzed reactions, by applying magnetic labeling techniques such as saturation transfer (29).

Phosphorous-31 MR spectroscopy has been extensively used for the study of cardiac energy metabolism. Initial animal studies were performed on a rapidly excised and cooled rat heart, and aimed at the characterization of normoxic and ischemic cardiac tissues (30). Subsequent studies were mostly carried out on a perfused working heart (31). Early examples of these types of experiments include the study of global and regional myocardial ischemia (32, 33, 34), the assessment of drug treatment of myocardial infarction (35), the observation of changes in high-energy phosphates at different phases of the cardiac cycle (36), assessment of the steady state rate of ATP synthesis (29), and creatine phosphokinase kinetics during ischemia and arrest (37).

The advent of high field, medium and large bore systems, and the concomitant development of localization techniques, have nowadays rendered possible the in vivo extension of previous studies (38). Very recently, first attempts of in vivo localized 31P spectroscopy of the human heart have been reported (28, 39, 40, 41, 42, 43).

Hydrogen-1 Spectroscopy

The feasibility of in vivo high resolution proton spectroscopy, at moderate magnetic field strength (1.5-2 Tesla), has been demonstrated in animal (44) and human brains (45, 46). This type of experiment is particularly difficult, in that one aims to detect metabolites which are present at concentrations that are typically four orders of magnitude smaller than the tissue concentration of water. Furthermore, the proton chemical shift range in biological tissue is small, so that the achievement of adequate spectral resolution in the proton spectrum would ideally require the use of high magnetic field strengths. This requirement is not met in the case of whole body imagers, for instance.

Despite these difficulties, several important metabolites, including phosphocreatine and creatine, lactate, and amino acids such as glutamine and N-acetyl-aspartate, could be identified in the spectra obtained in vivo from rabbit brain, at 1.9 Tesla (44). Also, the production and clearance of lactate during hypoxemia and recovery could be monitored with a time resolution of about 5 minutes.

The intrinsic sensitivity of the MR experiment is about 15 times larger for protons than for phosphorous-31 nuclei (at constant magnetic field [47]). The lactate concentration in the myocardium is known to increase from 1 mMol in healthy state to between 10 and 30 mMol in ischemic conditions (48). In other terms, the lactate methyl protons (which generate a single line in the proton spectrum) are present in the ischemic myocardium at concentrations ranging between 30 and 90 mMol. The comparison of these figures with the inorganic phosphate concentration in the myocardial cytosol (around 1 mMol), in combination with the intrinsic sensitivity argument, suggest that the lactate signal in the high resolution water suppressed proton spectrum, might constitute a more sensitive marker of myocardial ischemia than the inorganic phosphate signal in the phosphorous-31 spectrum (48). This statement has to be considered, however, in that it is difficult to compare the sensitivities of the phosphorous pH measurement (a frequency determination that constitutes an indirect measure of lactic acid production) and of the lactate proton signal intensity measurement. Besides, the complexity of the water suppressed proton experiment might further prove increased by the presence of lipids which also would obscure the lactate signal. In that case spectral editing methods (49) would have to be applied in addition to the localization and water suppression techniques. The application of these techniques to a moving organ such as the heart is undoubtedly at, or beyond, the limit of what currently may be considered feasible.

Carbon-13 Spectroscopy

At constant magnetic field intensity, the inherent MR sensitivity to carbon-13 nuclei is about one-sixtieth of that to protons (47). In addition, the natural abundance of the carbon-13 isotope hardly exceeds 1%. As a consequence, natural abundance carbon-13 signals from biological tissue are extremely weak. Only metabolites which are present at very high concentrations are detectable, at medium field strength, within clinically acceptable acquisition times.

Fatty acids in adipose tissues of the living rat (50) or hepatic glycogen in the living rabbit (51) have been detected within a few minutes by natural abundance carbon-13 spectroscopy at 1.9 Tesla. Optimization of the carbon-13 signal strength required gated proton decoupling, a technique whereby considerable RF power is dissipated within the tissues under study. It is not clear, as yet, whether these types of signal enhancement methods will be applicable to humans.

The MR detectability of glycogen is unexpected, in that glycogen is a high molecular weight polymer (about 100 Megadaltons). Hence, one would expect very broad MR lines, resulting from the lack of molecular mobility. In reality, appreciable intramolecular motion within the glycogen molecule is present, with correlation times of the order of 0.01 msec, as demonstrated by nuclear magnetic relaxation studies on rat liver, at 8.5 Tesla (52). These same studies have shown that intramolecular motions induce a 100% visibility of the glycogen carbon-13 nuclei in the high resolution MR spectrum.

The low natural abundancy of carbon-13 nuclei, in combination with the large chemical shift range spanned by these nuclei in biological tissue (200 ppm), has triggered the development of experiments with carbon-13 labelled substrates such as (1-13 C) glucose (53, 54). Initially applied with cellular suspensions (55) and perfused organs (56), these techniques have more recently found application in vivo (57, 58, 59, 60).

Carbon-13 MR spectroscopy has been used for the study of fuel metabolism in the heart (58, 59, 61). In vivo carbon-13 cardiac measurements on the open-chested guinea pig provided natural-abundance spectra with resonances which could be assigned to fatty acids. Natural-abundance glycogen could not be detected, however. During intravenous infusion of D-(1-13C) glucose and insulin, the time course of myocardial glycogen synthesis could be followed serially during four hours. Anoxia resulted in the degradation of the labeled glycogen within 6 minutes and in the appearance of the 13C label in the lactic acid. Simultaneous observation of the 31P MR spectrum demonstrated no change in the high energy phosphates, suggesting that carbon-13 experiments with labeled substrates really do provide a nondestructive tool for the study of cardiac fuel metabolism (58). To date, no carbon-13 experiments on the human heart have been reported.

In conclusion, MRS is currently an established research tool for the non-invasive assessment of metabolic processes in various organs, including the heart. In contrast to MRI, there is still a very long way to go, however, before MRS will have gained recognition as a clinical tool. Numerous difficulties must be overcome, some of which are related to the lack of sensitivity (or spatial resolution), to the necessary discrimination between tissues (spatial localization), to the lack of spectral resolution (especially true with 1H MRS), and to the presence of high intensity signals overlapping the spectral information arising from the metabolites of interest (water and lipid signal suppression technique).

REFERENCES

1. Mansfield P: Multi-planar image formation using NMR spin echoes. *J Phys C, 10:*155, 1977.

2. Mansfield P, Pykett IL: Biological and medical imaging by NMR. *J Magn Reson, 29:*355, 1978.

3. Kumar A, Welti D, Ernst RR: NMR Fourier Zeugmatography. *J Magn Reson, 18:*69, 1975.

4. Edelstein WA, Hutchison JMS, Johnson G, Redpath T: Spin warp NMR imaging and applications to human whole-body imaging. *Phys Med Biol, 25:*751, 1980.

5. Muir AL, Smith MA, Been M, Ridgway JP, Douglas RHB, Kean DM, Best JJK: Sequential changes in T_1 in man following acute myocardial infarction. *Soc Magn Reson Med, 86:*237, 1986.

6. Bottomley PA, Foster TH, Argersinger RE, Pfeifer LM: A review of normal tissue hydrogen NMR relaxation times and relaxation mechanisms from 1-100 MHz: Dependence on tissue type, NMR frequency, temperature, species, excision, and age. *Med Phys, 11:*425, 1984.

7. Higgins CB: Overview of MR of the heart (1986). *AJR, 146:*907, 1986.

8. Kaufman L, Crooks L, Sheldon P, Hricak H, Herfkens R, Bank W: The potential impact of nuclear magnetic resonance imaging on cardiovascular diagnosis. *Circulation, 67:*251, 1983.

9. Wehrli F, MacFall JR, Axel L, Shutts D, Glover GH, Herfkins RJ: Approaches to in-plane and out-of-plane flow imaging. *Noninvas Med Imag, 1:*127, 1984.

10. Bradley WG, Waluch V: Blood flow: Magnetic resonance imaging. *Radiology, 154:*443, 1985.

11. Moran PR: A flow velocity zeugmatographic interlace for NMR imaging in humans. *Magn Reson Imag, 1:*197, 1982.

12. van Dijk P: Direct cardiac NMR imaging of heart wall and blood velocity. *JCAT, 8:*419, 1984.

13. Waluch V, Bradley WG: NMR even echo rephasing in slow laminar flow. *JCAT, 8:*594, 1984.

14. Wendt RE, Murphy PH, Ford JJ, Bryan RN, Burdine JA: Phase alterations of spin echoes by motion along magnetic field gradients. *Magn Reson Med, 2:*527, 1985.

15. Wedeen VJ, Rosen BR, Chesler D, Brady TJ: MR velocity imaging by phase display. *JCAT, 9:*530, 1985.

16. Wedeen VJ, Meuli RA, Edelman RE, Geller SC, Frank LR, Brady TJ, Rosen BR: Projective imaging of pulsatile flow with magnetic resonance. *Science, 230:*946, 1985.

17. Feinberg DA, Crooks L, Heonninger J, Arakawa M, Watts J: Pulsatile blood velocity in human arteries displayed by magnetic resonance imaging. *Radiology, 153:*177, 1984.

18. Haase A, Frahm J, Matthaei J, Hanicke W, Merboldt KD: FLASH imaging: Rapid NMR imaging using low flip angle pulses. *J Magn Reson, 67:* 258, 1986.

19. Herfkens R, Utz J, Glover G, Fram E, Shimakawa A, Heinsimer J: Rapid dynamic NMR imaging of the heart: Initial clinical experience. *Soc Magn Reson Med, 86:*247, 1986.

20. Buxton RB, Edelman RR, Rosen BR, Wismer GL, Brady TJ: Contrast in rapid MRI: T_1 and T_2 weighted imaging. *JCAT* 1986, In press.

21. Doyle M, Chapman B, Turner R, Ordidge RJ, Cawley M, Coxon R, Glover P, Coupland RE, Morris GK, Worthington BS, Mansfield P: Real-time cardiac imaging of adults at video frame rates by magnetic resonance imaging. *Lancet*, September 20, 682, 1986.

22. Axel L: Fat-water phase contrast in rapid, small flip angle MR imaging. RSNA 1986, 184, 1986.

23. Dixon WT: Simple proton spectroscopic imaging. *Radiology, 153:* 189. 1984.

24. Reeves RC, Evanochko WT, Canby RC, McMillin JB, Pohost GM: 1H NMR spectroscopic detection of increased myocardial lipids in post-ischemic "stunned" myocardium. *Soc Magn Reson Med, 86:*WIP, 131, 1986.

25. Ackerman JJH, Grove TH, Wong GG, Gadian DG, Radda GK: Mapping of metabolites in whole animals by 31P NRM using surface coils. *Nature (London), 283:*167, 1980.

26. Aue WP: Localization methods for in vivo NMR spectroscopy. *Rev Magn Reson Med, 1:*21, 1986.

27. Gadian DG: *Nuclear Magnetic Resonance and its Applications to Living Systems.* Oxford: Oxford University Press, 1982.

28. Bottomley PA, Smith LS, Herfkens RJ, Bashore TM, Utz JA: Detecting human myocardial infarction with localized 31P NMR: Characterization of normal and ischemic tissue. *Soc Magn Reson Med, 86:*606, 1986.

29. Matthews PM, Bland JL, Gadian DG, Radda GK: The steady state rate of ATP synthesis in the perfused rat heart measured by 31P NMR saturation transfer. *Biochem Biophys Acta, 721:* 312, 1982.

30. Gadian DG, Hoult DI, Radda GK, Seeley PJ, Chance B, Barlow C: Phosphorous nuclear magnetic resonance studies on normoxic and ischemic cardiac tissue. *Proc Natl Acad Sci, USA, 73:*4446, 1976.

31. Jacobus WE, Taylor GJ, Hollis DP, Nunnally RL: Phosphorous nuclear magnetic resonance of perfused working rat hearts. *Nature, 265:* 756, 1977.

32. Hollis DP, Nunnally RL, Taylor GJ, Weisfeldt ML, Jacobus WE: Phosphorous nuclear magnetic resonance studies of heart physiology. *J Magn Reson, 29:*319, 1978.

33. Garlick PB, Radda GK, Seeley PJ: Phosphorous NMR studies on perfused heart. *Biochem Biophys Res Commun, 74:*1256, 1977.

34. Brooks WM, Willis RJ: 31P nuclear magnetic resonance study of the recovery characteristics of high-energy phosphate compounds and intracellular pH after global ischemia in the perfused guinea pig heart. *J Mol Cell Cardiol, 15:*495, 1983.

35. Nunnally RL, Bottomley PA: Assessment of pharmacological treatment of myocardial infarction by phosphorous-31 NMR with surface coils. *Science, 211:*177, 1981.

36. Fossel ET, Morgan HE, Ingwall JS: Measurement of changes in high-energy phosphates in the cardiac cycle of using 31P nuclear magnetic resonance. *Proc Natl Acad Sci, USA, 77:*3654, 1980.

37. Nunnally RL, Hollis DP: Adenosine triphosphate compartmentation in living hearts: A phosphorous nuclear magnetic resonance saturation transfer study. *Biochemistry, 18:*3642, 1979.

38. Nunnally RL: In vivo monitoring of metabolism with nuclear magnetic resonance spectroscopy. *Semin Nucl Med, 13:*377, 1983.

39. Whitman GR, Chance B, Bode H, Maris J, Haselgrove J, Kelley R, Clark BJ, Harken AH: Diagnosis and therapeutic evaluation of a pediatric case of cardiomyopathy using phosphorous-31 nuclear magnetic resonance spectroscopy. *JACC 5:*745, 1985.

40. Bottomley, PA: Noninvasive study of high-energy phosphate metabolism in human heart by depth-resolved 31P NMR spectroscopy. *Science, 229:*770, 1985.

41. Whitman GJR, Chance B, Bode H, Maris J, Haselgrove J, Kelley R, Clark BJ, Harken AD: Diagnosis and therapeutic evaluation of a pediatric case of cardiomyopathy using phosphorous-31 nuclear magnetic resonance spectroscopy. *JACC, 5:*745, 1985.

42. Styles P, Blackledge MJ, Oberhaensli R, Galloway G, Radda GK: Localization techniques for the routine examination of human brain, liver and heart by 31P NMR spectroscopy. *Soc Magn Reson Med, 86:*1085, 1986.

43. Bottomley PA, Smith LS, Herfkens RJ, Bashore TM, Utz JA: Detecting human myocardial infarction with localized 31P NMR: Characterization of normal and ischemic tissue. *Soc Magn Reson Med, 86:*606, 1986.

44. Behar KL, Rothman DL, Shulman RG, Petroff OAC, Prichard JW: Detection of cerebral lactate in vivo during hypoxemia by 1H NMR at relatively low field strengths (1.9 T). *Proc Natl Acad Sci, USA, 81:*2517, 1984.

45. Luyten PR, den Hollander JA: Observation of metabolites in the human brain by MR spectroscopy. *Radiology, 161:*795, 1986.

46. Bottomley PA, Edelstein WA, Foster TH, Adams WA: In vivo solvent-suppressed localized hydrogen nuclear magnetic resonance spectroscopy: A window to metabolism? *Proc Natl Acad Sci, USA, 82:*2148, 1985.

47. Lee K, Anderson WA: Nuclear spins, moments, and magnetic resonance frequencies. In: *The Handbook of Chemistry and Physics,* Weast RC (Ed.). Cleveland: The Chemical Rubber Company, 1978.

48. Barrett EJ, Alger JR, Zaret BL: Nuclear magnetic resonance spectroscopy: Its evolving role in the study of myocardial metabolism. *JACC 6:*497, 1985.

49. Williams SR, Gadian DG, Proctor E, Sprague DB, Talbot DF: Proton NMR studies of muscle metabolites in vivo. *J Magn Reson, 63:*406, 1985.

50. Canioni P, Alger JR, Shulman RG: Natural abundance carbon-13 nuclear magnetic resonance spectroscopy of liver and adipose tissue of the living rat. *Biochemistry, 22:*4974, 1983.

51. Alger JR, Behar KL, Rothman DL, Shulman RG: Natural-Abundance 13C NMR measurement of hepatic glycogen in the living rabbit. *J Magn Reson, 56:*334, 1984.

52. Sillerud LO, Shulman RG: Structure and metabolism of mammalian liver glycogen monitored by carbon-13 nuclear magnetic resonance. *Biochemistry, 22:*1087, 1983.

53. Shulman RG: NMR Spectroscopy of living cells. *Scien Amer, 248:* 76, 1983.

54. Alger JR, Shulman RG: Metabolic applications of high resolution 13C nuclear magnetic resonance spectroscopy. *Brit Med Bull, 40:*160, 1984.

55. Ugurbil K, Brown TR, den Hollander JA, Glynn P, Shulman RG: High resolution 13C nuclear magnetic resonance studies of glucose metabolism in Escherichia coli. *Proc Natl Acad, USA, 75:*3742, 1978.

56. Cohen SM, Shulman RG, McLaughlin AC: Effects of ethanol upon alanine metabolism in perfused mouse liver studied by 13C NMR. *Proc Natl Acad Sci, USA, 76:*4808, 1979.

57. Alger JR, Sillerud LO, Behar KL, Gillies RJ, Shulman RG, Gordon RE, Shaw D, Hanley PE: In vivo carbon-13 nuclear magnetic resonance studies of mammals. *Science, 214:*660, 1981.

58. Neurohr KJ, Barrett EJ, Shulman RG: In vivo carbon-13 nuclear magnetic resonance studies of heart metabolism. *Proc Natl Acad Sci, USA, 80:*1603, 1983.

59. Neurohr KJ: An experimental setup for carbon-13 NMR studies of heart metabolism in live guinea pigs. *J Magn Reson, 59:*511, 1984.

60. Cross TA, Pahl C, Oberhaensli R, Aue WP, Keller U, Seelig J: Ketogenesis in the living rat followed by 13C NMR spectroscopy. *Biochemistry, 23:*6398, 1984.

61. Bailey IA, Gadian DG, Matthews PM, Radda GK, Seeley PJ: Studies of metabolism in the isolated perfused rat heart using 13C NMR. *FEBS Letters, 80:*1603, 1983.

62. Heelan RT, Martini N, Westcott JW, Bains MS, Watson RC, Caravelli JF, Berkmen YM, Henschke CI, McCormack CM, McCaughan BC, Zaman MB: Carcinomatous involvement of the hilum and mediastinum: Computed tomographic and magnetic resonance evaluation. *Radiology, 156:*111-115, 1985.

63. Martini N, Heelan R, Westcott J, Bains MS, McCormack P, Caravelli J, Watson R, Zaman M: Comparative merits of conventional, computed tomographic, and magnetic resonance imaging in assessing mediastinal involvement in surgically confirmed lung carcinoma. *J Thorac Cardiovasc Surg, 90:*639-648, 1985.

64. Brown JJ, Peck WW, Gerber KH, Higgins CB, Strich G, Slutsky R: Nuclear magnetic resonance analysis of acute and chronic myocardial infarction in dogs: Alterations in spin-lattice relaxation times. *Am Heart J, 108:* 1292-1297, 1984.

65. McNamara MT, Higgins CB: Magnetic resonance imaging of chronic myocardial infarcts in man. *AJR, 146:*315-320, 1986.

66. Eichstaedt HW, Felix R, Doughterty FC, Langer M, Rutsch W, Schmutzler H: Magnetic resonance imaging (MRI) in different stages of myocardial infarction using the contrast agent gadolinium-DTPA. *Clin Cardiol, 9:* 527-535, 1986.

67. Florentine MS, Grosskreutz CL, Chang Wei, Hartnett JA, Dunn VD, Ehrhardt JC, Fleagle SR, Collins SM, Marcus ML, Skorton DJ: Measurement of left ventricular mass in vivo using gated nuclear magnetic resonance imaging. *J Am Coll Cardiol, 8:*107-112, 1986.

68. Cohen MD, McGuire W, Cory DA, Smith JA: MR appearance of blood and blood products: An in vitro study. *AJR, 146:*1293-1297, 1986.

69. Underwood SR, Ress RSO, Savage PE, Klipstein RH, Firmin DN, Fox KM, Poole-Wilson PA, Longmore DB: Assessment of regional left ventricular function by magnetic resonance. *Br Heart J, 56:*334-340, 1986.

70. Valk PE, Hale JD, Crooks LE, Kaufman L, Roos MS, Ortendahl DA, Higgins CB: MRI of blood flow: Correlation of image appearance with spin-echo phase shift and signal intensity. *AJR 146:*931-939, 1986.

71. Didier D, Higgins CB: Estimation of pulmonary vascular resistance by MRI in patients with congenital cardiovascular shunt lesions. *AJR, 146:* 919-924, 1986.

72. Fletcher BD, Jacobstein MD: MRI of congenital abnormalities of the great arteries. *AJR, 146:*941-948, 1986.

73. Dinsmore RE, Wismer GL, Guyer D, Thompson R, Liu P, Stratemeier E, Miller S, Okada R, Brady T: Magnetic resonance imaging of the interatrial septum and atrial septal defects. *AJR, 145:*697-703, 1985.

74. Didier D, Higgins CB, Fisher MR, Osaki L, Silverman NH, Cheitlin MC: Congenital heart disease: Gated MR imaging in 72 patients. *Radiology, 158:*227-235, 1986.

75. Jacobstein MD, Fletcher BD, Riemenschneider, TA: Magnetic resonance imaging in patients with hypoplastic right heart syndrome. *Am Heart J, 110:*154-158, 1985.

76. Klipstein RH, Firmin DN, Longmore DB: Color display of quantitative blood flow and cardiac anatomy in a single magnetic resonance cine loop. *Br J Rad, 60:*105-111, 1987.

77. Axel L: Blood flow effects in magnetic resonance imaging. *AJR, 143:*1157-1166, 1984.

78. Sechtem U, Tcholakoff D, Higgins CB: MRI of the normal pericardium. *AJR, 147:*239-244, 1986.

79. Sechtem U, Tcholakoff D, Higgins CB: MRI of the abnormal pericardium. *AJR, 147:*245-252, 1986.

80. Tomoda H, Hoshiai M, Furuya H: Evaluation of pericardial effusions with CT. *Am Heart J, 109:*701-706, 1985.

81. Stark DD, Higgins CB, Lanzer P: Magnetic resonance imaging of the pericardium. Normal and pathologic findings. *Radiology, 150:*469-474, 1984.

82. Guttierez FR, Shakelford GD, McKnight RC, Levitt RG, Hartmann A: Diagnosis of congenital absence of left pericardium by MRI. *J Comp Asst Tomog, 9(3):*551-553, 1985.

83. Underwood SR, Rees RS, Savage PE, *et al.*: Assessment of regional left ventricular function by magnetic resonance. *Br Heart J, 56:*334-340, 1986.

84. Fletcher BD, Jacobstein MD: MRI of congenital abnormalities of the great arteries. *AJR, 146:*941-948, 1986.

85. Buckwalter KA, Alsen AM, Dilworth LR, Mancini GBG, Buda AJ: Gated cardiac MRI: Ejection fraction determination using the right anterior oblique view. *AJR, 147:*33-37, 1986.

86. Dooms GC, Higgins CB: MR imaging of cardiac thrombi. *JCAT, 10:* 145, 1986.

87. Conces DJ, Vix VA, Klatte EC: Gated MR imaging of left atrial myxomas. *Radiology, 156:*445-447, 1985.

88. Poon PY, Bronskill MJ, Henkelmann, RM, *et al.*: Magnetic resonance imaging of the mediastinum. *J Can Ass Rad, 37:*173-181, 1986.

89. Dinsmore RE, Liberthon RR, Wismer GL, *et al.*: Magnetic resonance imaging of thoracic aneurysm: Comparison with other imaging methods. *AJR, 146:*309-314, 1986.

90. Dinsmore RE, Wedeen VJ, Miller SW, *et al.*: MRI of dissection of the aorta: Recognition of the intimal tear and differential flow velocities. *AJR 146:*1286-1288, 1986.

91. Boxer RA, LaCorte MA, Singh S, *et al.*: Evaluation of the aorta in the Marfan syndrome by MRI. *Am Heart J, 111.5:*1001-1002, 1986.

92. Tscholakoff D, Higgins CB, Sechtem U, Caputo G, Derugin N: MRI of reperfused myocardial infarcts in dogs. *AJR 146:*925-930, 1986.

93. Brown JJ, Peck WW, Gerber KH, *et al.*: Nuclear magnetic resonance analysis of acute and chronic myocardial infarction in dogs. *Am Heart J, 108.5:*1292-1297, 1984.

94. Nishimura DG, Macovsky A, Pauly JM: Magnetic resonance angiography. IIEE Transactions on medical imaging, *MI–5,* 140-151, 1986.

95. Meuli RA, Wedeen VJ, Geller SC, Edelman RR, Frank LR, Rosen BR: MR gated substraction angiography. Evaluation of lower extremities. *Radiology, 159:*411-418, 1986.

5
Mediastinal Lesions

The mediastinum is a difficult area for diagnostic imaging due to a variety of densities compiling its structures. On conventional x-ray films, distinction between the air-filled lungs and the mediastinal soft tissues can usually be achieved. The trachea and the proximal bronchial system can also be relatively accurately outlined. Further details can be obtained by the use of complex motion tomography, but delineation of intra-mediastinal pathology generally remains poor. Conventional radiography lacks the ability to establish the topographic relationship of mediastinal mass lesions to the bronchovascular tree. Furthermore, the above technique is time consuming and rather tiresome for the patient who has difficulty remaining still during the whole length of the examination combined with a high irradiation penalty to the patient.

With the advent of computed tomography, cross-sectional (transverse) images of the mediastinum can be obtained in a simple manner. The ability of CT to detect small differences in tissue density permits a precise diagnostic evaluation of the different mediastinal soft tissue components; namely, its contrast sensitivity allowing distinction between air, fat, and soft tissue density. With CT imaging systems of the last generations, a superior spatial resolution can be obtained due to very short exposure times. Nevertheless, in many instances injection of a high dose of iodinated contrast medium is necessary to enable the distinction between mass lesions and vessels.

Unlike CT however, MRI has the unique capability to provide three-dimensional imaging of the mediastinum with inherent high signal intensity contrast between bronchial and vascular structures. The patient is not exposed to the risk of penetrating irradiation or to the injection of contrast media to generate high contrast images of the mediastinum. Comparative studies have demonstrated that vascular compression or obstruction can be more accurately demonstrated with MRI than is usually achieved with contrast-enhanced CT (1).

The superiority of CT over conventional radiography in defining normal anatomical structures, detecting pathological mediastinal masses, differentiating solid from cystic or vascular lesions, and in the staging of bronchogenic and esophageal carcinoma has been demonstrated (2). MRI is adding a new and noninvasive imaging modality to the diagnostic examination scheme of mediastinal pathology. The clinical indications for MRI studies of the mediastinum have still to be more precisely defined. Advantages and shortcomings of this new imaging modality have not yet been thoroughly evaluated.

MEDIASTINAL ANATOMY AND MRI

The mediastinum is the portion of the thorax lying between the right and left pleural sacs, bounded ventrally by the sternum and dorsally by the vertebral bodies of the thoracic spine. The mediastinum is subdivided into parts related to the pericardial sac. Several authors (3, 4, 5) propose different ways of dividing the mediastinum in relation to anatomical, pathogenetic, and diagnostic criteria. Since MRI has the unique possibility to demonstrate the mediastinal morphology three-dimensionally and with high detail, we believe that a rigid subdivision into different spaces is not of primary importance in the diagnostic evaluation of mediastinal pathology by MR imaging. For tumor localization purposes, we think that the simple division into superior, anterior, middle, and posterior mediastinum (6) is accurate enough to define the topography of a lesion mass in relation to other mediastinal structures.

The superior mediastinum extends above a line drawn from the sternal angle to the lower rim of the fourth thoracic vertebra. Below this plane it is divided into the anterior mediastinum, which is anterior to the pericardial sac, the middle mediastinum containing the pericardial sac and its contents, and the posterior mediastinum occupying the space behind the pericardial sac.

In the analysis of the superior mediastinum by MR images, identification of the aortic arch should first be made since it is constantly and unequivocably shown as a low signal intensity structure surrounded by variable amounts of mediastinal fat (Figures 5.1 and 5.2). Both brachiocephalic branches can be clearly recognized with the veins being ventrally located in relation to the arteries. The left brachiocephalic vein is seen in front and above the aortic arch (Figure 5.3) and its junction with the right brachiocephalic vein to form the superior vena cava. This may occasionally be outlined on coronal MR images. The proximal portion of the left common carotid artery, the subclavian vessels, the jugular veins, the trachea, and remnants of the thymus may also be well visualized by MRI.

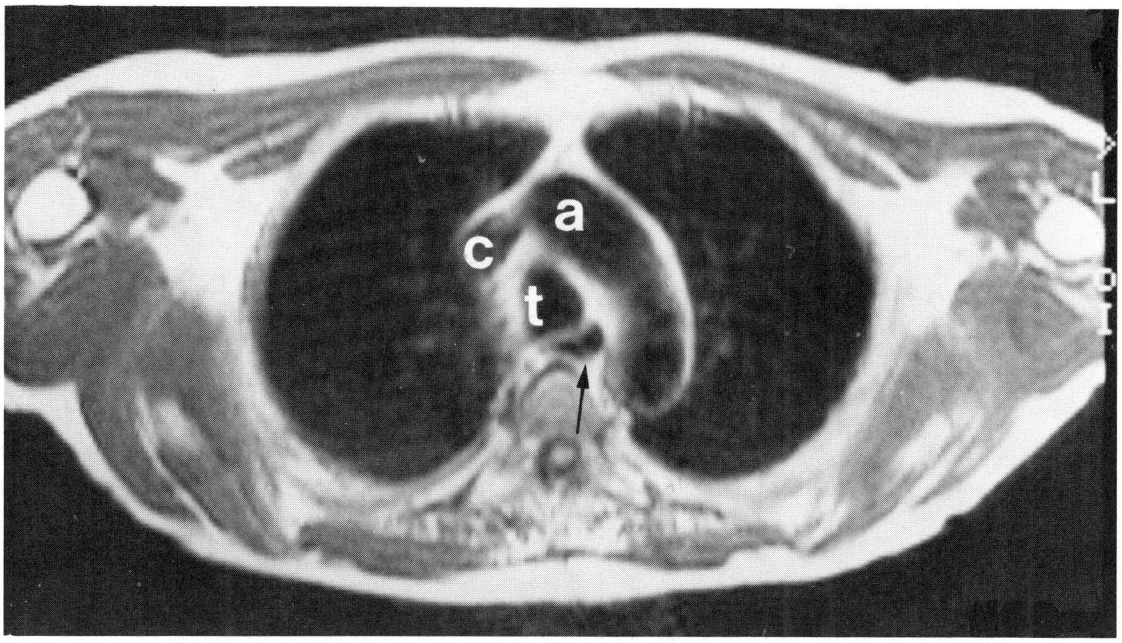

Figure 5.1. Transverse SE image (TR 500 ms) delineates very clearly the aortic arch (a), superior vena cava (c), trachea (t), and air containing esophagus (arrow) due to surrounding mediastinal fat.

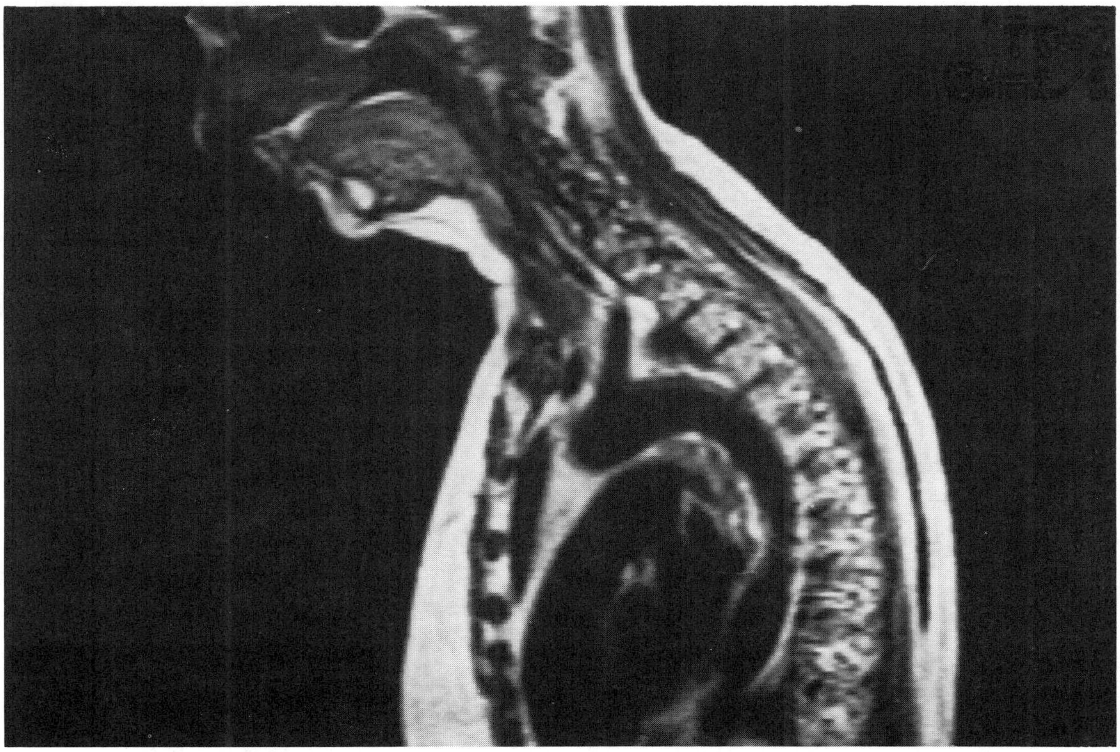

Figure 5.2. Sagittal SE image shows segmental length of the aorta surrounded by fatty tissue. Origin of brachio-cephalic artery well shown.

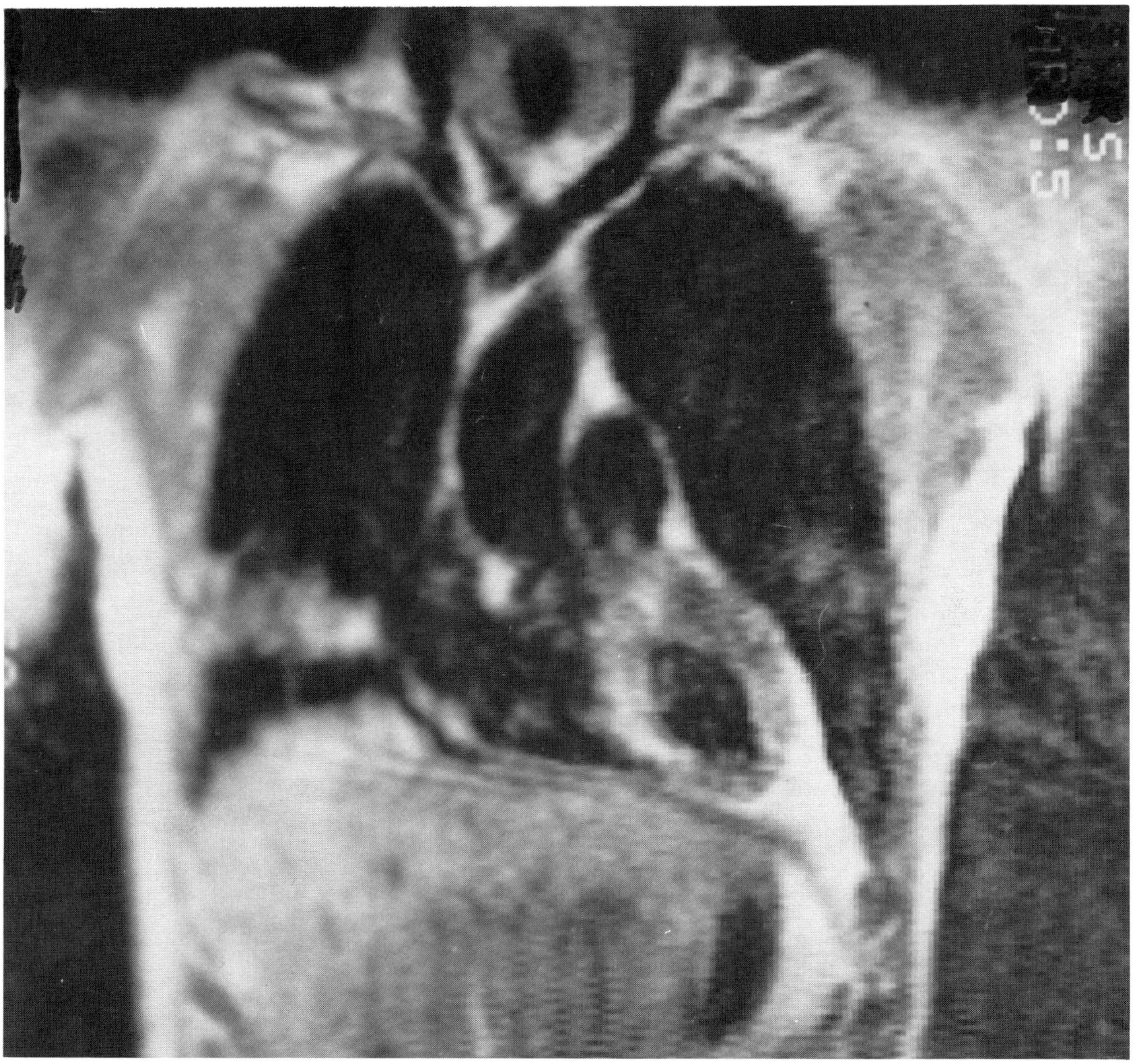

Figure 5.3. MRI in the coronal plane outlines left brachio-cephalic vein in front and above the aortic arch. Both jugular veins and a short segment of the right brachio-cephalic vein equally demonstrated.

The anterior mediastinum contains only a few fascia, lymph nodes, and vessels. The middle mediastinum contains the heart and pericardial sac. Segmental length of the ascending aorta and of the terminal part of the superior vena cava with the azygos vein draining into it can be delineated. The efferent pathways of the right ventricle and the pulmonary trunk with its dividing branches are easily identified because they are embedded in epicardial fatty tissue (Figure 5.4). The terminal portions of the right and left pulmonary veins and the right atrium are usually well shown by

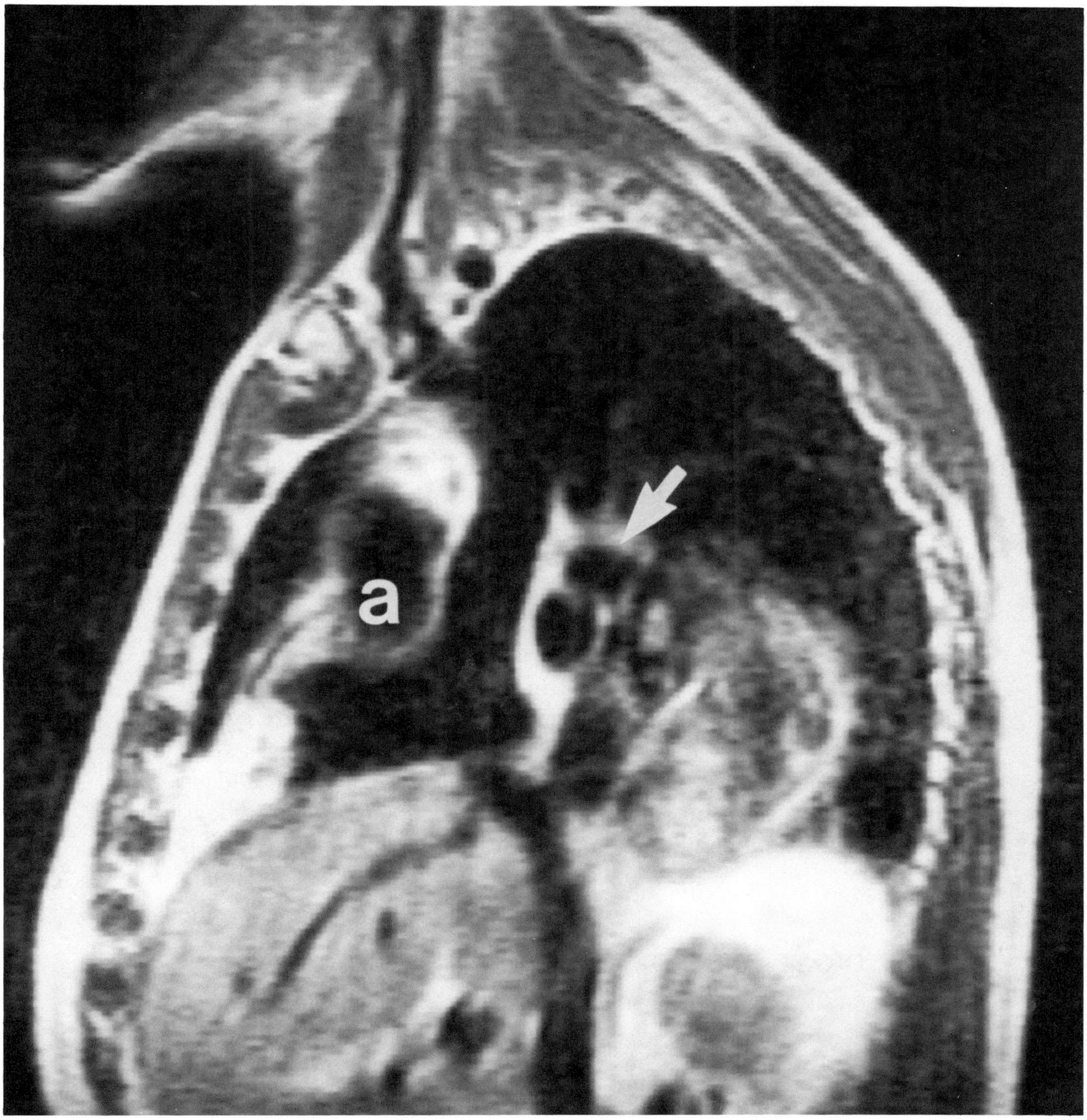

Figure 5.4. Sagittal SE image using cardiac gating shows with superb anatomical detail the inferior vena cava, the right atrium and a small portion of the right ventricle, the superior vena cava, the brachio-cephalic and jugular vein. Notice ascending aorta (a) and main pulmonary vessels posteriorly (arrow).

MRI. The posterior mediastinum contains the descending aorta, the tracheal bifurcation with the main left and right bronchi, the azygos and hemiazygos veins and many lymph nodes. These structures can be most accurately delineated by MRI. The vagus and splanchnic nerves are not visualized by MRI. In many instances, it is difficult to identify the esophagus which may be misinterpreted as a pathological lymph node by inexperienced radiologists (7).

Space-occupying lesions located in the mediastinum may affect or compress any of the prementioned mediastinal structures. For this reason, a precise knowledge of mediastinal anatomy with special reference to topography and interrelationship of its compiling structures is of primary importance whenever pathology in this area is under study. Three-dimensional representation of mediastinal pathology as routinely provided by MRI facilitates interpretation, but it also demands a three-dimensional understanding of mediastinal anatomy. As coronal or sagittal images have the potential to delineate whole longitudinal segments of the main vascular branches and of the trachea, pathology affecting these structures may be investigated more easily. Abnormalities extending over longer portions of the main mediastinal vessels can be more accurately outlined and some indications as to their etiology and nature may be obtained. With CT scanning, this type of pathology can only be understood by the serial study of contiguous axial slices. Coronal and sagittal CT images of the mediastinum may only be generated through indirect reformatting, which limits their spatial resolution. Although transverse images alone are sufficient to establish a correct diagnosis in the vast majority of cases, we believe that direct coronal and sagittal imaging provide incremental information about the precise topography and extension of mediastinal masses. In agreement with Aronberg *et al.* (7), we think that this statement is mainly true in the investigation of the aorto-pulmonary window, in imaging the aorta and great vessels, and in defining the relationship of a posterior mediastinal mass to the spinal canal.

INDICATIONS FOR MRI OF THE MEDIASTINUM

1. Evaluation of the mediastinum having an abnormal appearance on standard radiographs and the inability to investigate the mediastinal lesion in a satisfactory manner by CT scanning due to streak artifacts or other technical problems.
2. Evaluation of extension and localization of mediastinal tumor masses, especially in cases where bronchial and vascular compression and/or invasion are suspected.
3. Three-dimensional evaluation of a mass or enlarged lymph nodes located in the aorto-pulmonary window.
4. Defining the relationship of a mass discovered in the posterior mediastinum to the spinal canal.
5. MRI may be used as a complementary diagnostic tool to CT scanning in the TNM staging of bronchogenic carcinoma.

6. Hilar tumors extending into the mediastinum or alternatively mediastinal masses involving the hilar region may be well investigated by MRI.

7. Tissue characterization of mediastinal lesions, to differentiate between solid, cystic or lipomatous structures.

8. In patients with a widened mediastinum, MRI is capable of demonstrating if this enlargement is due to lipomatosis or enlarged mediastinal vessels.

9. Evaluation of pathological conditions sitting just above the diaphragm and whenever extension of the disease across the thoraco-abdonimal junction is suspected. Images in the coronal and sagittal planes are especially valuable in the study of these conditions.

10. The study of the cardiovascular system. This aspect is discussed in detail in Chapter 4.

TECHNICAL CONSIDERATIONS

It has already been stated that one of the main advantages of MRI over CT scanning is its capability to provide three-dimensional representations of pathology. Therefore we recommend carrying out all investigations in three planes: transverse, sagittal, and coronal. In the study of lymphadenopathy within the aorto-pulmonary window, the examination may exceptionally be complemented by oblique sections. If an extremely elongated atherosclerotic mediastinal vessel is present, motion artifacts due to vascular beating can be obtained. For this reason, we strongly recommend the use of cardiac gating in every patient showing prominent mediastinal vessels on conventional x-ray films. Cardiac gating should be used in all cases where the main interest is in the heart or in the mediastinal vessels. T_1 and T_2 weighted images should be routinely performed.

We start the MRI investigation of the mediastinum with a pulse sequence in the sagittal plane using a short TR (300 ms), a short TE (32 ms), 2 data acquisitions and a 1 cm slice thickness. The midline slice of this series is used as a "scout" to perform subsequent coronal and transverse imaging. Then, images in the coronal plane using a TR 500 ms, a TE 32 ms, 4 data acquisitions and 1 cm slice thickness are generated. Finally, the examination is completed by a series in the transverse plane using a long TR (3000 ms), 4 delayed echos (32, 64, 96, and 128 ms) and a 1-1.5 cm slice thickness. This T_2 weighted pulse sequence using a long TR provides complete examination of the mediastinum and upper abdomen in the transverse direction since 14 to 16 images can be generated (Table 1).

TABLE 1
EXAMINATION PROTOCOL OF THE MEDIASTINUM

	First Sequence	*Second Sequence*	*Third Sequence*
Receiver coil	Body		
Patient position	Supine		
Imaging plane	Sagittal	Coronal	Transverse
Slice thickness	1 cm	1 cm	1-1.5 cm
Interleave gap	0.5 cm	0.5 cm	0.5 cm
Pulse parameters	TR 350 ms TE 32 ms	TR 500 ms TE 32 ms	TR 3000 ms TE 32, 64, 96, 129 ms
Number of slices	5	9	14
Data acquisitions	2	4	2
Cardiac gating	Routinely done in the study of cardio-vascular pathology and in the distorted mediastinum following pneumonectomy.		
Surface coils	Used for imaging of pathology in the posterior mediastinum involving the spine. A 192 x 256 matrix, 4 data acquisitions and a 0.5 cm slice thickness were used.		

In Chapter 2, we already stated that T_1 weighted images are most valuable in differentiating mediastinal mass lesions from the broncho-vascular system on one side and from mediastinal fat on the other side. Pathological nodes appear as structures with intermediate signal intensity when compared to the high signal intensity of mediastinal fat and in comparison with the very low signal intensity of mediastinal vessels and airways. Masses can be very accurately separated from surrounding structures on T_1 weighted images. Images with long TR intervals (T_2 weighted) produce significant differential change of the signal intensity of pathological tissues in such a way that they may easily be differentiated from normal structures. The signal contrast between tumor and mediastinal fat decreases as the intensity of the tumor increases more than the intensity of fat. However, the signal to noise ratio usually improves on images at longer TRs. This explains why a pathological mass is generally not less clearly visualized than on T_1 weighted images and that its heterogeneous consistency may even become more prominent (8). Considerable information can be obtained by comparing images at a short repetition time with those obtained at a long repetition time and observing the difference between them.

MRI IN PATHOLOGY OF THE MEDIASTINUM

Mediastinal Widening

Mediastinal widening is a frequently encountered diagnostic problem usually detected on plain films of the chest. It may be due to a normal variant, such as abundant fat deposition (mediastinal lipomatosis) or to a tortuous vessel. Pathological widening of the mediastinum may be vascular in etiology (such as aneurysm). It may also be caused by primary tumors, metastatic masses, and enlarged lymph nodes. CT is a very accurate technique capable of differentiating vascular from nonvascular causes of mediastinal enlargement, providing a conclusive diagnosis about its etiology and nature in many instances. Nevertheless, CT has a few shortcomings in the diagnostic work-up of mediastinal lesions. Even with a dynamic CT technique using a rapid high-dose injection of contrast, differentiation between various tissue components having similar attenuation values remains difficult. In some cases, the contrast enhancement within some vessels may be insufficient and separation between vascular structures and pathological masses is still impossible. Detection of pathological lymph nodes can be difficult and a very precise knowledge of CT anatomy of the mediastinum is mandatory.

MRI is able to show mediastinal mass lesions without having to inject iodinated contrast material and without using ionizing radiation. Five tissue properties may affect the created images: proton density, T_1 and T_2 relaxation times, blood motion, and the chemical composition of the molecules containing the protons (9). Images may be weighted towards any one of these properties by changing the radio frequency pulses. Structures like mediastinal fat with high proton density and short T_1 produce the brightest signal. Benign fat accumulation within the mediastinum is commonly associated with obesity, corticosteroid treatment, and Cushing's syndrome. In many of these patients, none of the prementioned etiological factors may be discovered. Computed tomography confidently separates an innocent mediastinal lipomatosis from truly pathological conditions in a simple way, obviating the need for further investigation. Homogeneous low density areas surround the great vessels in the superior mediastinum on transverse CT images (10). MRI remains an expensive diagnostic tool not yet available in most clinical centers. For this reason, we consider CT to be still the primary diagnostic technique in the investigation of mediastinal lipomatosis. Nevertheless, MRI may be preferred to CT scanning in young patients or whenever irradiation has to be restricted in patients having already undergone several radiological investigations. Mediastinal fat is always

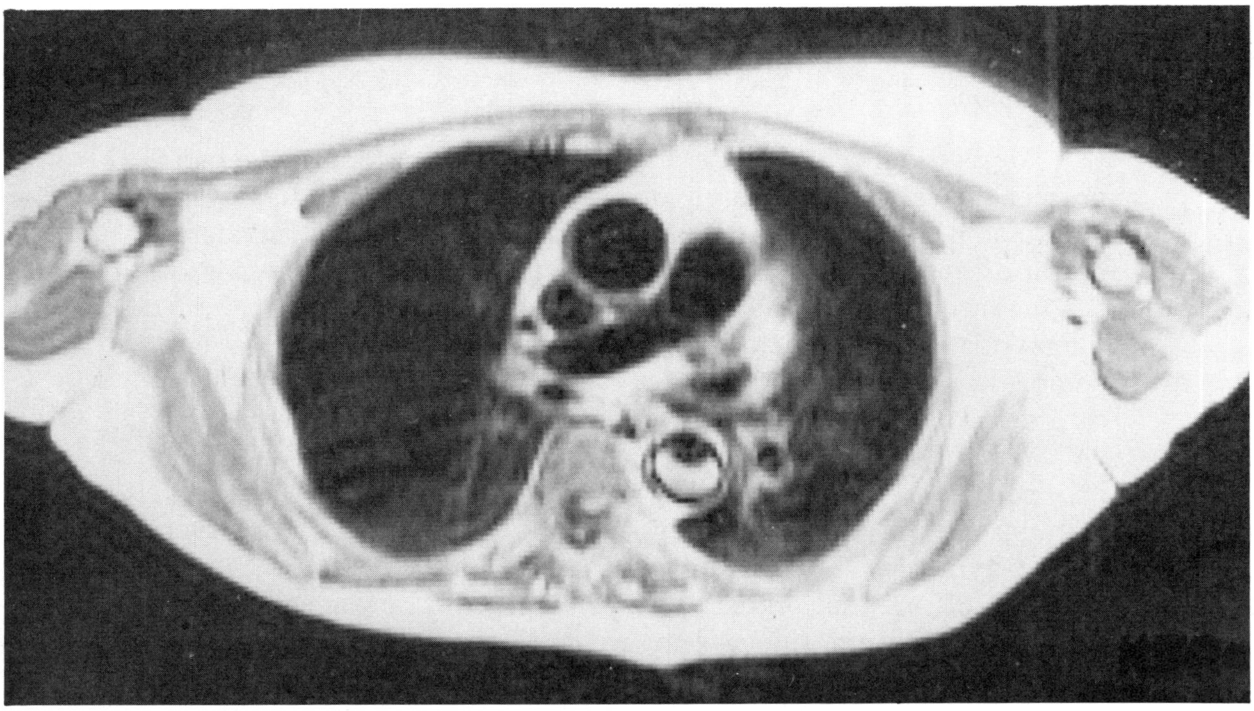

Figure 5.5. Due to relatively important fatty mediastinal deposits, low signal intensity structures of the broncho-vascular system are particularly well demonstrated by MRI.

visualized as a very high signal intensity structure independent of the pulse sequence parameters that may be used with MR imaging. As a side effect, mediastinal vessels may be particularly well demonstrated in patients presenting relatively important lipomatous deposits in the mediastinum (Figure 5.5).

In elderly patients, mediastinal widening as seen on plain chest films is most commonly caused by tortuous atherosclerotic vessels displacing the superior vena cava or right innominate vein laterally. Dissection and aneurysms of the aorta represent other etiological causes for mediastinal widening. As there is an intrinsic signal intensity difference between rapidly flowing blood and the wall of the vessel, the main mediastinal and pulmonary vessels are shown with superb anatomical detail. Vascular occlusion or thrombosis may be diagnosed with MRI without the use of contrast injection (11). Mills *et al.* (12) reported that the use of different technical parameters helps to differentiate pathologic alterations in blood flow patterns. It has been stated that distinction between slowly flowing and stationary blood is possible depending on signal intensity variations between the first and second delayed echo (12). Vascular occlusion may be recognized as high intensity signal on the first echo that diminishes somewhat on the second delayed echo. In the case of slowly flowing blood, the signal intensity will be equal or higher on the second delayed echo.

In Chapter 2 we already mentioned that, due to a phenomenon termed "paradoxical enhancement," slowly flowing blood may produce a higher signal intensity than stationary blood. In order to obtain accurate MRI studies in pathology of the main mediastinal vessles, cardiac gating is mandatory. Figure 5.6 shows a patient presenting an elongated arch, the descending aorta crossing around the anterior aspect of the thoracic spine towards the right side (Figure 5.6 A,B,C,). Obvious aortic dissection together with enlargement of the descending aorta was found on the right side (Figure 5.6 D). Within the dissected aortic wall, intermediate and high signal intensity areas could be seen (Figure 5.6 E). The main disadvantage of MRI in the study of vascular abnormalities is its inability to depict calcium deposits within the wall of the vessels. Nevertheless, we think that MRI may play a major role in the diagnostic evaluation of various congenital vascular disorders.

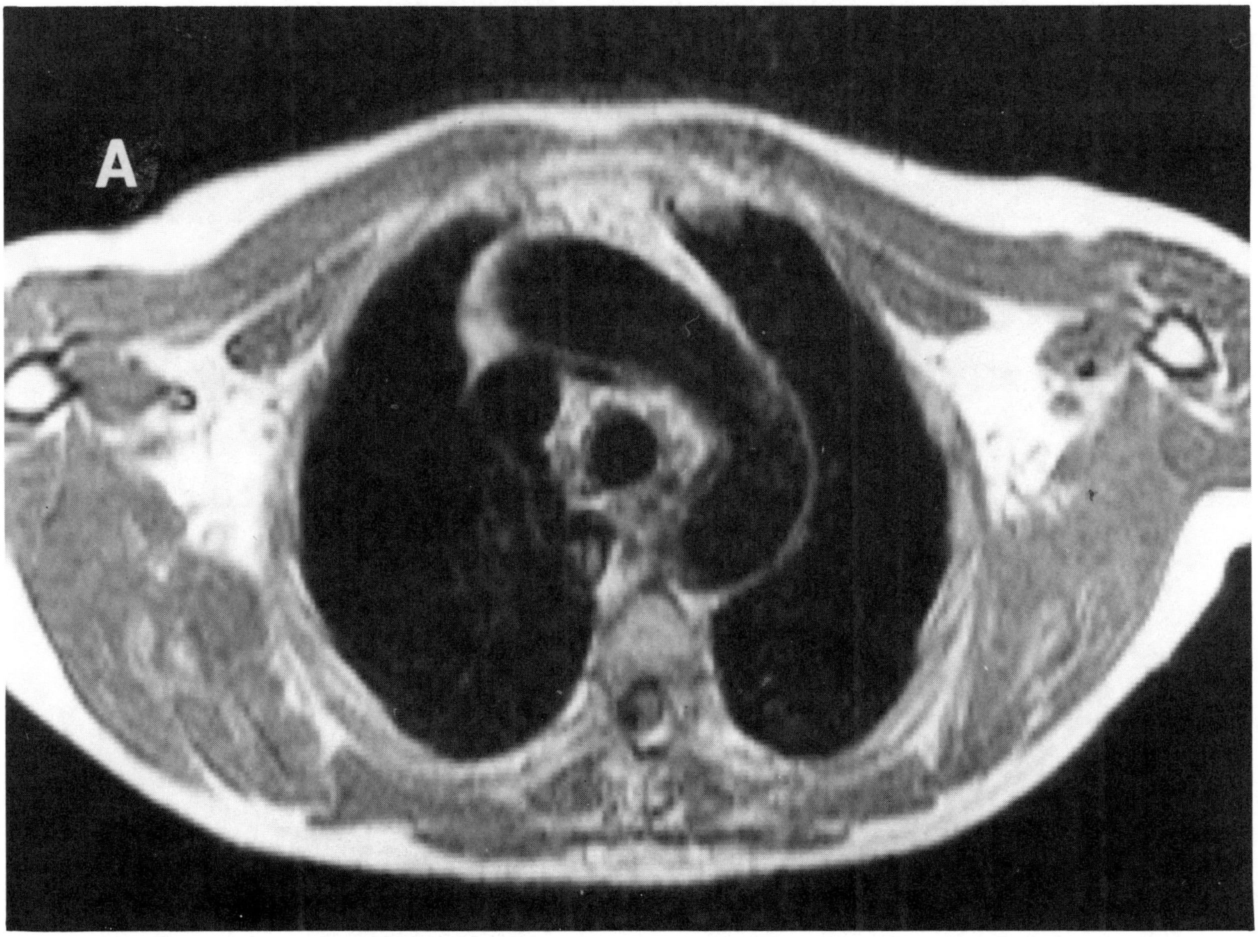

Figure 5.6 (A,B,C,D,E). SE images carried out with cardiac gating. Elongated aortic arch (A) and descending aorta crossing around anterior aspect of the thoracic spine towards the left side (B and C) well shown. Aortic dissection (D) containing high signal intensity area (E) due to thrombosis obviously demonstrated.

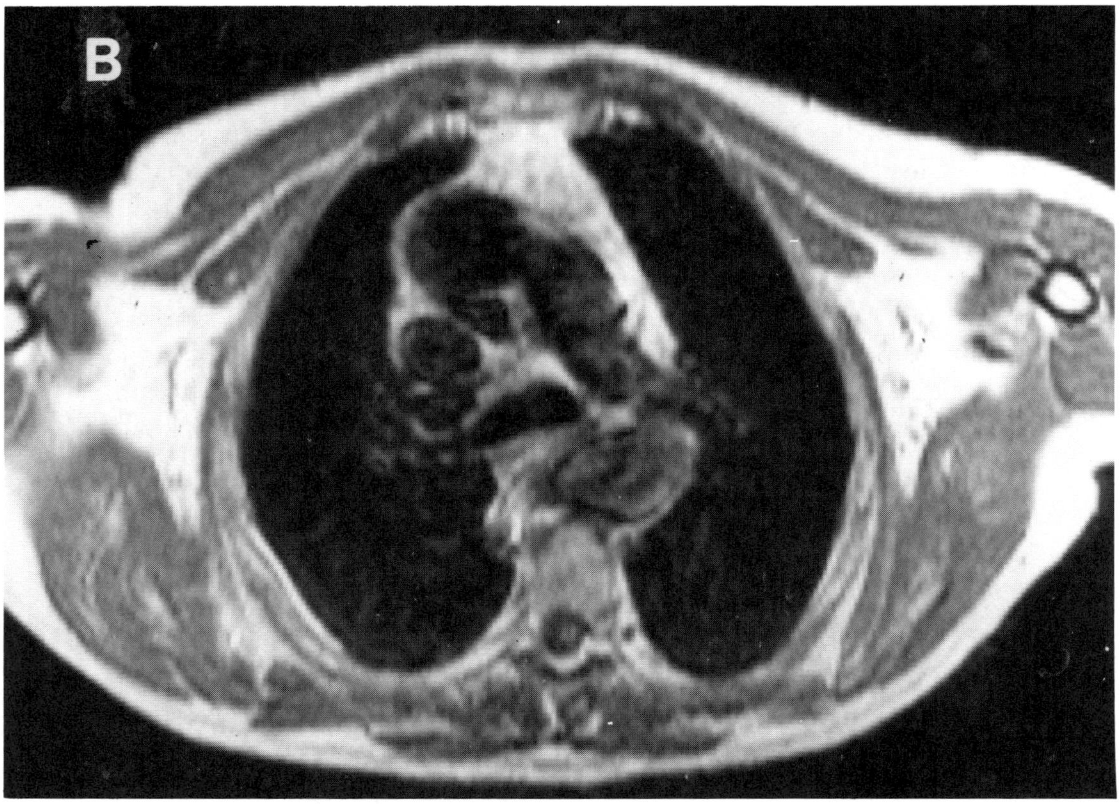
B

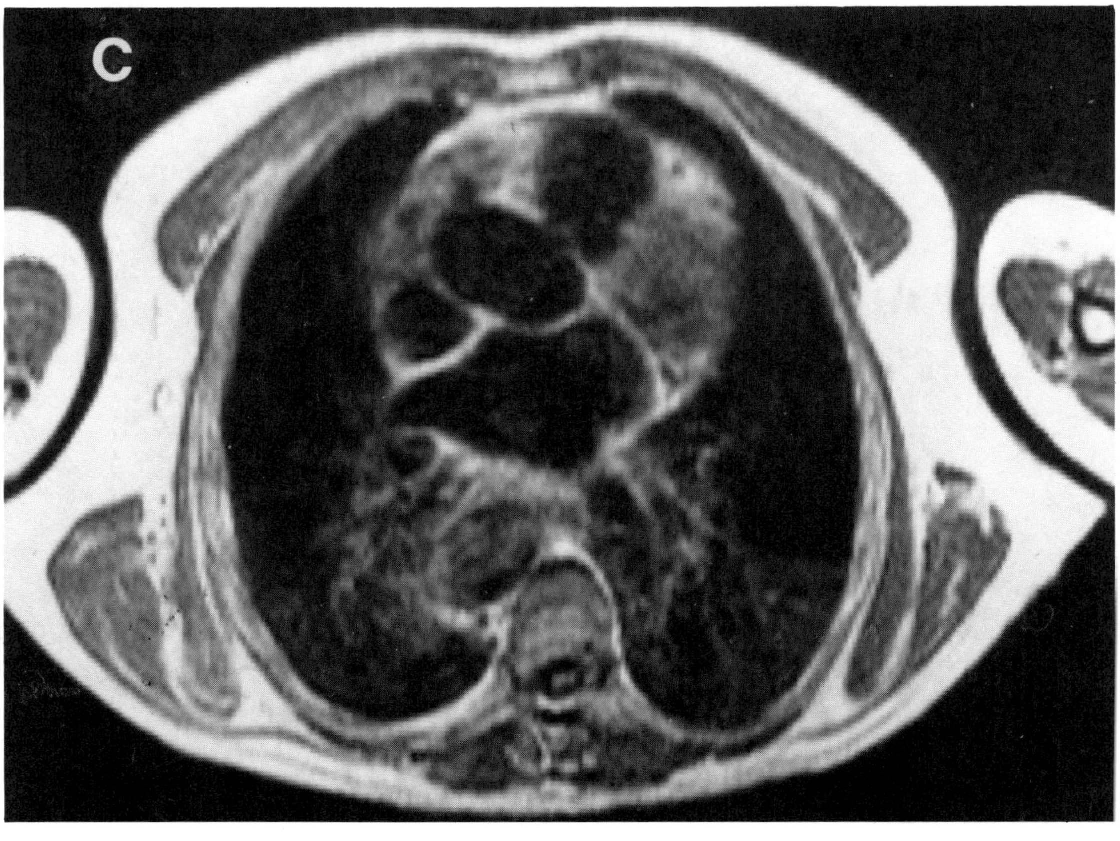
C

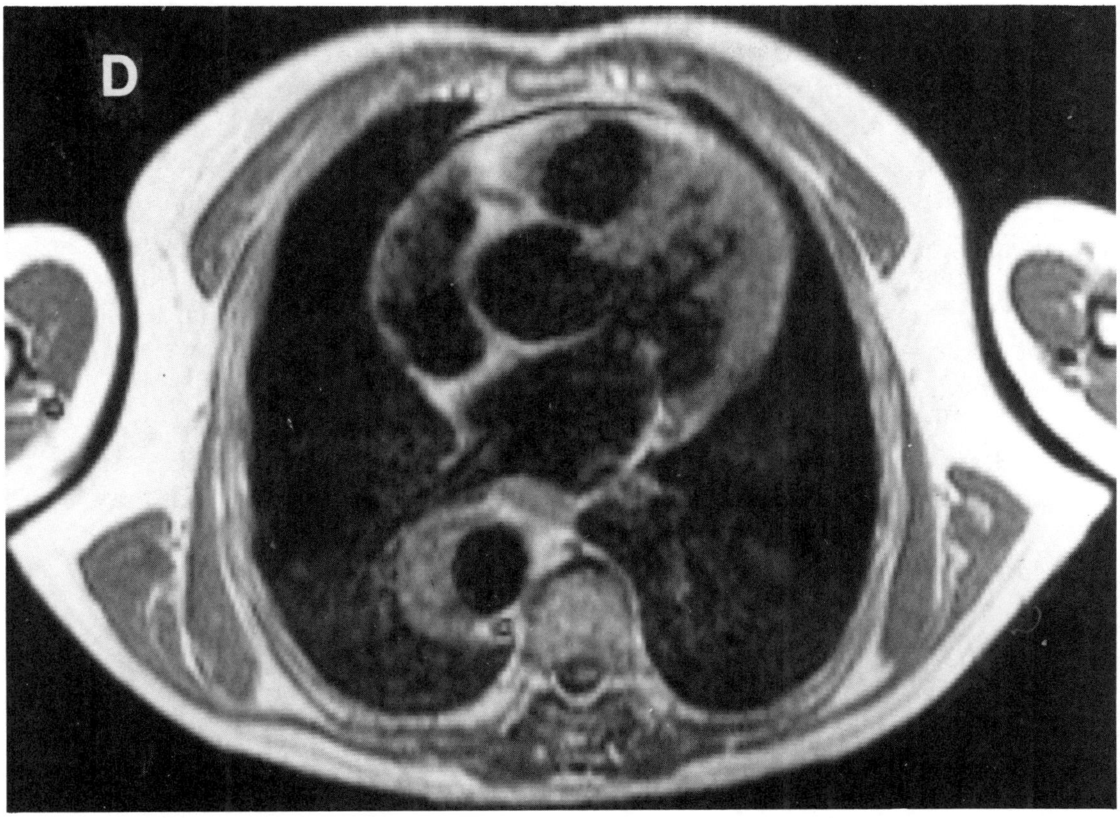
D

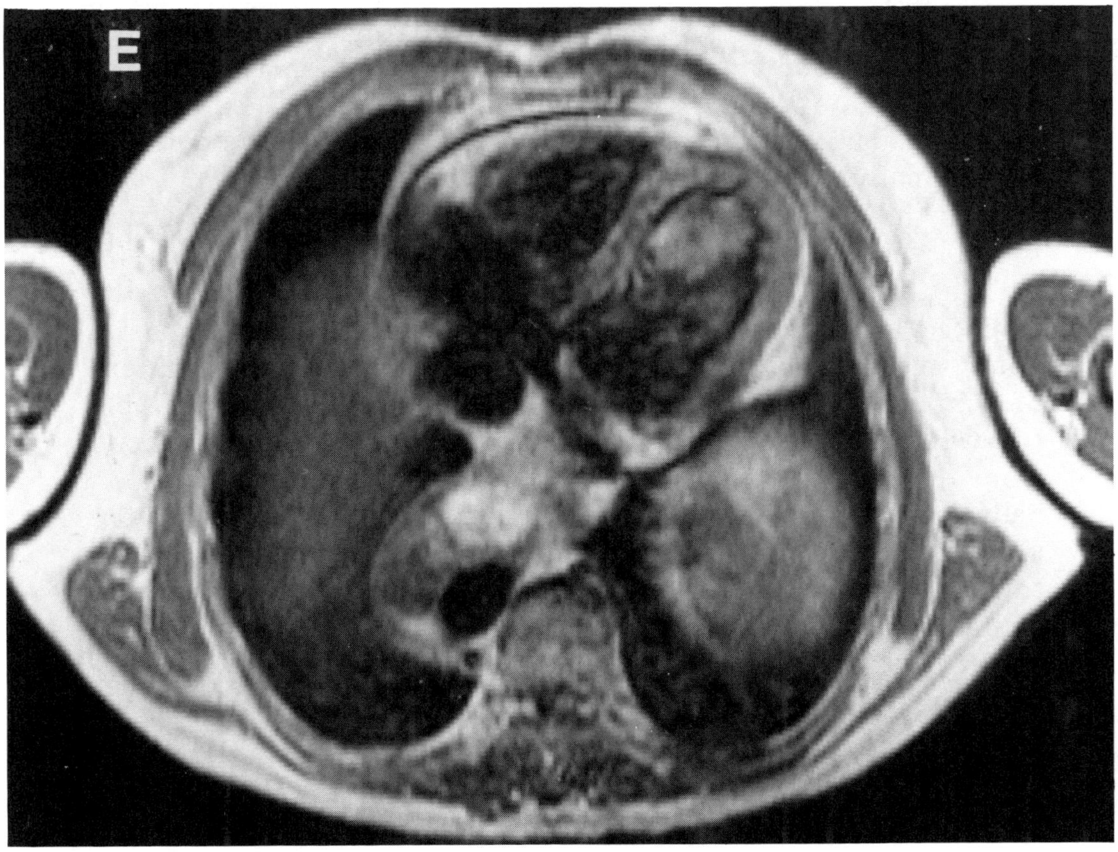
E

Mediastinal enlargement as seen on chest x-rays may also be due to a variety of pathological disorders occurring in the thymus. Thymomas are solid neoplasms which occur at any age, but the highest incidence is in the fourth decade of life. The malignant or invasive form with infiltration of adjacent tissues is about as frequent as the benign variant. A thymoma is found in 15% of patients with myasthenia gravis. A benign thymoma as shown by MRI has been reported (8). A mass lying in front of the pulmonary artery showed a very heterogeneous consistency and the boundaries between the mass and the mediastinum were ill defined.

Thymic hyperplasia occurs preferentially in adolescence and should always be considered in the differential diagnosis with thymomas. In Grave's disease, a true thymic hyperplasia may occur. Thymic persistence rarely leads to a large mass. Usually, small retrosternal nodules are found (13). Infiltration of the thymus by lymphoreticular neoplasms may occur. A young boy showing enlargement of the anterior mediastinum on plain chest x-rays was referred to our Clinic for further evaluation by MRI. Images obtained with a short TR (500 ms) displayed an enlarged thymic gland within the anterior mediastinum (Figure 5.7 A). This mass showed smooth boundaries and did not appear to involve any of the surrounding structures. MR images using a long TR (3000 ms) showed definitely increased signal intensity within the thymus, but no heterogeneous or cystic areas could be detected within the mass (Figure 5.7 B). The diffuse and homogeneous enlargement of the thymic gland appeared to be due to lymphomatous infiltration.

In the past, the use of CT scanning has been recommended in the presence of strong clinical indications. At the present time, we believe that for diagnostic assessment of thymic pathology MRI may be a better diagnostic choice as most of these patients are still young and they should not unnecessarily be exposed to the hazard of ionizing radiation. Endothoracic goiters may be responsible for widening of the upper mediastinum. They usually originate from the lower parts of the thyroid lobes and extend retrosternally in front of the trachea. More rarely, they originate from the posterior portion of the thyroid gland and extend behind the trachea. Ectopic mediastinal goiters are rare. Since incorporation of radionuclides in the ectopic thyroid lobe occurs only in a minority of the cases, CT or MRI clarification of the relationship between the thyroid and the mass is very important. The diagnosis of an endomediastinal goiter is highly probable when a communication between both parts can be demonstrated.

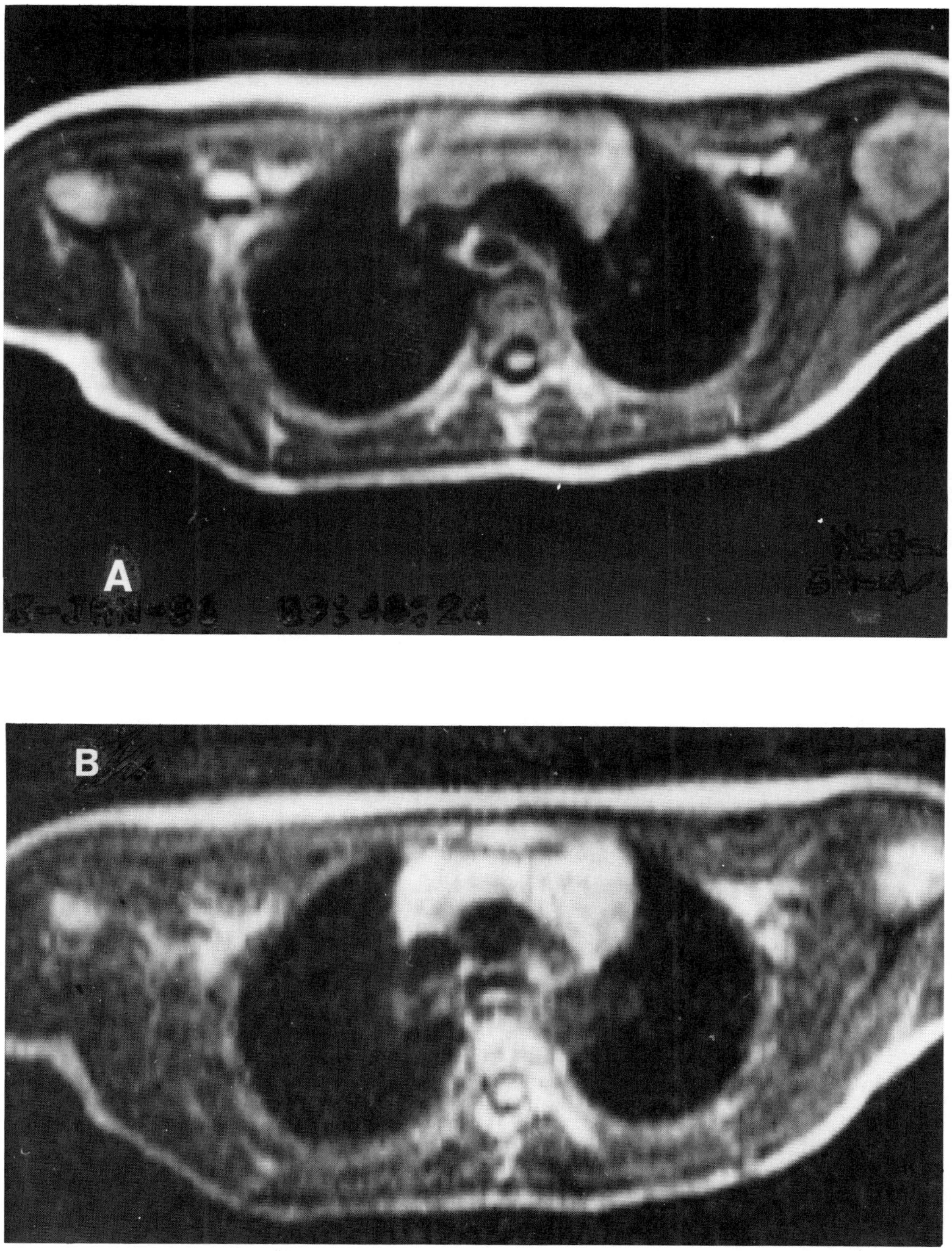

Figure 5.7 (A, B). Mediastinal widening due to lymphomatous infiltration of the thymus found in an 8-year-old boy. T_1 MR image (TR 500 ms) shows enlarged thymic gland as a structure of intermediate signal intensity bounded by high signal intensity rim due to fatty tissue (A). T_2 weighted images (TR 3000 and a delayed echo at 64 ms) demonstrates a significantly increased signal intensity, but no cystic or necrotic areas were detected (B).

On spin-echo (SE), MR images through the intrathoracic goiter, solid and cystic areas may be visualized. The presence of calcifications, however, may not be documented by MRI. Using longer TR and TE values, both solid and cystic parts of the goiter show an obvious increase in signal intensity (Figure 5.8). Gamsu *et al.* reported a case in which a colloid cyst demonstrated even a higher signal intensity than subcutaneous fat on a T_2 weighted image (8). Discrimination between fat, water and soft tissue densities requires the viewing of multiple MR images using different pulse sequences.

Hypertrophic lymph nodes due to malignant lymphomas are a relatively frequent etiology for mediastinal widening. MRI displays physico-chemical properties of tissues unrelated to electron density and the general belief existed at an early stage in the experience with MRI that distinction between malignant and benign solid mediastinal masses would be possible with this modality. However, tissue characterization using T_1 and T_2 relaxation times for differentiating various pathological conditions offers quite poor tissue specificity. It has been stated that there is a considerable overlap between the T_1 and T_2 relaxation values of the different pathologies and the derived intensity data do not appear to be specific for individual pathologic states. The reason for this overlap between pathological lymph nodes of different etiologies may be explained by the fact that T_1 and T_2 relaxation times depend mainly on the water content of the lymph nodes. According to the degree of inflammatory reaction, necrosis or fibrosis, the water content in benign and malignant lymph nodes may vary greatly. Dooms *et al.* (15) stated, however, that discrimination between benign and malignant lymph nodes in the same patient seems to be feasible by using T_1 and T_2 relaxation times as the values obtained were higher in pathological nodes. Another reason may be found in the fact that MRI has inherent lower spatial resolution due to long scanning times, patient motion and a relatively large slice thickness which cause volume averaging with the surrounding fat. This explains why large variations in relaxation times are found whenever measurements are done in nodes smaller than 10 mm in diameter (15). It is our hope that with improvements in the spatial resolution of MRI and the reduction in the section thickness used with MRI the problem of partial volume averaging may be overcome. Motion artifacts may be reduced by more sophisticated gating techniques. Furthermore, all the studies reported up to date were performed on different MRI devices, varied techniques of mediastinal examination and perhaps varying levels of expertise in interpretation. The sensitivity of MRI may be even further restricted in patients presenting normal-sized medias-

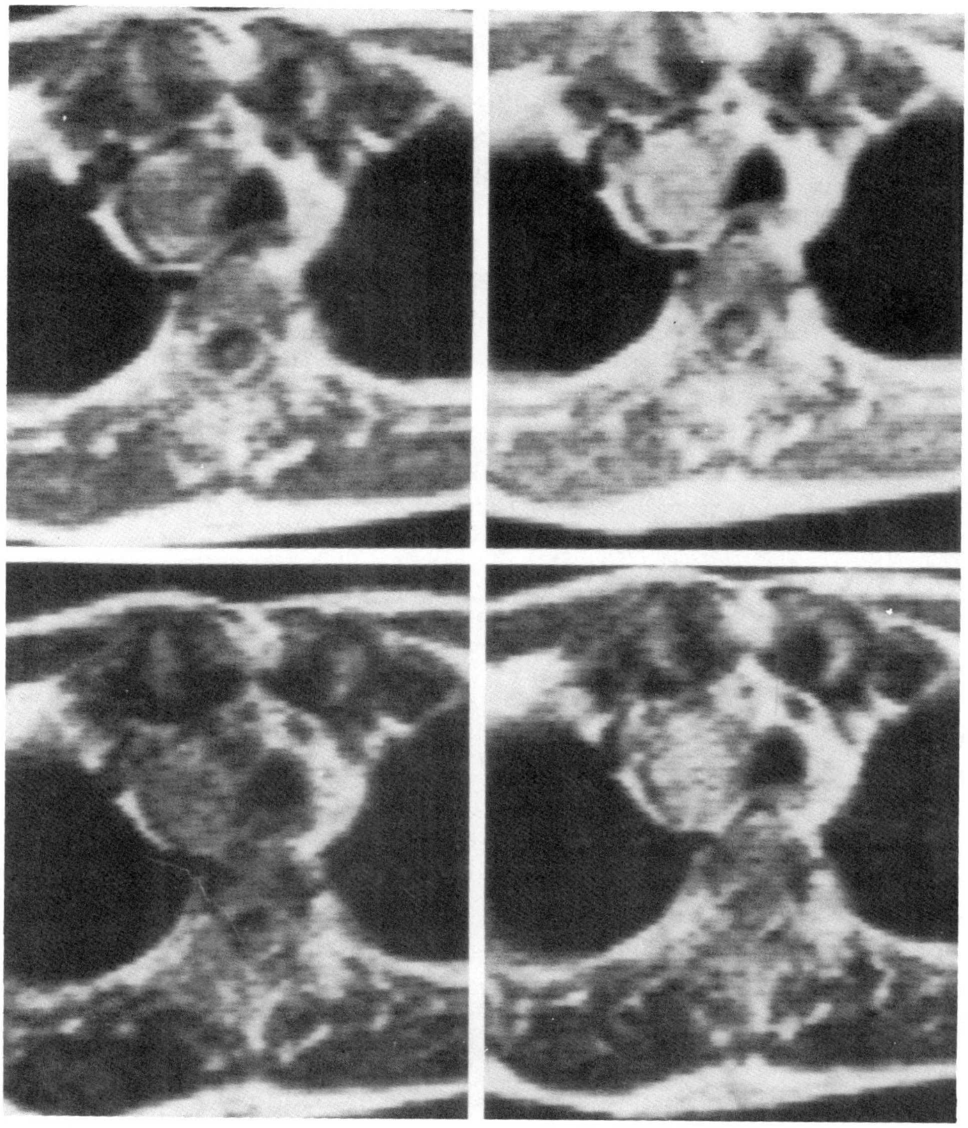

Figure 5.8. Mediastinal extension of a goiter. Four MR spin echo images are at a TR of 500 ms (left side) and 1000 ms (right side), and TE of 28 ms (upper panel) and 56 ms (lower panel). The intensity of the right paratracheal mass increases markedly with both a longer TR and TE (used with permission reference 8).

tinal lymph nodes that contain tumor (16). Consequently, characteristic features or criteria for benignity or malignancy cannot yet be established using MRI (17). Only by combining image information such as location, size, contour and homogeneity of a lesion with the patient's clinical data, more indications as to the etiology of an encountered hypertrophic lymph node may be derived.

In our series, we found a patient showing obvious mediastinal widening on conventional x-rays due to a mass bulging out of the left mediastinal silhouette (Figure 5.9 A). CT was carried out before and after injection of intravenous contrast. A quite large anterior mediastinal mass lesion was found on the left side (Figure 5.9 B) which showed a small calcified rim. There was apparent malignant infiltration of the anterior chest wall (Figure 5.9 B). Transverse MRI images using a short TR (500 ms) showed the mass with superb anatomical detail. It was outlined as a relatively low signal intensity structure sitting within the anterior portion of the left mediastinum and it was delineated by surrounding mediastinal fat (Figure 5.9 C). Its close relationship to the main pulmonary vessels on the left side was clearly demonstrated, but the peripheral rim was not visualized by MRI. Furthermore, the involvement of the anterior thoracic wall was less clearly shown with MRI than on CT images. On coronal images obtained with a long TR (2000 ms), the mass showed only minimal increase in signal intensity (Figure 5.9 D). Sagittal MR images located the anterior mediastinal mass above the cardiac silhouette and posteriorly to the chest wall, but involvement of the thoracic wall was not delineated (Figure 5.9 C). This mass could easily have been misdiagnosed as recurrent Hodgkin's disease on MR images. The patient's clinical history taught us that she had been operated and treated for a chondrosarcoma on the left side and the mass was representing tumor recurrency. MRI provided a three-dimensional imaging of the lesion and showed with high detail its topographic location to surrounding structures. This information is very useful for treatment planning whenever radiotherapy is contemplated. But, no indication as to the etiology of the lesion could be obtained by MRI. Its eventual primary origin from the chest wall was more clearly indicated by CT imaging.

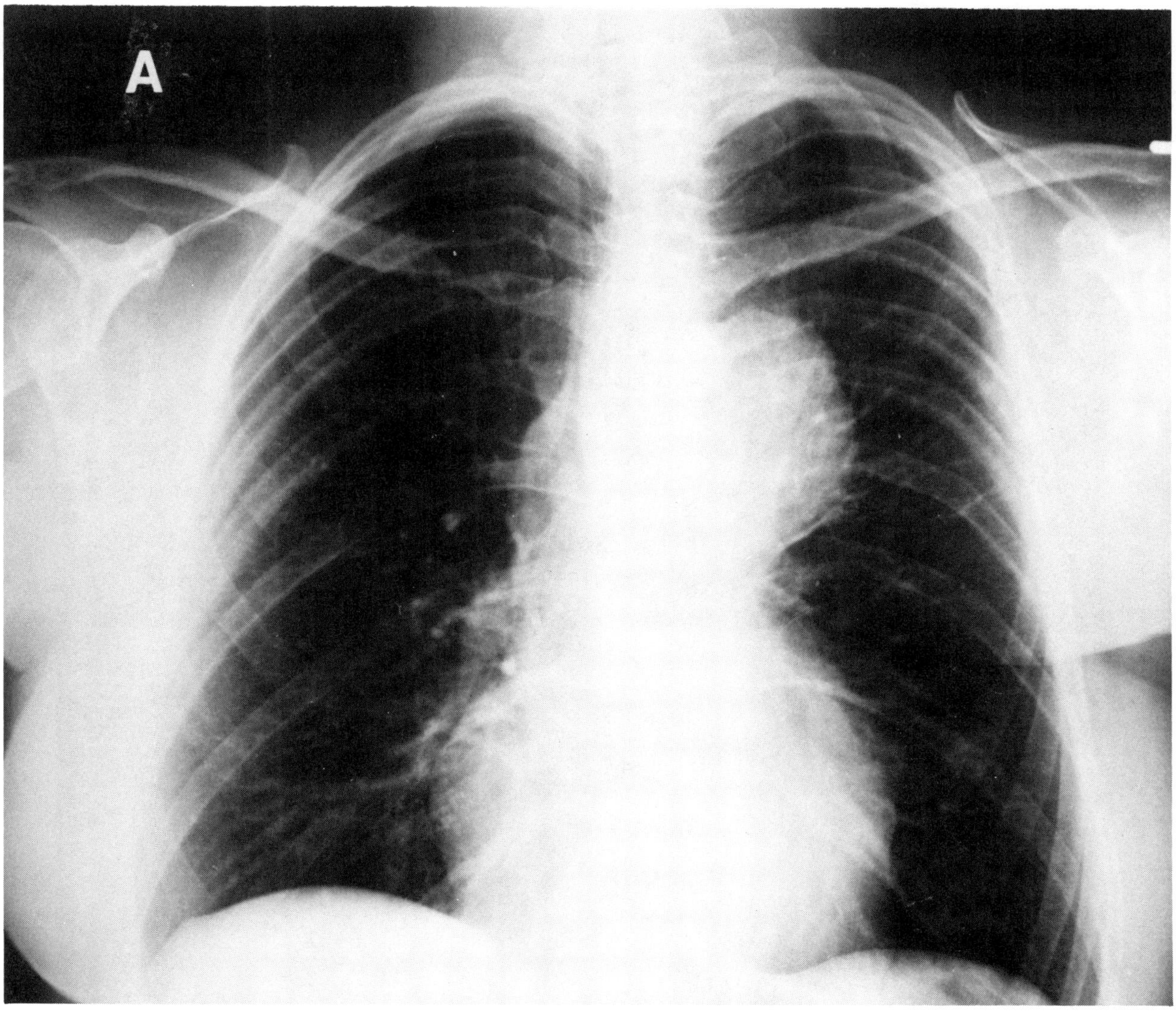

Figure 5.9 (A,B,C,D,E). Conventional film of the chest shows gross enlargement of the left mediastinal contour due to a bulging mass (A). Contrast enhanced CT scan demonstrates mass sitting within the anterior mediastinum on the left (B). Notice small rim calcifications (arrowhead) and involvement of anterior wall of the chest (arrow). MRI using a short TR outlines a well circumscribed mass of relatively low signal intensity, its medial portion being surrounded by mediastinal fat (C). Rim calcification not visualized. Coronal images using a long TR (2000 ms) shows some increase of signal intensity of the mass (D). Sagittal imaging localized the mass above the cardiac silhouette and behind the sternum, but involvement of the chest wall could not be visualized (E).

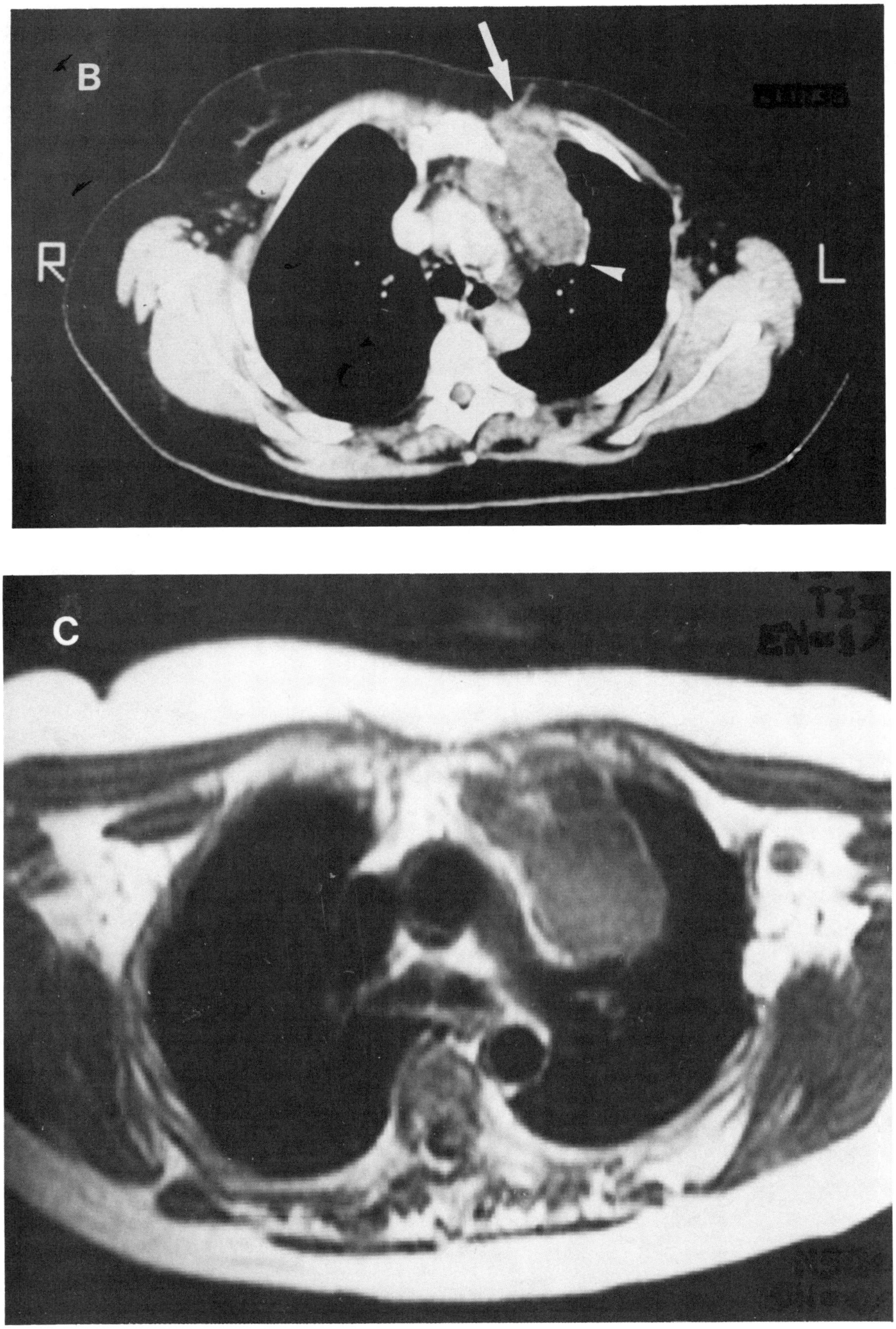
B
R
L
C

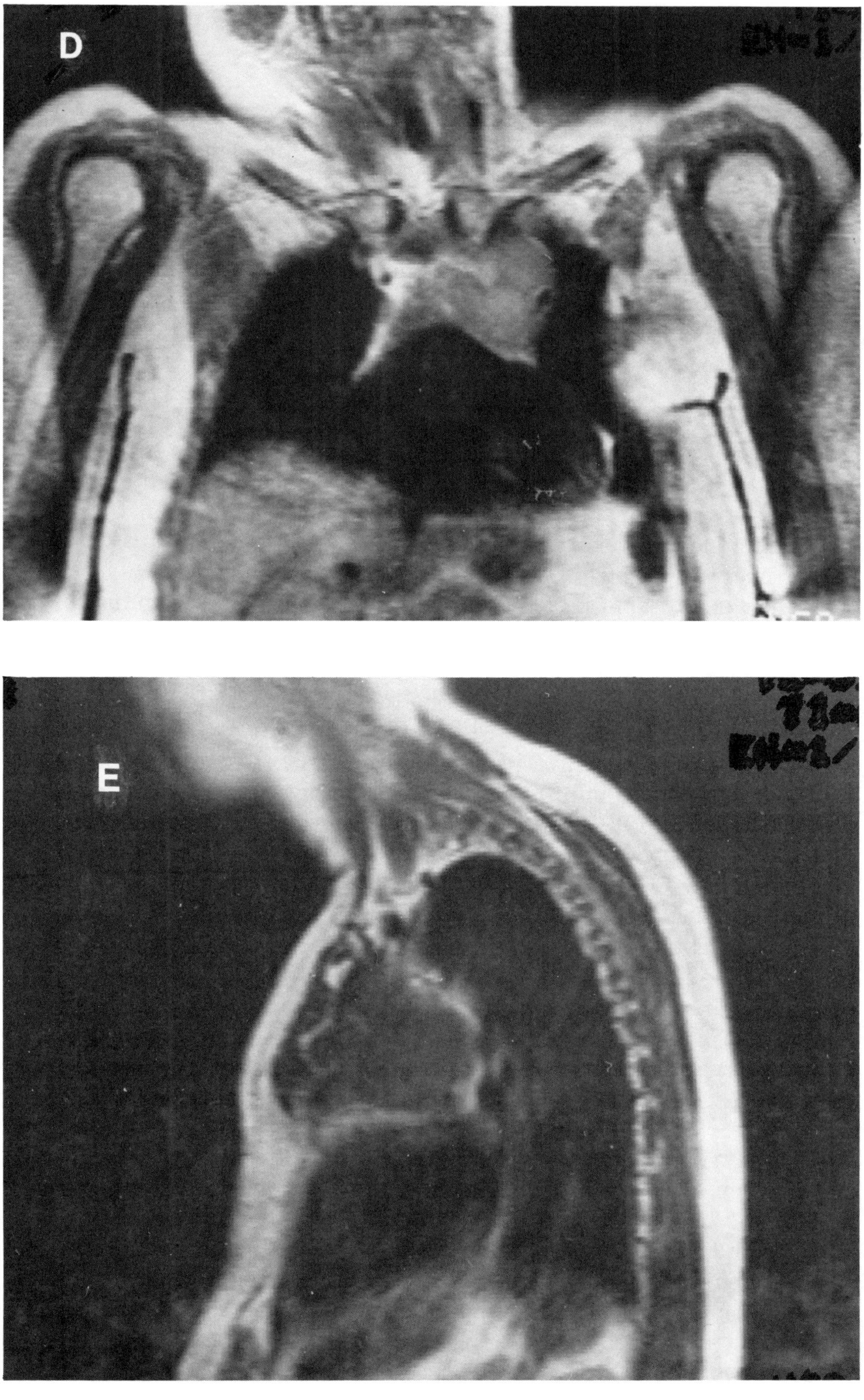
D
E

Evaluation of Abnormalities or Questionable Lesions Discovered on Conventional Radiographic Studies

On standard radiographs, multiple lesions have the tendency to blend in with the surrounding mediastinal components, making their evaluation and accurate localization impossible. Transverse imaging as provided by CT scanning permits precise separation of the various mediastinal components from the suspected abnormality (10). These lesions may have various etiologies: tumorous (benign or malignant), granulomatous or metastatic. Epstein *et al.* reported on a series of 45 patients which had undergone MRI of the mediastinum for various pathological conditions (2). The MRI results were retrospectively compared to CT images and correlation with available pathological and clinical information was done. MRI and CT findings were evaluated in respect to identification of normal and abnormal anatomy and to their ability to provide useful clinical information. In 63% of the cases, MR and CT images were considered to be comparable. Delineation of soft tissue abnormalities from vascular structures was satisfactory with CT imaging provided contrast injection had been given, while MRI provided the same information without requiring intravenous contrast administration. The major shortcoming with both techniques is their inability to predict histology and to distinguish benign from malignant disease. The major disadvantages with MRI in the study of the mediastinum were:

1. Calcifications within a lung nodule, which provide evidence of a benign lesion on CT or plain radiography, can be missed by using MRI only. The presence of calcification is very difficult to be identified on T_1 weighted images, particularly when calcifications are located adjacent to a region of low or intermediate signal intensity.

2. The relatively poor spatial resolution on MR images in comparison to CT. It is mainly due to long imaging sequences and respiration movements. On MR images, small-sized structures and also the margins of large mediastinal masses may not easily be recognized. As a consequence, in many instances it may be impossible to separate a single from a cluster of mediastinal lymph nodes by MRI.

3. Volume averaging may result in significant interpretation problems with MRI if only a single pulse sequence is performed. Volume averaging of mediastinal fat, which has high signal intensity, and low intensity flowing blood may produce a region of intermediate signal intensity that simulates a mediastinal mass or lymphadenopathy (17). Volume averaging can only be separated from a true mass by imaging with different TR values. When a long TR (2000–3000 ms) is used, the signal intensity of a mass will

increase relatively to fat, while a volume averaging does not change its relative intensity. Nevertheless, T_1 weighted images allow detection of most, if not all, mediastinal nodes that are borderline in size (1-1.5 cm) or enlarged (1). In some cases, mediastinal lymph nodes that are visible on MRI are difficult to see with CT due to streak artifacts. Due to their inherently reduced spatial resolution, lymphadenopathy is more difficult to be identified on T_1 weighted images.

In our experience with MRI of the mediastinum, we were able to evaluate several mediastinal mass lesions of different etiologies which had initially been found on chest films: mediastinal lymph node spread from bronchogenic carcinoma (Figure 5.10), a posterior mediastinal lymph node abscess due to tuberculosis (Figure 5.11), a paraesophageal tumor due to Hodgkin's disease (Figure 5.12), and a posterior mediastinal bronchogenic cyst (Figure 5.13). By comparing the MRI results with CT images we found that differentiation of mediastinal mass lesions from surrounding structures was superior on MR images than on CT scans in some of the cases (Figure 5.12). The degree of compression of broncho-vascular structures was also much more accurately outlined (Figure 5.10 and 5.13), while tumor contours were more sharply delineated by CT scanning (Figure 5.12). A bronchogenic cyst showed definitely higher signal intensity than subcutaneous fat due to its viscid mucoid content. The cyst showed very smooth borders and some compression of the right pulmonary artery was demonstrated (Figure 5.13). Another patient had a mass lesion (Figure 5.14) in a similar location as the lesion shown in Figures 5.11 and 5.13. This lesion also had smooth contours and a morphologic appearance very similar to the bronchogenic cyst shown in Figure 5.13, but it had definitely lower signal intensity. On the other hand, its signal intensity was very similar to the lymph node abscess in Figure 5.11 which had a quite different morphological appearance. In fact, the abnormality shown in Figure 5.14 was due to an enterogenic esophageal cyst. The three cases illustrate the relatively low tissue specificity provided by spin-echo MR images. Size, site and extension of the lesions are well demonstrated, but only little information about their etiology may be derived from T_1 and T_2 weighted images, as the signal intensity variations cannot be considered to be specific for determined pathologic conditions.

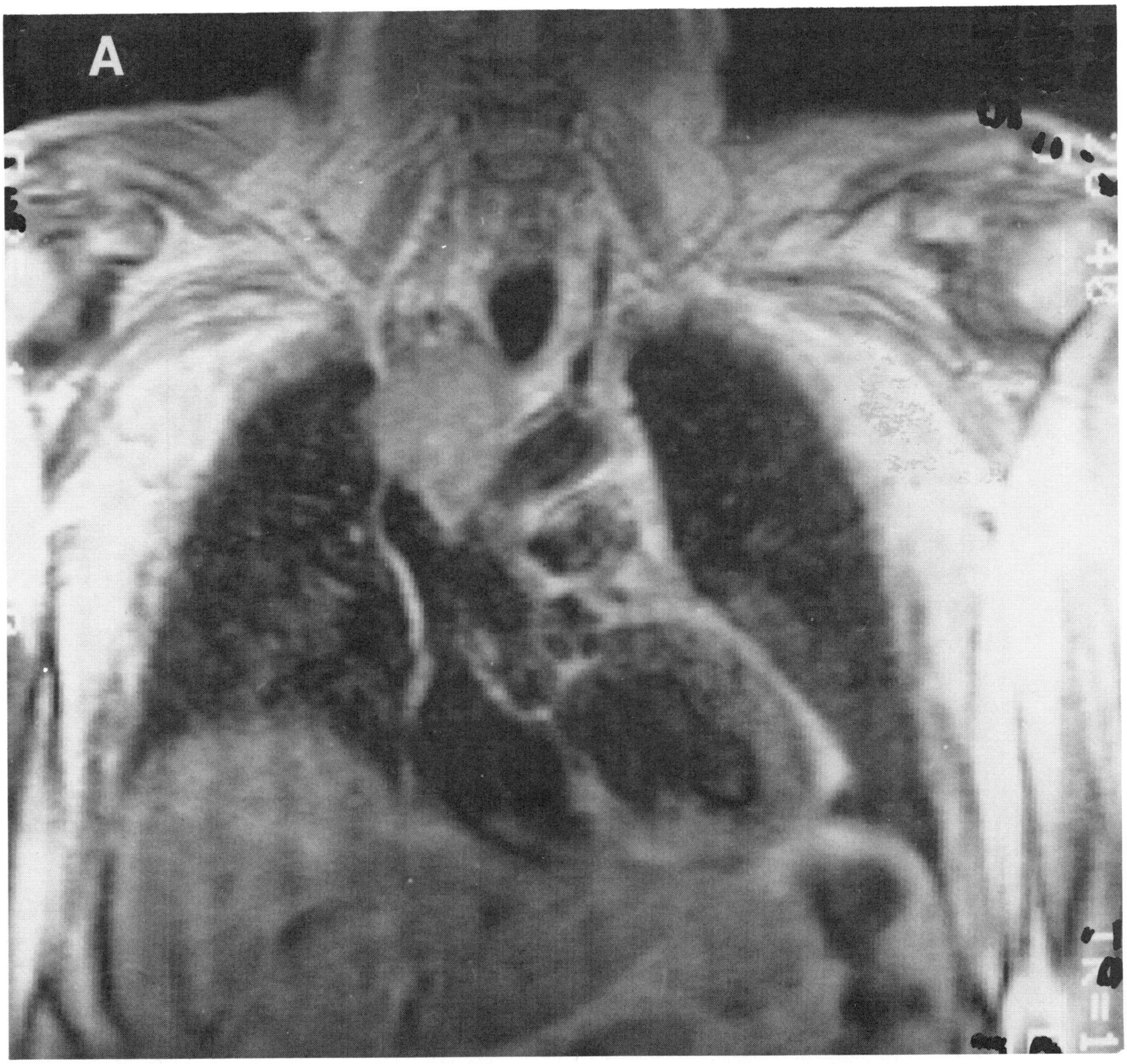

Figure 5.10 (A,B,C,D). Lung carcinoma on the right side with mediastinal metastases. Coronal images using a TR 1500 ms and two delayed echos demonstrate large metastatic seeding in the right upper mediastinum compressing the superior vena cava with some tracheal deviation to the left. This node of intermediate signal intensity can be accurately separated from the broncho-vascular structures (A). On the delayed echo (64 ms) there is some increase in signal intensity and a more homogeneous appearance of the mass (B). Transverse slice using a short TR demonstrates relationship of mass to surrounding vessels (C) while with T_2 weighted imaging the signal intensity of the mass increases in such a way that it can less sharply be separated from mediastinal fat (D). Note gross intraparenchymal tumor.

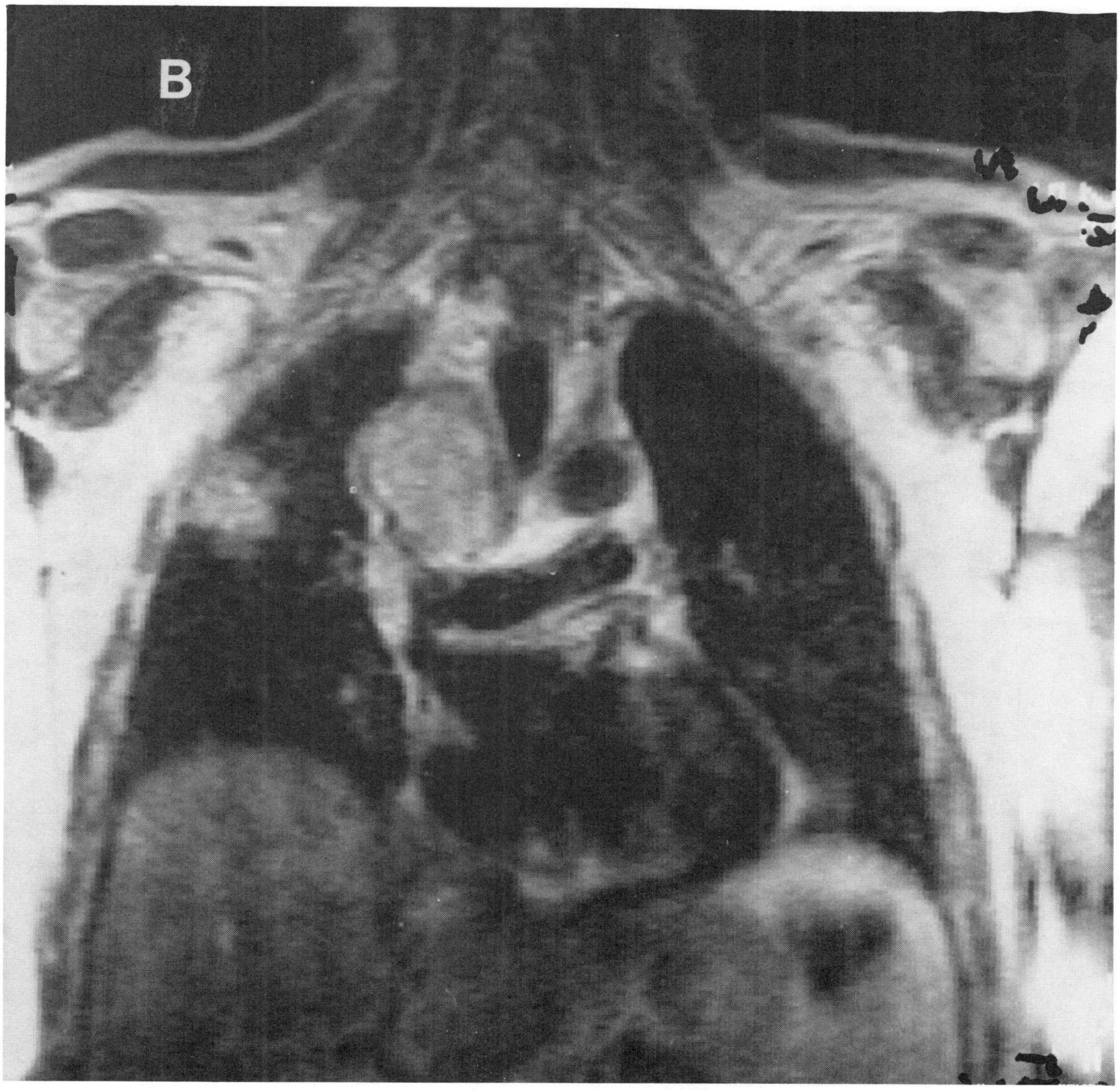
B

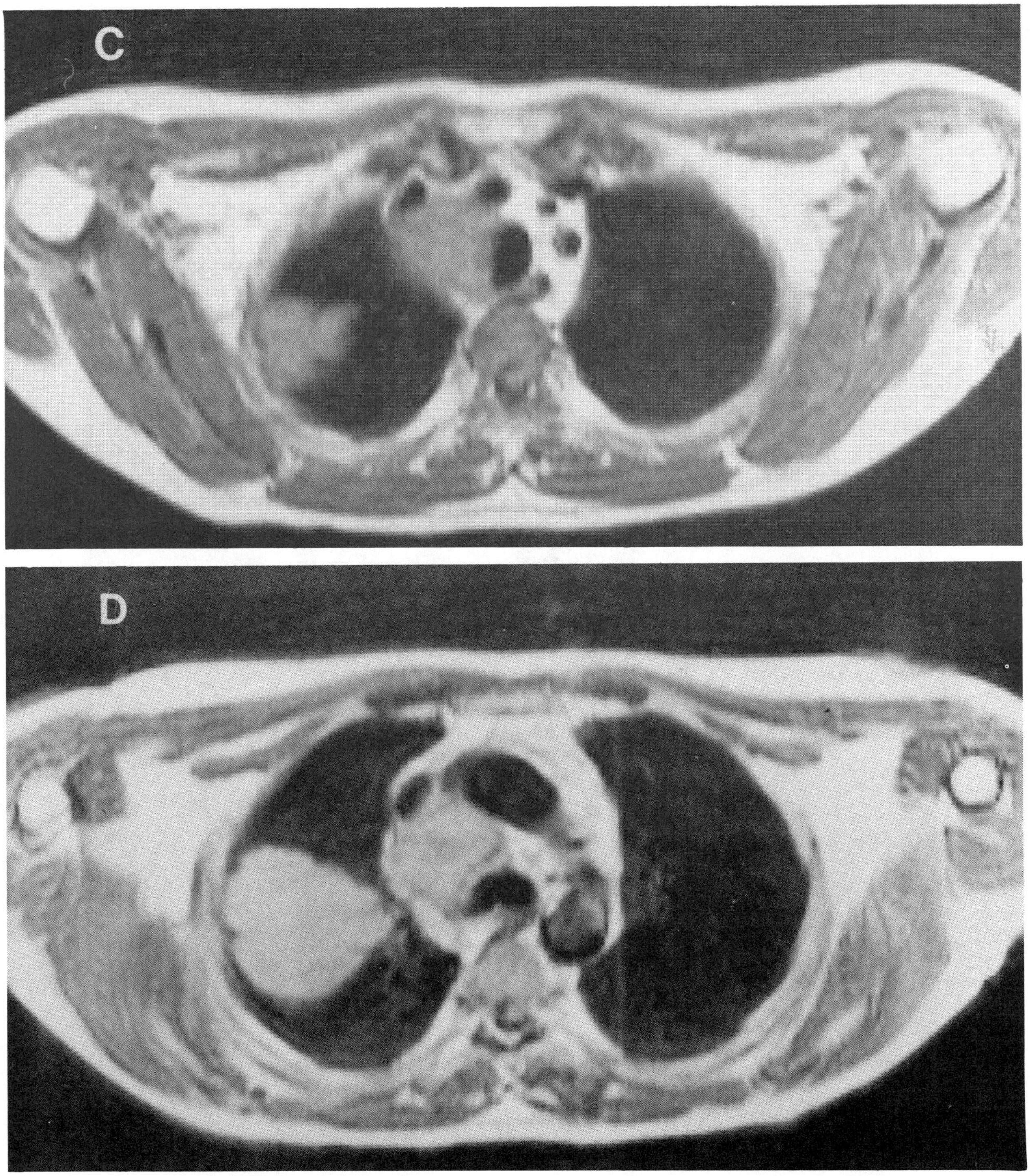

Figure 5.11 (A,B). A young man presented with motoric deficit in both lower limbs. MRI of the lumbar spine showed obvious thickening in the conus medullaris together with an area of increased signal intensity (A). As the suspicion of an enlarged paravertebral line was raised on conventional films of the spine, the MRI examination was extended to the lower thoracic region. Transverse MR images (TR 500 ms) show a right paravertebral mass of intermediate signal intensity due to a lymph node abscess.

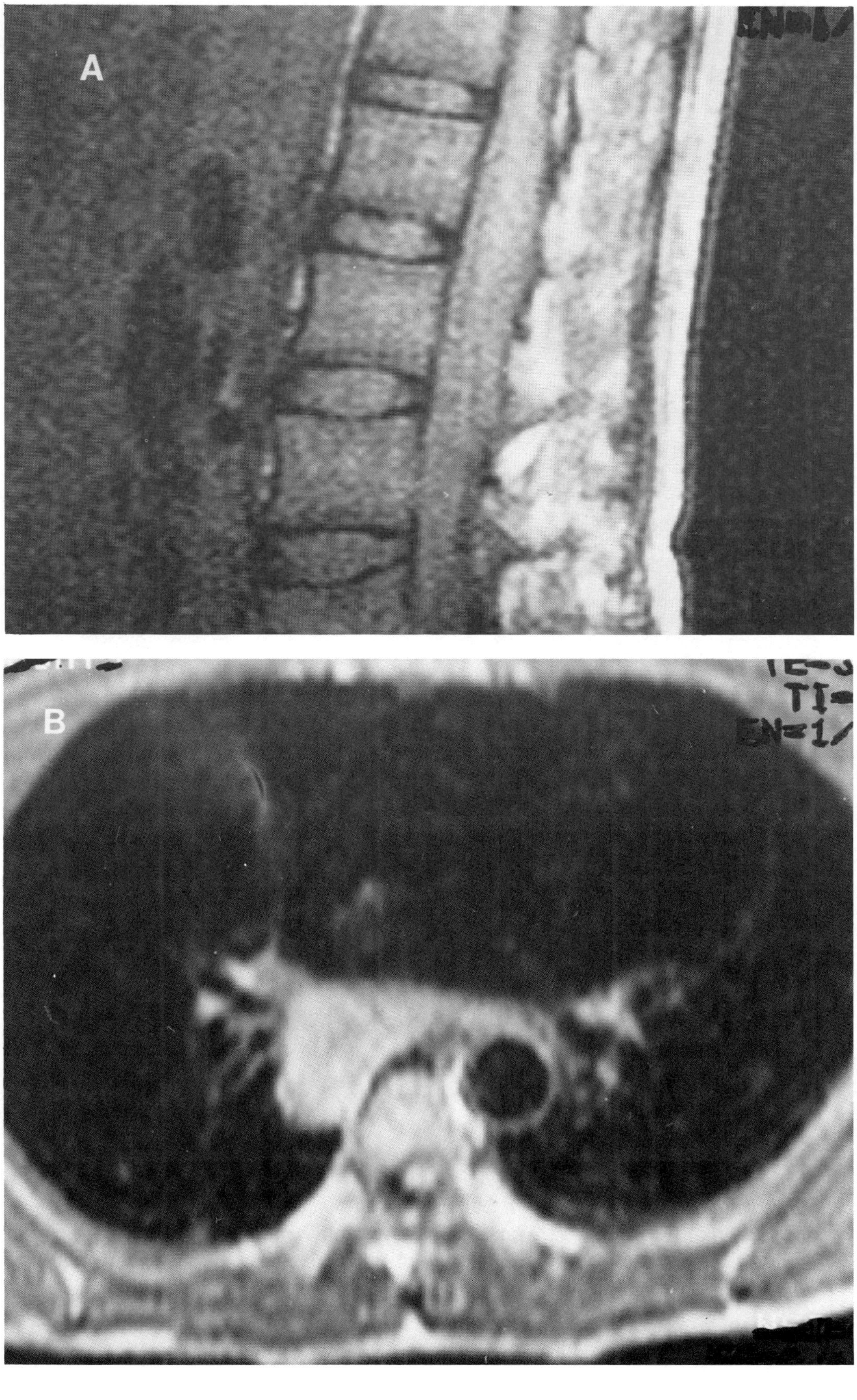
A
B

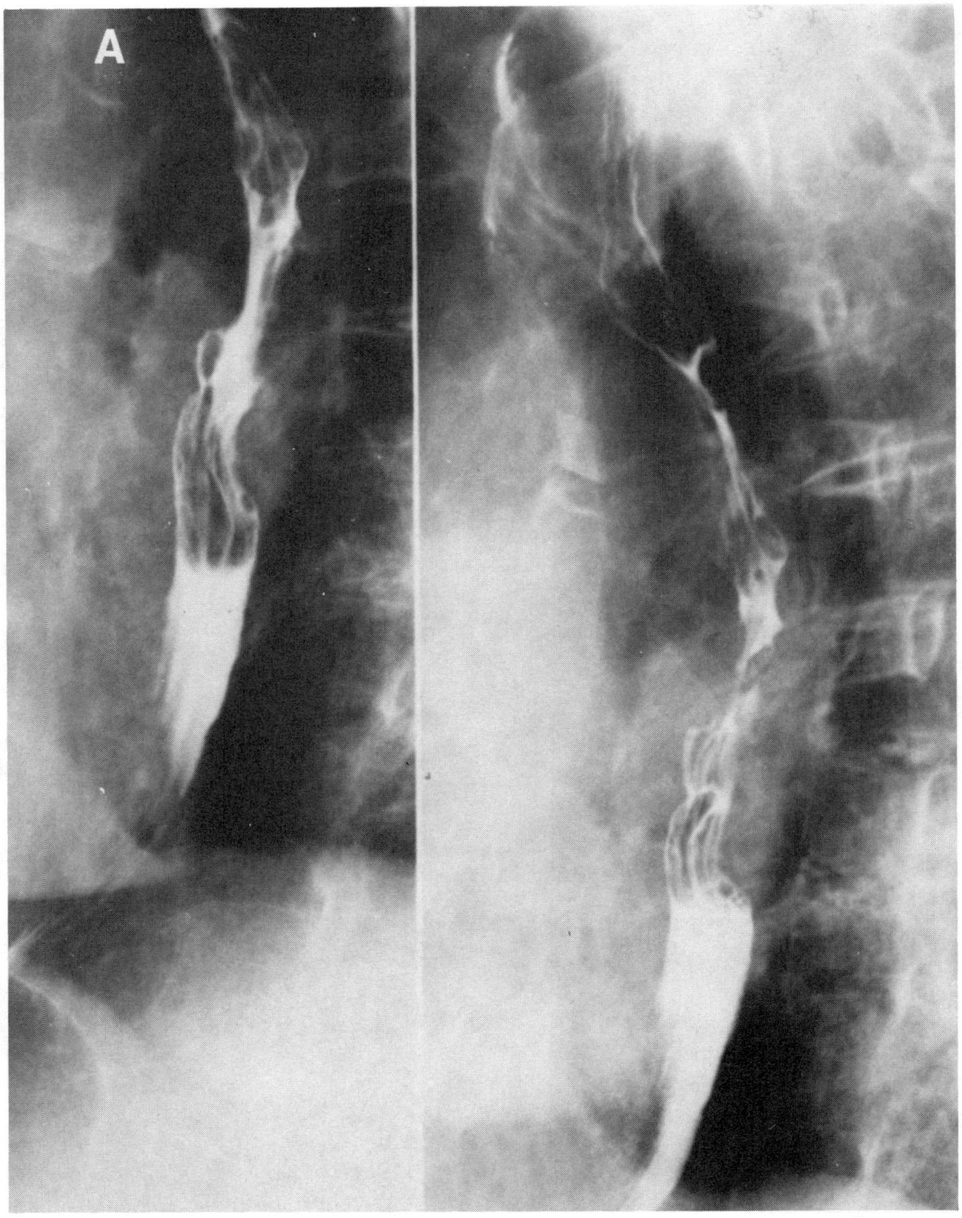

Figure 5.12. Barium swallow demonstrates extensive compression on the esophagus from an extrinsic mass (A). Axial CT scans at the level of carinal bifurcation demonstrate soft tissue mass in the posterior mediastinum mimicking an esophageal tumor. Notice the presence of enlarged lymph nodes within the anterior mediastinal fat (B). On the contrary coronal MRI using a short TR (500 ms) outlines the exact extension of the disease as a large process showing relatively low signal intensity was also found in the right mediastinum (C). On T_2 weighted images using a TR 3000 ms and a TE 64 ms the signal intensity of this mass increases significantly and it also seems to surround the trachea, therefore explaining the fact that the patient initially presented with stridor (D).

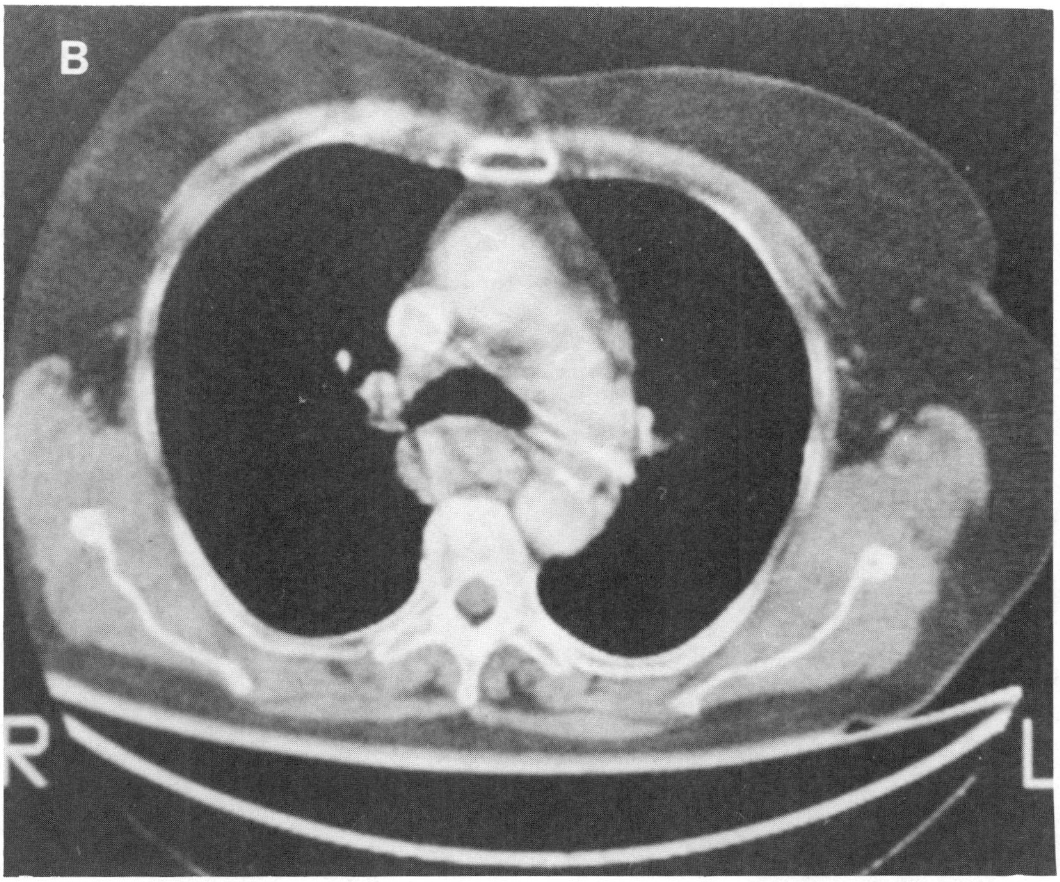
B
R
L

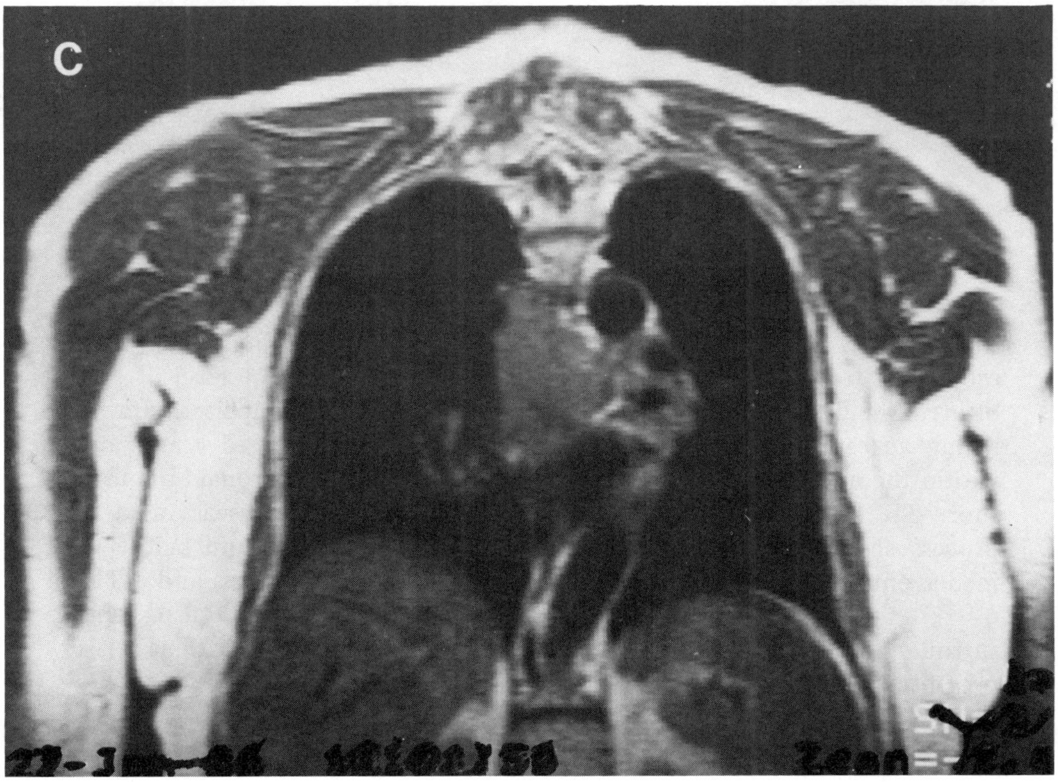
C

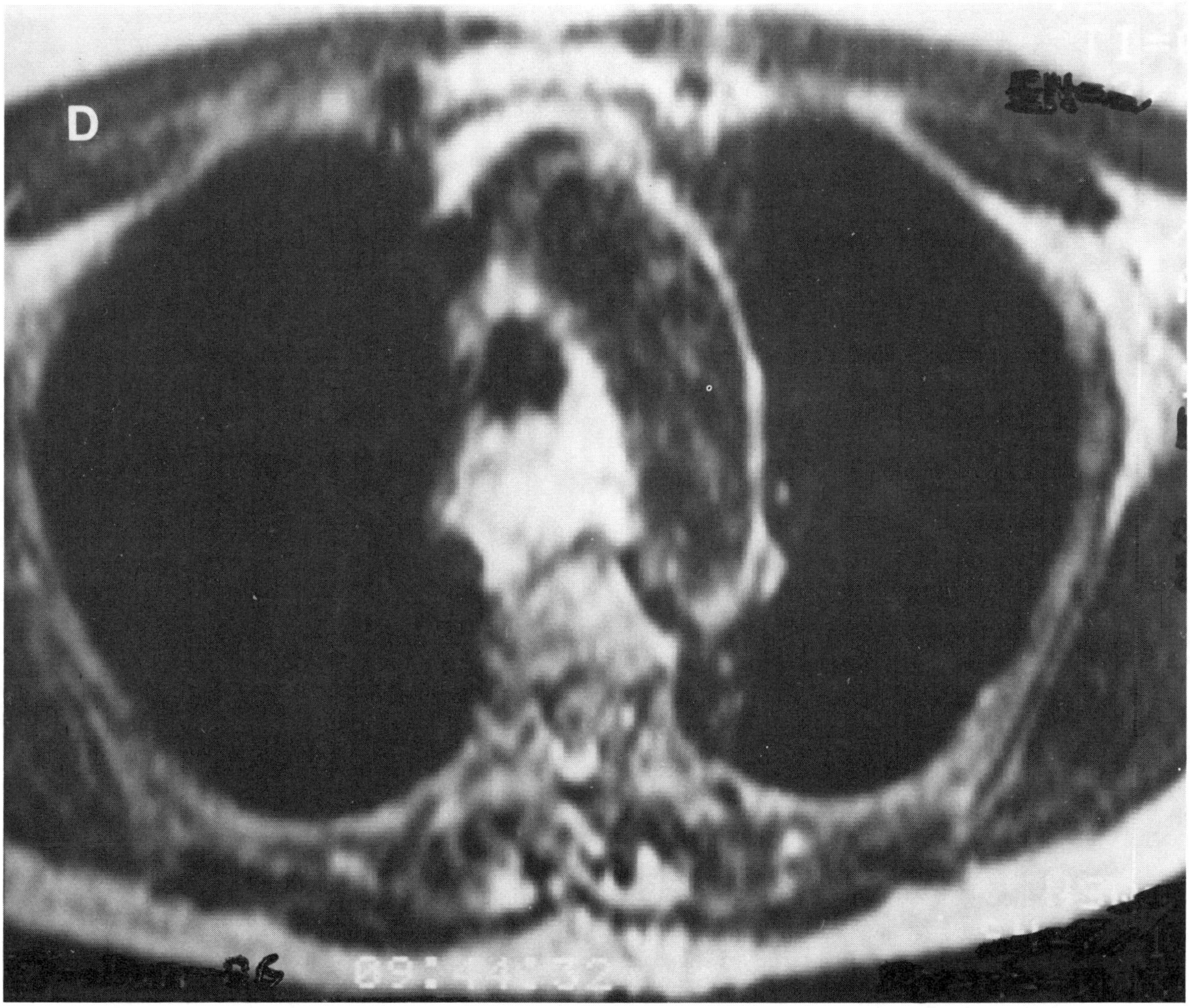
D

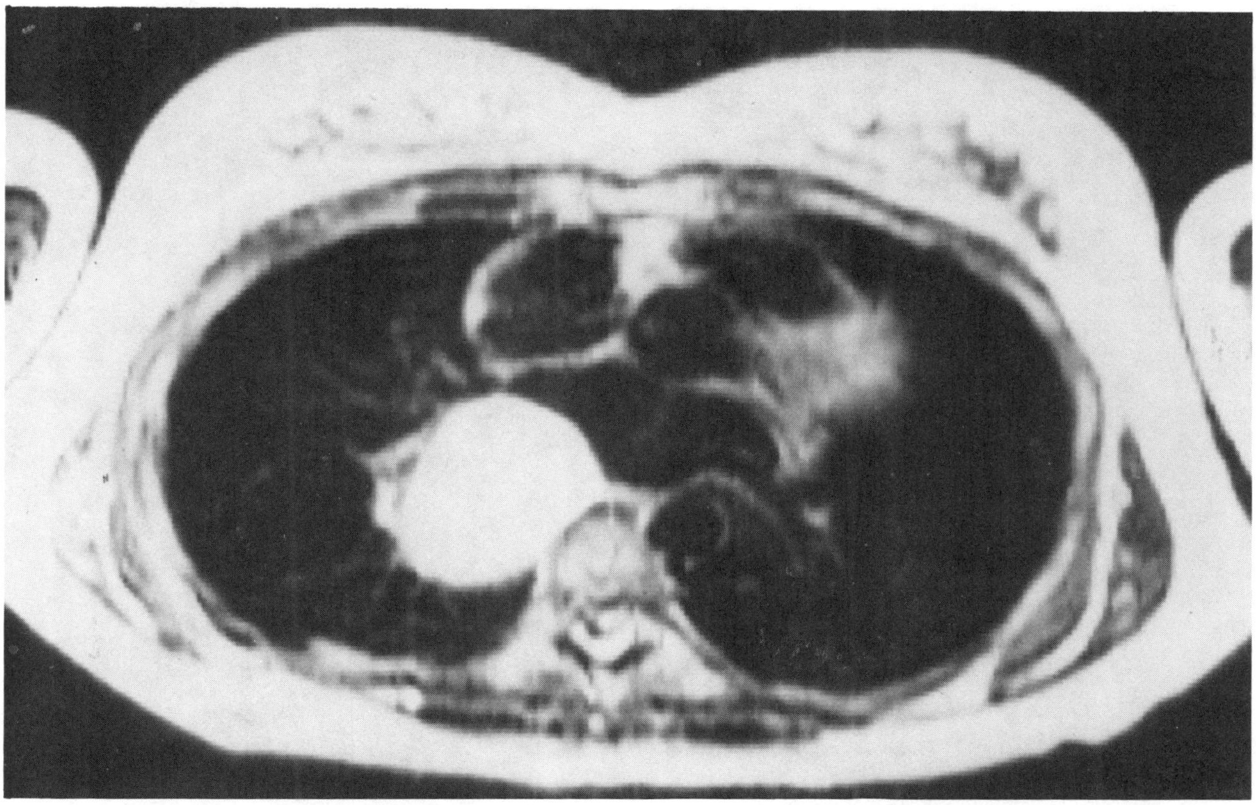

Figure 5.13. Young patient with sharply marginated lesion in the posterior mediastinum on the right side compressing the pulmonary artery (arrow). On all SE images the lesion showed very high signal intensity due to its viscid-mucoid content. The lesion represented a bronchogenic cyst.

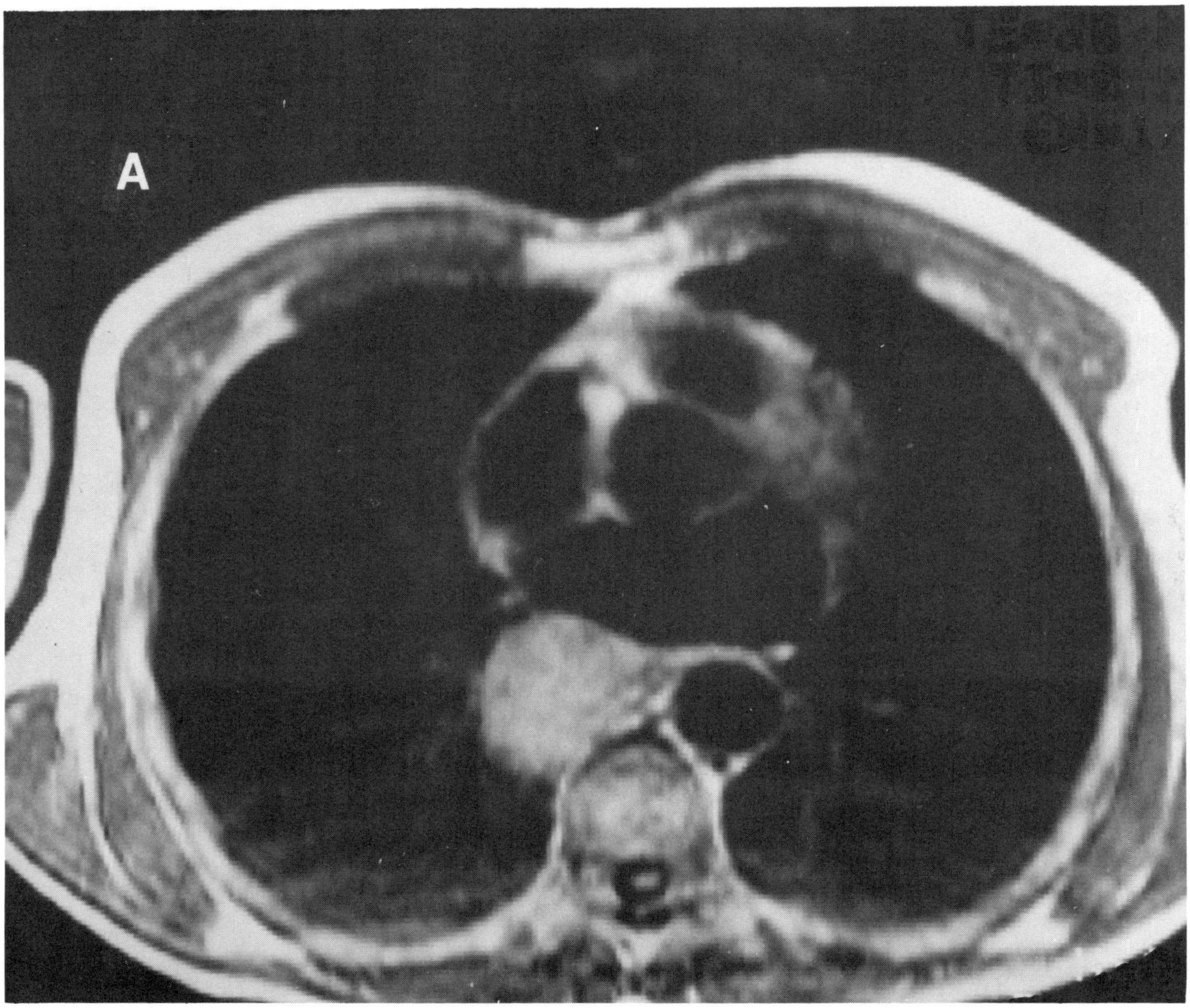

Figure 5.14 (A,B). MRI in a patient with a lesion located in the posterior mediastinum on the right. Mass is smoothly marginated and has a quite similar morphological appearance as the lesion shown in Figure 5.13, but it has obvious lower signal intensity (A). Coronal imaging shows its location in the right paravertebral gutter (B). The mass was due to an enterogenic esophageal cyst.

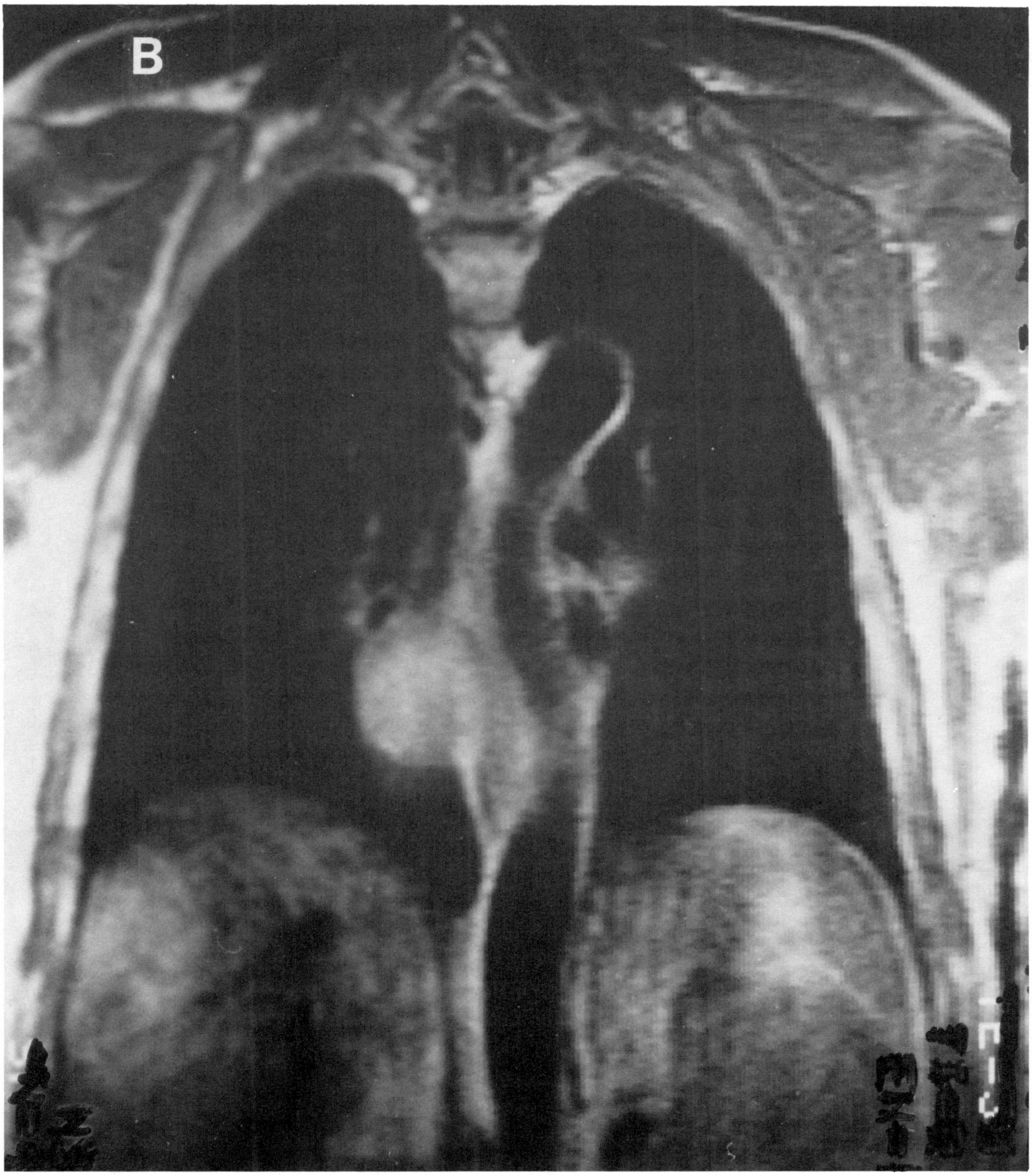
B

By using cardiac gating, accurate visualization of the heart and of the pericardial space may be obtained. Moderate pericardial effusion missed by CT scanning may easily be diagnosed on MR images (16). With MRI we investigated a patient showing an obviously abnormal posterior contour of the heart on chest films (Figure 5.15A) in which further diagnostic evaluation was requested. A large aneurysm of the posterior wall of the left ventricle was clearly outlined (Figure 5.15 B). Intramural thrombi and myocardial infarction may also be diagnosed with MRI (19). A more detailed report about MRI of the heart and pericardial space is provided in Chapter 4.

MRI OF THE MEDIASTINUM IN BRONCHOGENIC CARCINOMA

The presence of lymph node spread in carcinoma of the lung is known to affect prognosis in a significant way. If mediastinal nodes are involved, fewer than 10% of patients live five years after surgery, whereas apparent complete resection in patients without mediastinal metastases may provide a five-year survival rate ranging between 30 and 45%. It is very important to find such metastatic involvement during the preoperative work-up as in some cases surgery may be contraindicated. It is generally admitted that contralateral mediastinal lymph node metastases rule out surgery. Contralateral spread occurs most frequently from a left sided tumor to the right side, but right to left drainage is also known to occur. If high ipsilateral nodal involvement is present, surgery may be disregarded in most of the cases.

Consequently, preoperative TNM staging of bronchogenic carcinoma is extremely important in selecting patients for surgery. Conventional radiography including tomography is able to demonstrate mediastinal nodes only at a relatively advanced stage. Computed tomography significantly improved the diagnostic work-up in these patients as an overall accuracy of 81% in evaluating mediastinal nodes has been reported (16). Nevertheless, some areas like the aorto-pulmonary window remain difficult for preoperative evaluation and false-positive and false-negative interpretations may occur. Mediastinoscopy is an important diagnostic tool to view and biopsy accessible mediastinal masses and lymph nodes. The areas that may be inspected by mediastinoscopy are somewhat limited, mainly the anterior mediastinum and the aorto-pulmonary window are not within the range of view.

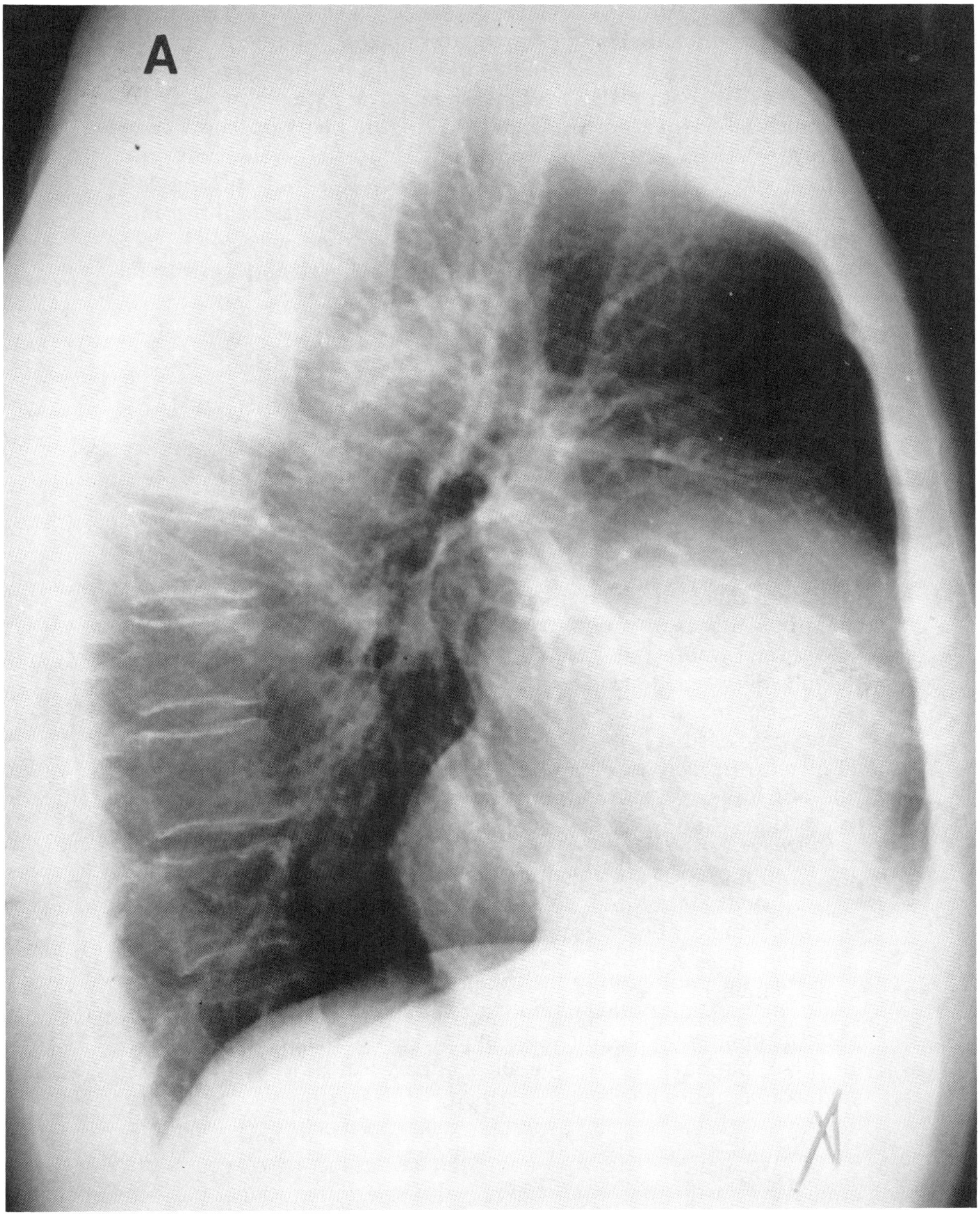

Figure 5.15 (A,B). Lateral film of the chest shows very prominent posterior contour of the heart (A). Transverse MRI using cardiac gating demonstrated a large aneurysm of the left ventricle together with marked thickening of the posterior myocardial wall (B).

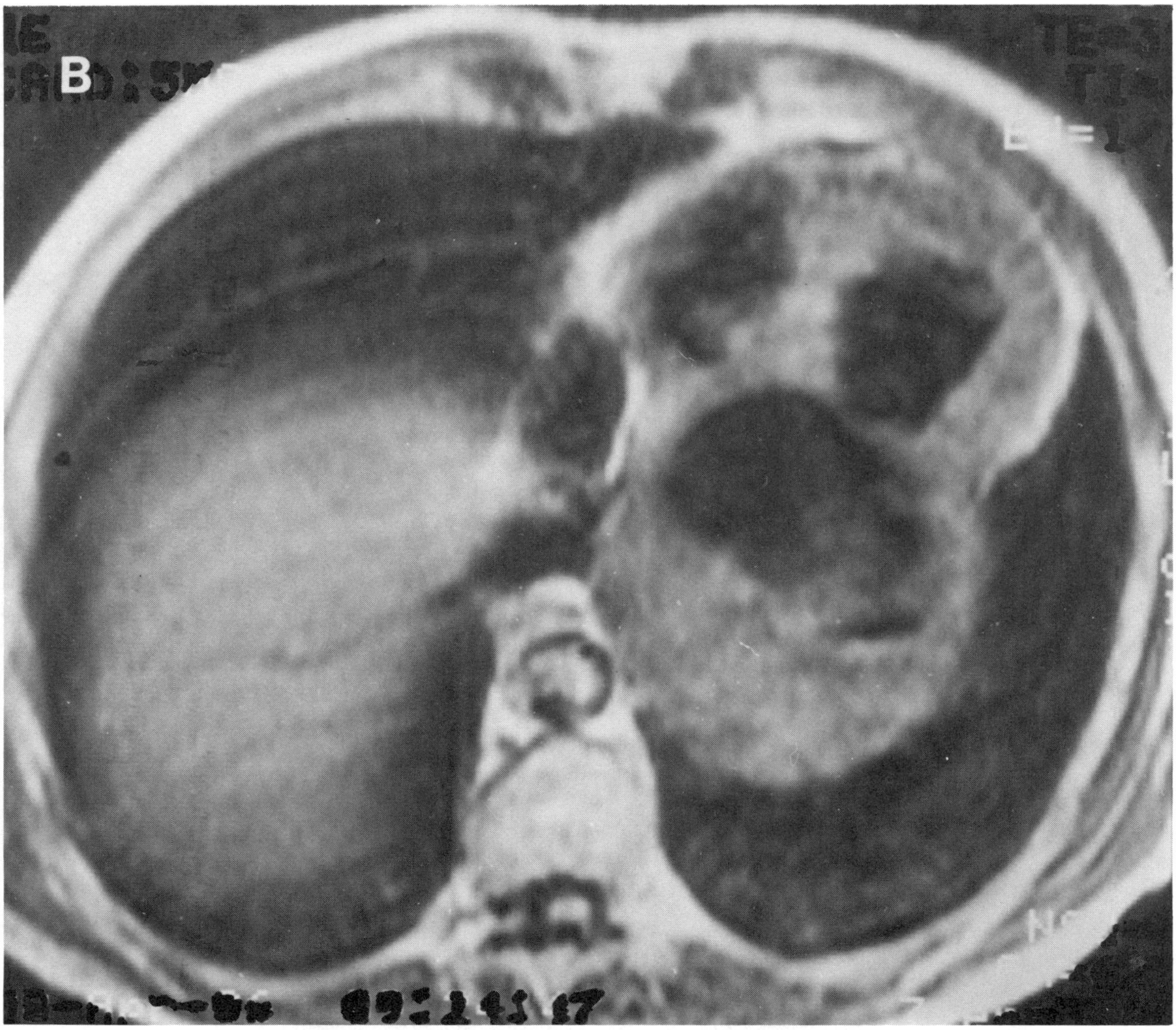

The more recent advent of MRI of the human body raises the possibility that this modality may prove to be superior to CT in the assessment of mediastinal metastases. In our experience, T_1 weighted images are most helpful in delineating mediastinal lymph nodes which may be clearly seen as masses of intermediate signal intensity within the high signal intensity of mediastinal fat. As the main broncho-vascular structures are clearly visualized by MRI as low density structures, the relationship of pathological nodes to these structures can be accurately assessed. Broncho-vascular compression and/or invasion may be confirmed or excluded (Figure 5.16). We believe that CT and MRI are going to play complementary roles in the preoperative work-up of lung cancer patients and that the rate of false-negative and false-positive results can still be reduced by the impact of MR imaging. In whis way, invasive procedures such as mediastinoscopy and exploratory thoracotomy may be obviated in the future in numerous patients.

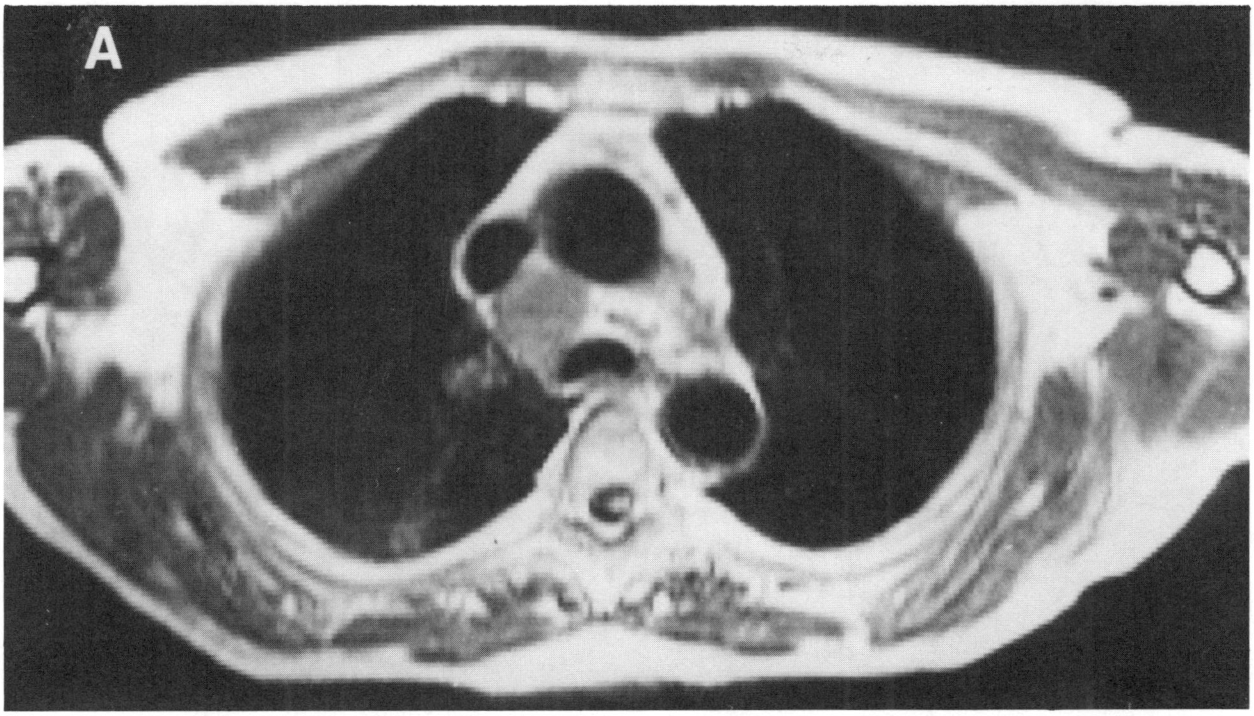

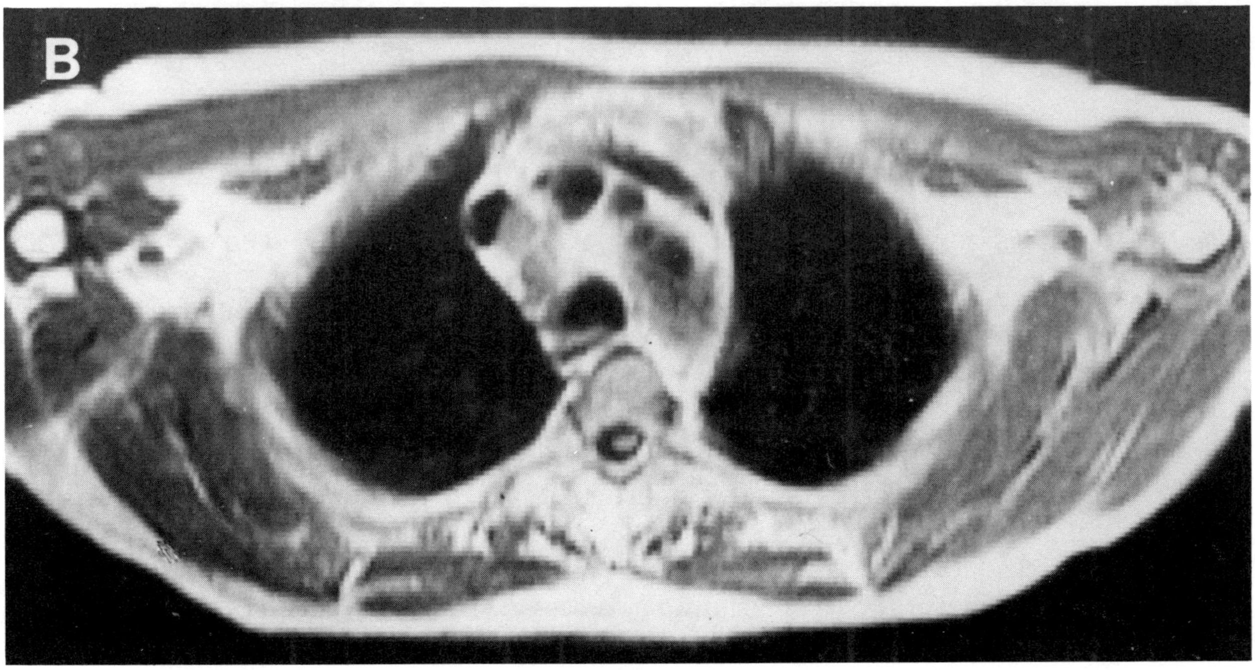

Figure 5.16 (A,B,C). Transverse MRI images using a short TR (500 ms) and respiratory gating demonstrate small lesion in the right lung posteriorly (arrow) and mediastinal lymph node metastasis with intermediate signal intensity (A). Some compression of the superior vena cava by the pathological lymph nodes delineated (B). Coronal imaging using cardiac gating show precise relationship of the mass to trachea and right pulmonary vessels (C).

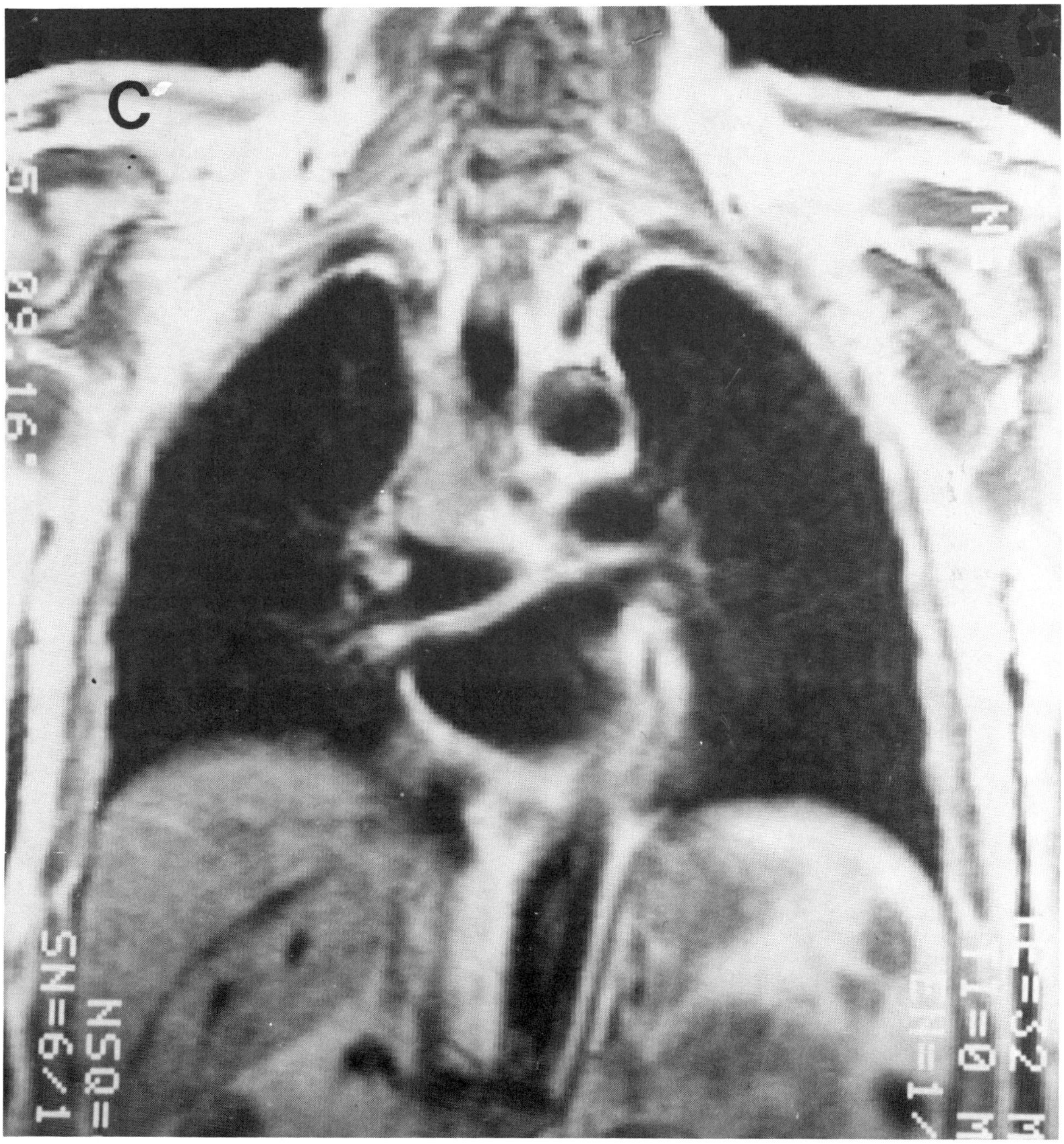

Heelan *et al.* (16) reported on 20 patients with primary lung tumors in which the results of CT and MRI were correlated with surgical findings and histopathological evaluation. Both imaging modalities showed a similar ability to detect hilar and mediastinal tumor. There were false-positive interpretations by CT examinations in three patients and in five cases MR investigations provided false-positive findings, but there were no false-negative findings by either modality. Both modalities had false-positive interpretations in the same three patients (Table 2). But it should be kept in mind that we are still expanding our diagnostic capabilities with MRI, while the principles of CT scanning have been established for some time. Pitfalls in MRI evaluation of the mediastinum have been described (20). The esophagus may be misinterpreted as an enlarged retrotracheal lymph node unless serial scans are studied. Several adjacent small lymph nodes shown individually by CT may appear as a single enlarged lymph node by MRI due to partial volume averaging (20). The combined use of CT and MRI should allow detection of tumor recurrences and mediastinal lymph node metastases at an early stage in patients having undergone pneumonectomy. Due to shifting and rotation of the cardio-mediastinal structures towards the affected side, conventional radiography is not an appropriate diagnostic method in the postoperative follow-up of these patients. Transverse CT imaging provides important diagnostic information about the cardio-mediastinal structures and malignant involvement of the mediastinum may be detected at a much earlier stage. We believe that for this particular purpose, MRI represents a major diagnostic tool to detect mediastinal masses in post-pneumonectomy patients due to its inherent high contrast sensitivity allowing a most accurate separation between pathological mediastinal nodes from the distorted broncho-vascular tree. Figure 5.17 shows a post-pneumonectomy patient presenting massive tumor recurrency within the mediastinum. T_1 weighted images demonstrated the mass as a structure of intermediate signal intensity causing partial compression of the superior vena cava and of the aortic arch (Figure 5.17 A–C). On T_2 weighted images, it was almost impossible to separate tumor from mediastinal fat due to a relatively higher increased signal intensity of tumor in comparison to fatty tissue (Figure 5.17 D). Coronal MR images showed very clearly the intramediastinal growth of the tumor and its relation to broncho-vascular structures (Figure 5.17 E).

TABLE 2
INTERPRETATION OF CT AND MRI FINDINGS IN MEDIASTINUM AND CORRELATION WITH PATHOLOGIC FINDINGS

Patient No.	*Pathology*	*CT*	*MR*	*Comment*
1	—	—	—	
2	—	+ (FP)	+ (FP)	Enlarged anthracotic mediastinal nodes
3	+	+	+	
4	—	—	—	
5	+	+	+	At pathology - direct invasion of mediastinum not mentioned on CT or MR image.
6	—	—	+ (FP)	At pathology - enlarged mediastinal lymph nodes with foci of fibrosis and histoplasma.
7	+	+	+	CT and MR led to diagnosis of direct spread into mediastinum.
8	—	+ (FP)	+ (FP)	CT and MR:direct extension. Pathology-tumor extends to, not through, pleura.
9	—	—	—	
10	+	+	+	CT, MR: direct tumor extension to mediastinum. Pathology: no direct extension; benign pleural plaque at medial lung right upper lobe.
11	—	—	+ (FP)	MR - suspicion for direct extension. Pathology - tumor extends to pleura not through; fibrous pleural exudate with thickening at this site.
12	+	+	+	(1) Pericardial nodules (2) MR led to diagnosis of pericardial effusion, confirmed at surgery, missed by CT.
13	+	+	+	
14	—	+ (FP)	+ (FP)	Pathology: enlarged anthracotic and fibrotic mediastinal nodes.
15	+	+	+	
16	—	—	—	
17	+	+	+	
18	—	—	—	Multiple small lung nodules: present on CT scans not on MR images.
19	+	+	+	
20	+	+	+	

FP = False positive

With permission reference 16.

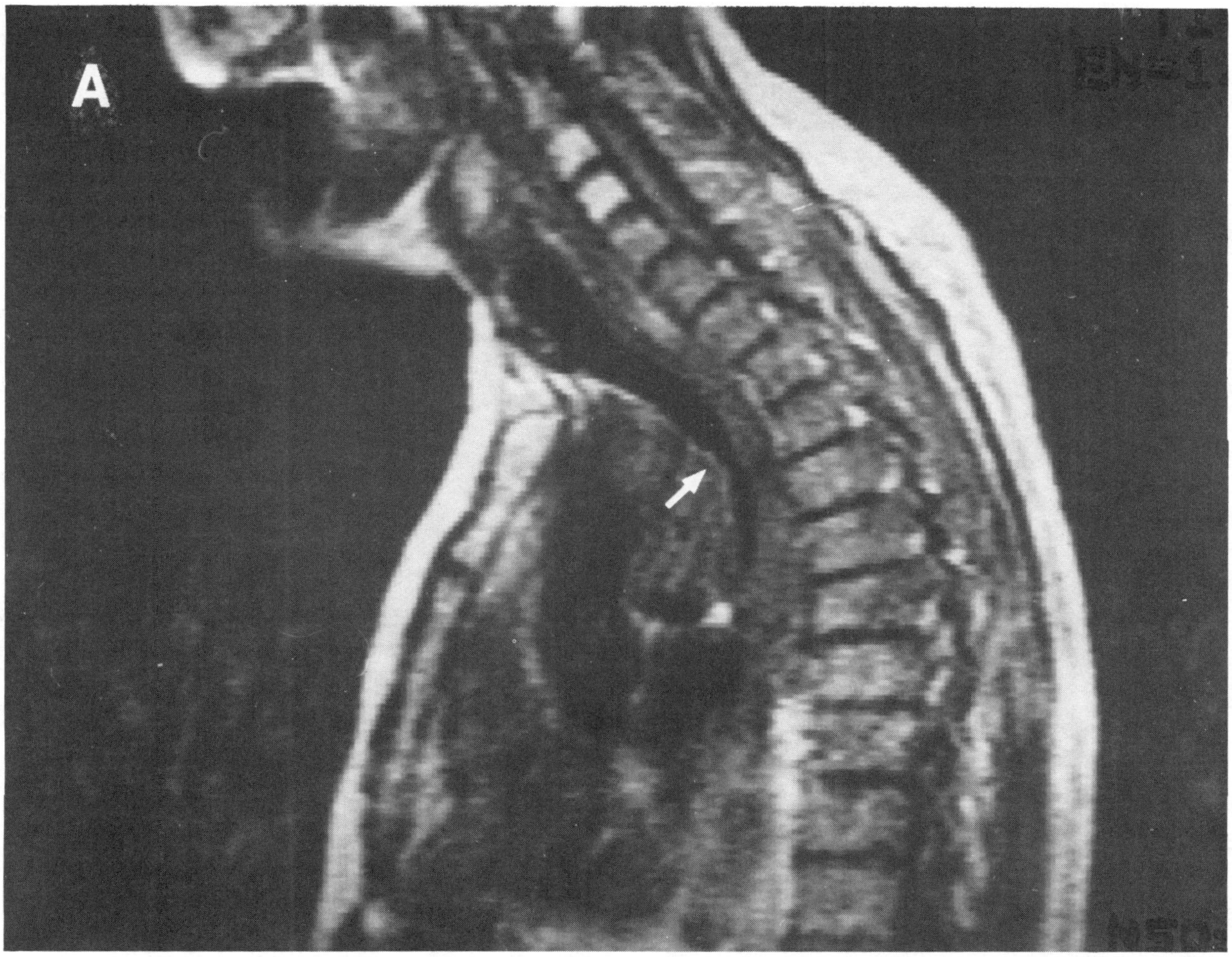

Figure 5.17 (A,B,C,D,E). Post-pneumonectomy patient shows large mediastinal mass on sagittal "Scoutview" deviating the trachea posteriorly (arrow) (A). T_1 weighted transverse MRI sections show very well tumor recurrency within mediastinal fat (B & C). Notice compression of aortic arch and deviated trachea (B) as well as compressed superior vena cava (arrowhead) (C). On T_2 weighted images using a long TR (3000 ms) tumor recurrency could not be separated from mediastinal fat (D). Coronal images using a TR 500 ms (T_1 weighted) showed the intramediastinal growth of the tumor and its relation to broncho-vascular structures (E).

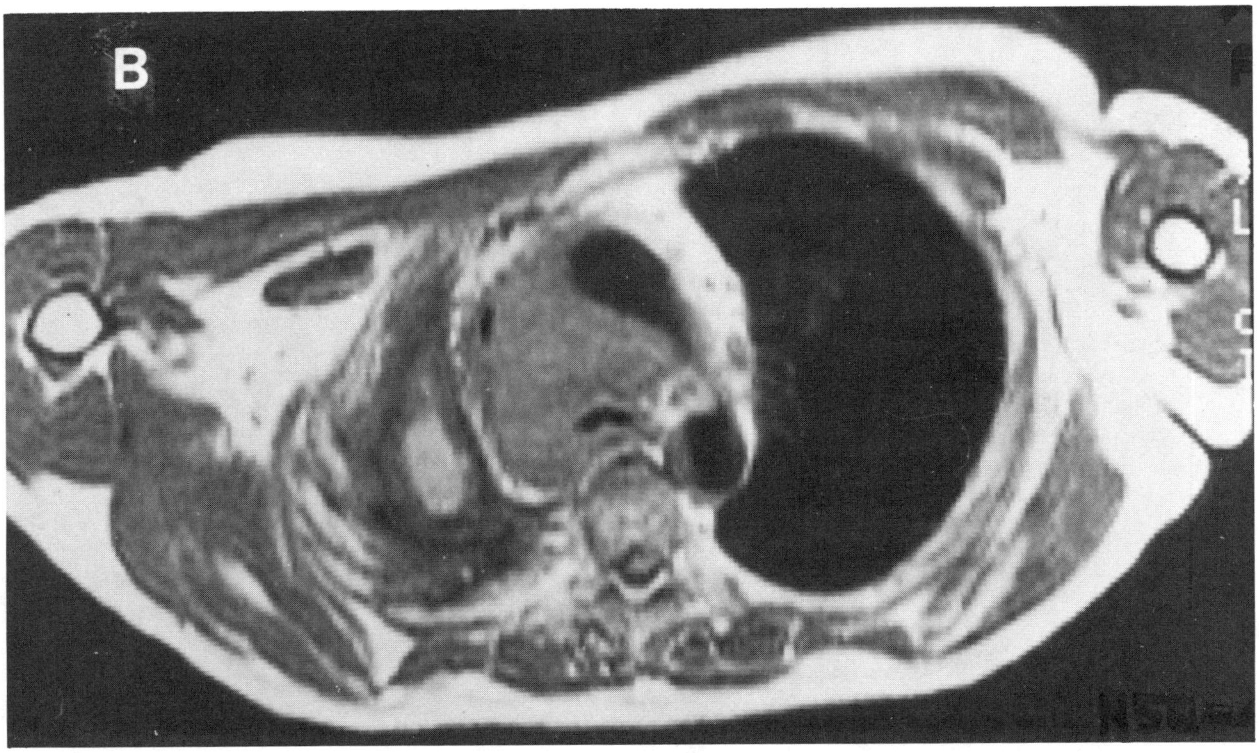
B

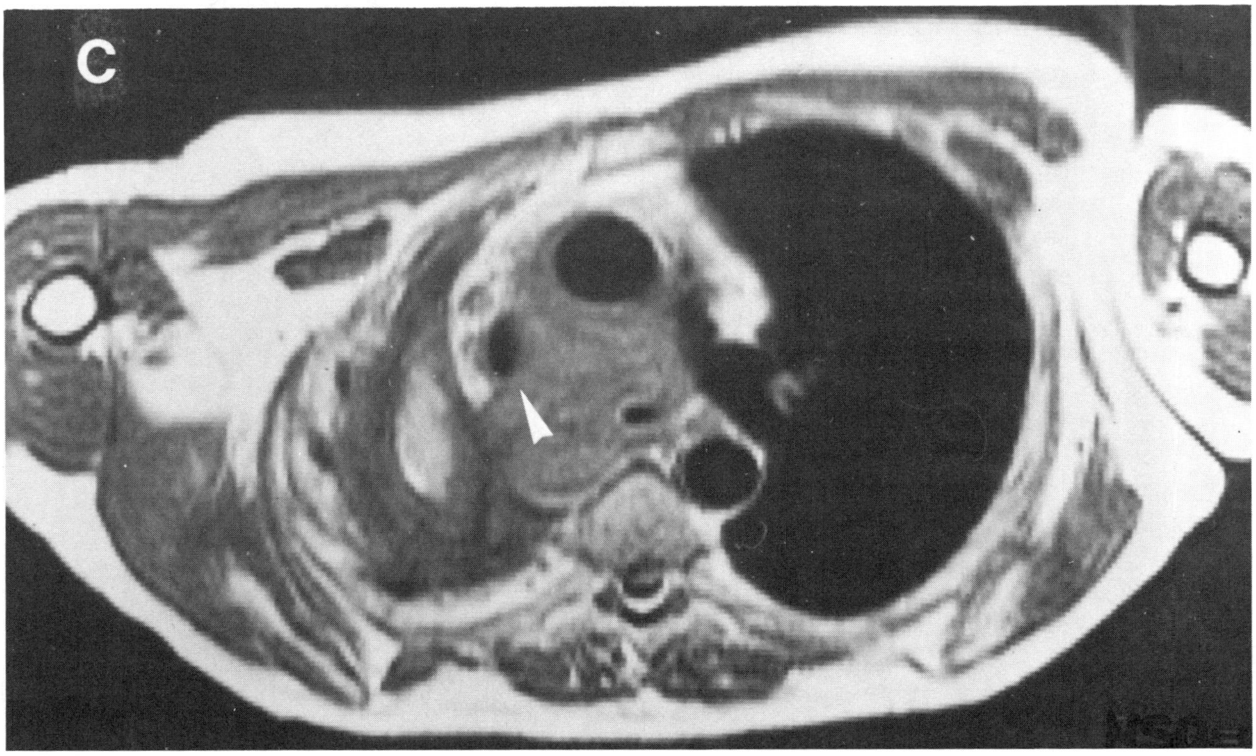
C

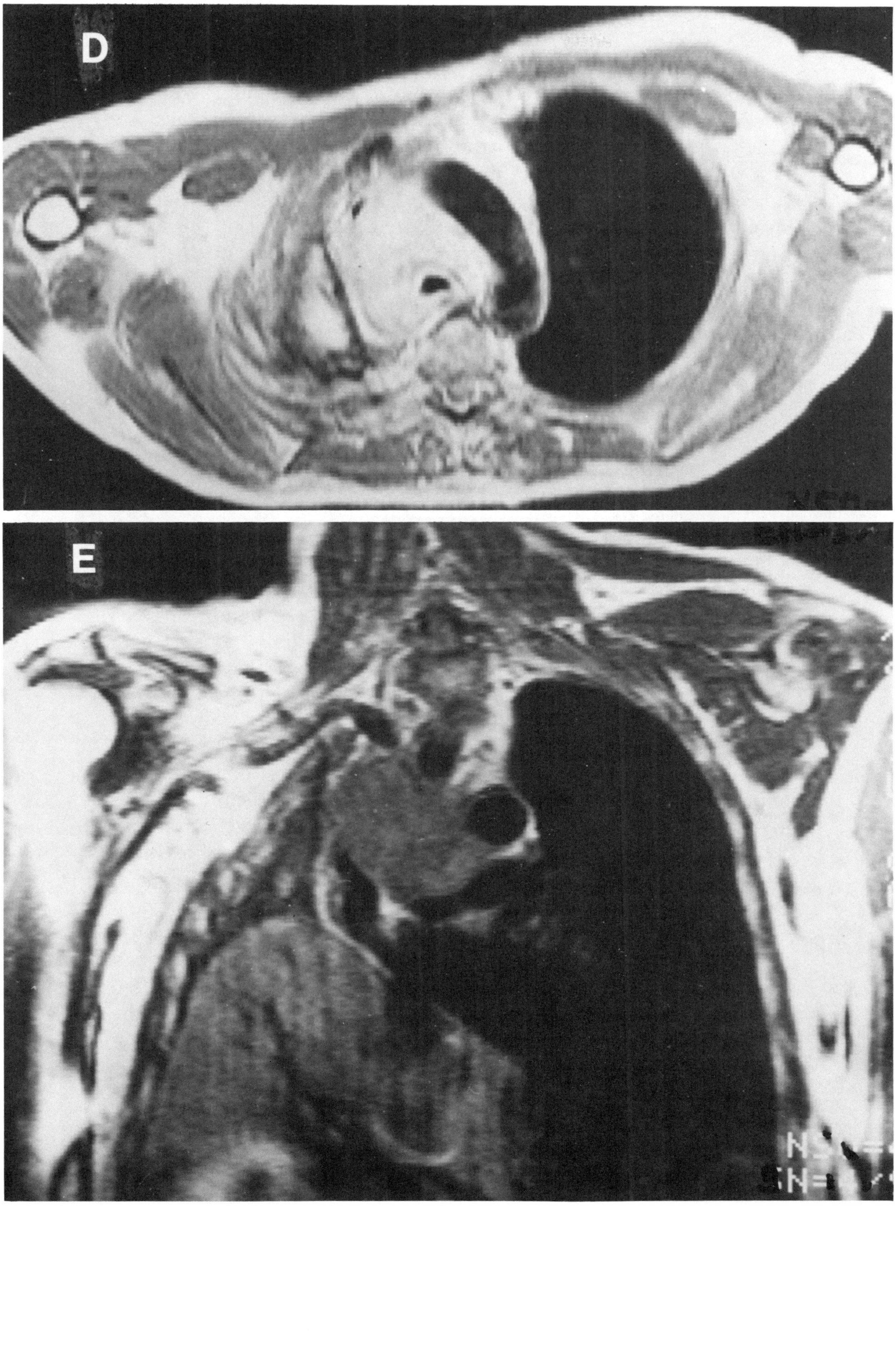
D
E

POSTERIOR MEDIASTINAL MASSES AND THEIR RELATIONSHIP TO THE SPINE

Ganglioneurinomas and neuroblastomas are mainly encountered in childhood, while neurinomas and neurofibromas are usually discovered in young adults. Phaeochromocytomas are very rare tumors in the posterior mediastinum. The paravertebral localization of these solid neurogenic tumors may readily be demonstrated by MRI as well as erosions or destructions of the spinal bone and adjacent ribs. Widening of the spinal canal and of the foramina may be equally well demonstrated.

Cystic lesions such as meningoceles and neurenteric cysts may rarely be encountered in the posterior mediastinum. MRI easily defines the cystic nature of these lesions and almost constantly demonstrates eventual communication with the intraspinal contents.

The thoracic spine is a frequent target for metastatic seeding from numerous primary neoplasms of the body. These spinal metastases may sometimes reach a considerable size. They may invade the paravertebral gutter or the posterior mediastinal space in an anterior direction. In a posterior direction, the spinal canal and the intraspinal contents may be infiltrated (Figures 5.18 and 5.19). Direct invasion of the spine by primary lung neoplasms is also possible (Figure 5.19). In the prementioned conditions, we would like to recommend the use of surface coils, as the main interest in these patients is on the spine. Due to the small size of surface coils, their limited field of view and their proximity to the area being imaged, the signal-to-noise ratio may be increased in such a way that the spatial resolution may be nearly equivalent to that achieved by CT scanners (21). Surface coils are also compatible with multiplanar, multiecho-imaging techniques and 4 mm slice thickness can be used on our MRI device. We used a 192 x 256 matrix. The spine as well as the posterior mediastinum were accurately visualized on all examinations. As shown in Figures 5.18 and 5.19, sagittal and coronal images are most valuable in demonstrating the relationship of a mediastinal mass to the spine and spinal canal. This may be explained by the fact that in the transverse plane the spine has a relatively small caliber when compared to the size of the body and that the main axis of the spine lies within the longitudinal plane. The metastatic process in Figure 5.18 was due to spread from an adrenal tumor. Anterior extension of the process in the direction of the aortic wall was clearly shown on sagittal images (Figure 5.18B), while invasion of the spine and spinal cord as well as the large left-sided paraverte-

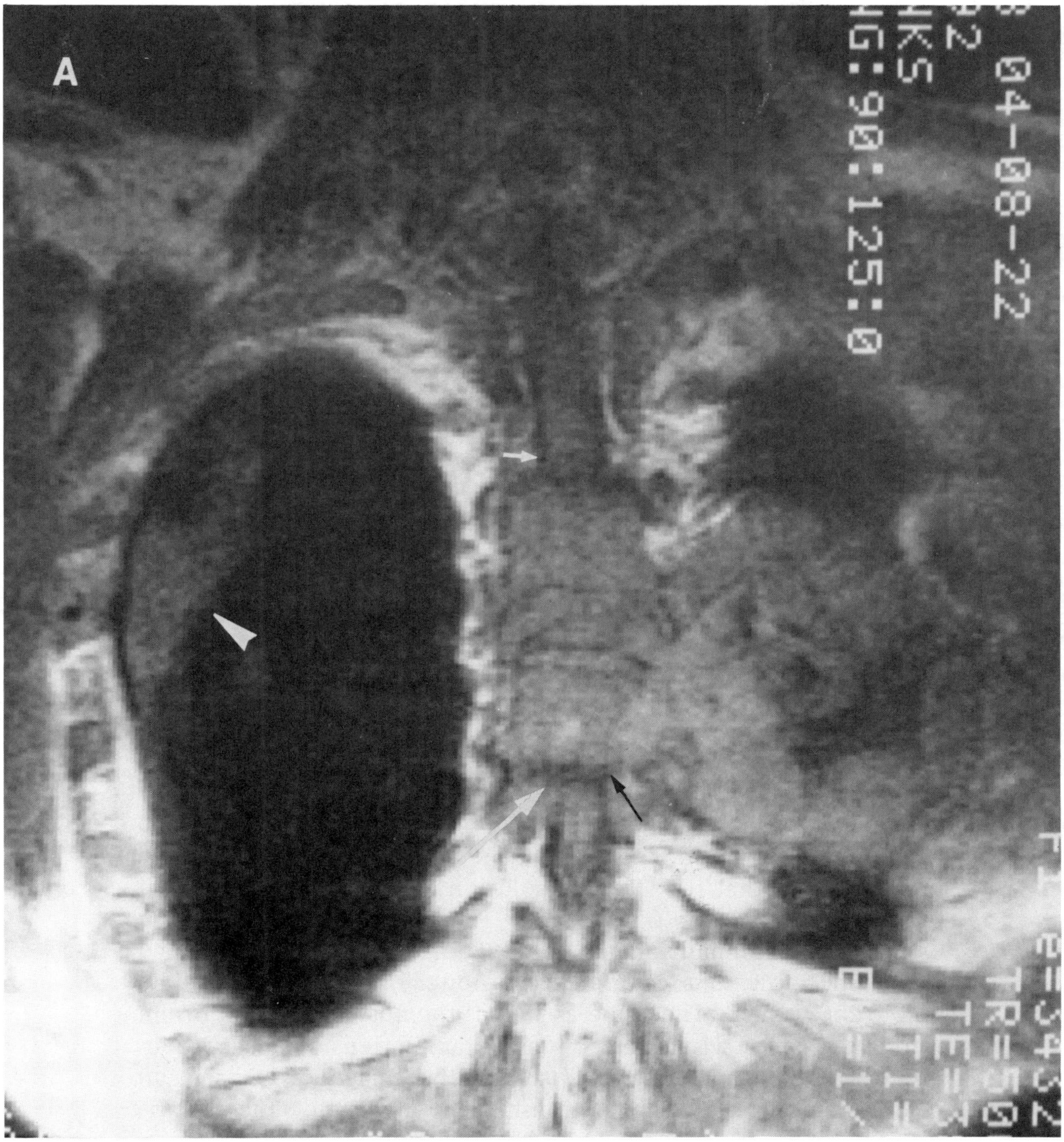

Figure 5.18 (A,B). Metastatic spread to the thoracic spine from adrenal tumor. Malignant infiltration of vertebral bodies together with compression of the cord (arrows) well outlined. Large mass located in the left paravertebral gutter. Arrowhead points to edge artifacts induced by the surface coil (A). Sagittal image demonstrates gross tumor mass extending towards the posterior aortic wall (B). Mass outlined as structure having intermediate signal intensity.

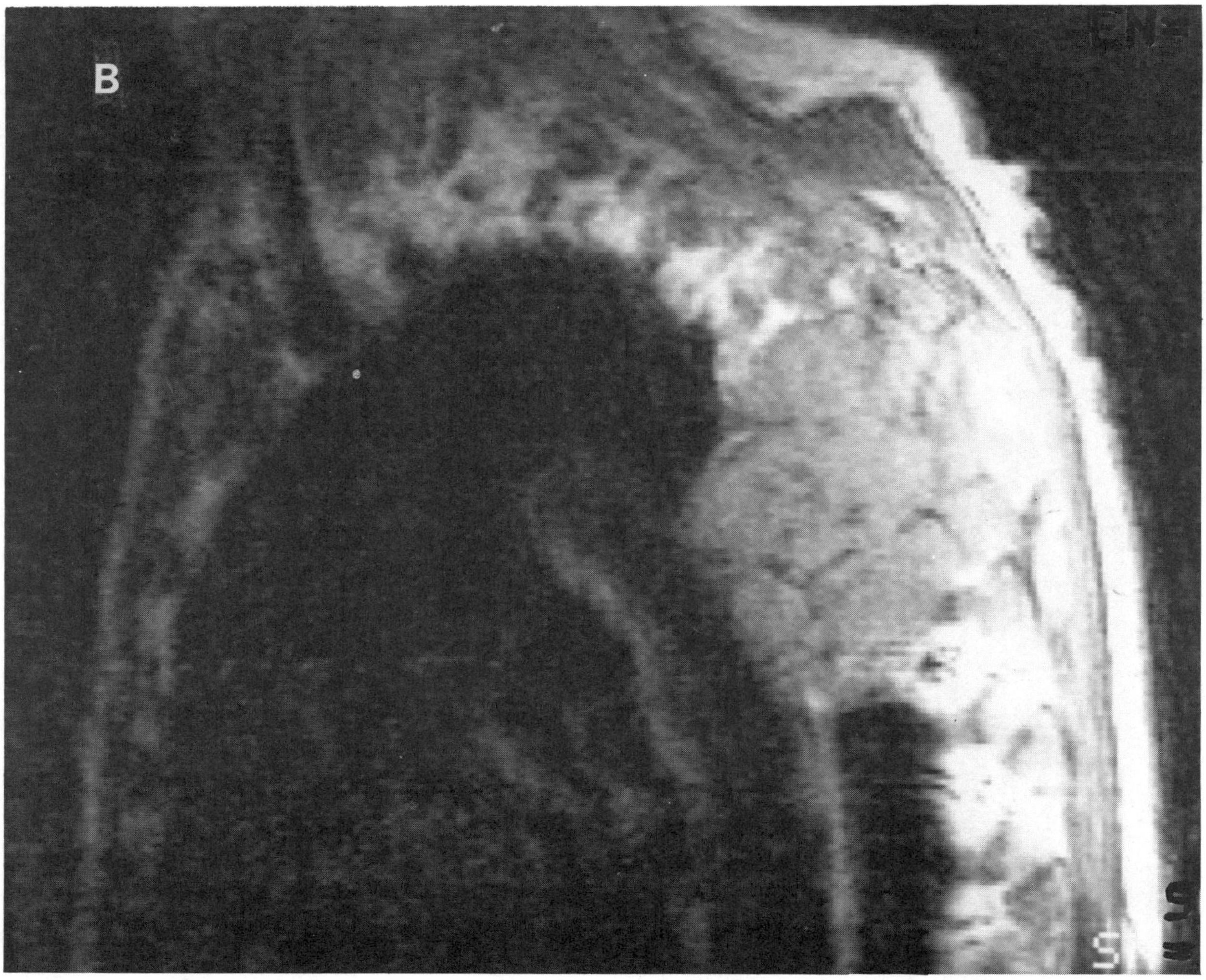

bral mass were mainly demonstrated on coronal images (Figure 5.18 A). The major disadvantage of using surface coils in the study of the thorax is due to the fact that they induce quite important artifacts on the edge of the image which could easily be misdiagnosed as an intraparenchymal tumor. These artifacts may result from a nonuniform RF field.

In Figure 5.19 C, a malignant lesion of the apex of the left lung was seen invading the upper thoracic spine with outgrowth towards the right side as obvious paravertebral thickening was present. Sagittal MR images clearly showed the malignant destruction of two vertebral bodies with definite compression of the thoracic cord (Figure 5.19 A,B). Transaxial MR images used to be less useful in these cases. The images contained per slice generated less information and the relationship between the metastatic process and the spine was not so well appreciated than on the coronal and sagittal images.

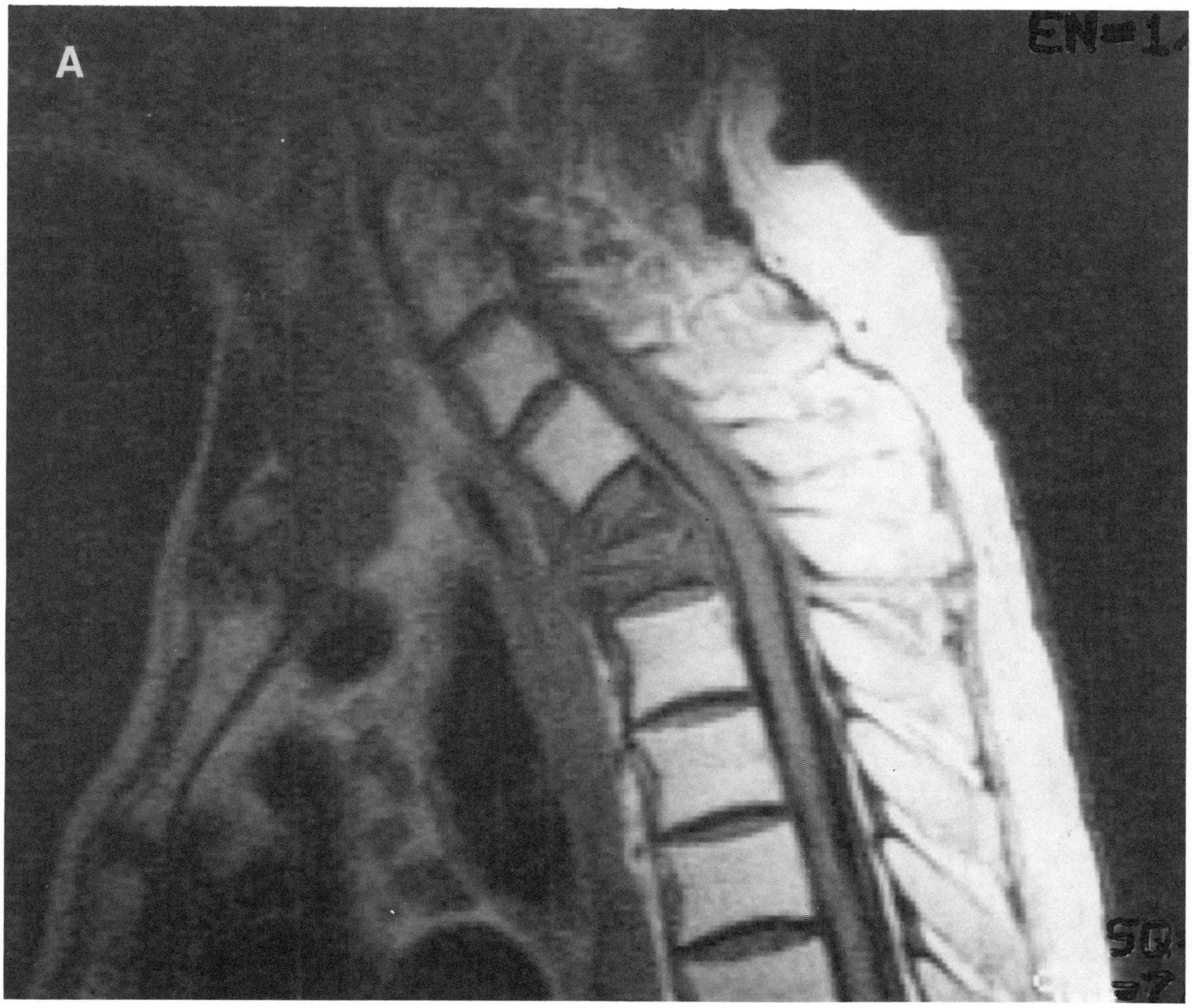

Figure 5.19 (A,B,C). Surface coil images using a 192 x 256 matrix, four data acquisitions and a 0.5 cm slice thickness. Neoplastic destruction of two vertebral bodies with some compression of the thoracic cord shown on sagittal MR image (A). Sagittal images through the left paravertebral area showed a large mass above and posteriorly to the aorta, there was no obvious compression or infiltration of the aortic wall (B). Coronal images show large intraparenchymal process in the upper lobe of the left lung invading the spine. Note paravertebral thickening on the right side (arrow) and important edge artifacts (C).

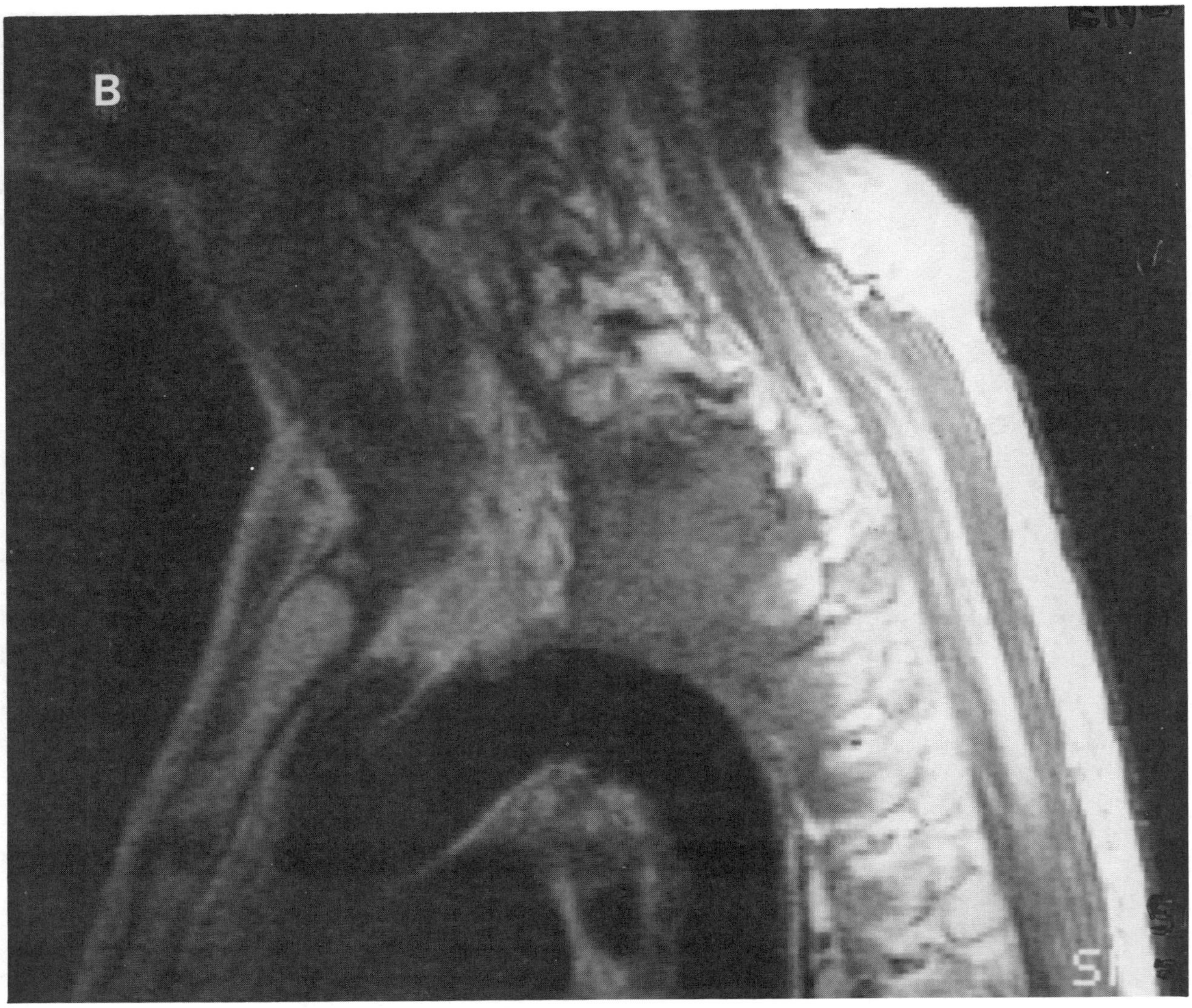
B

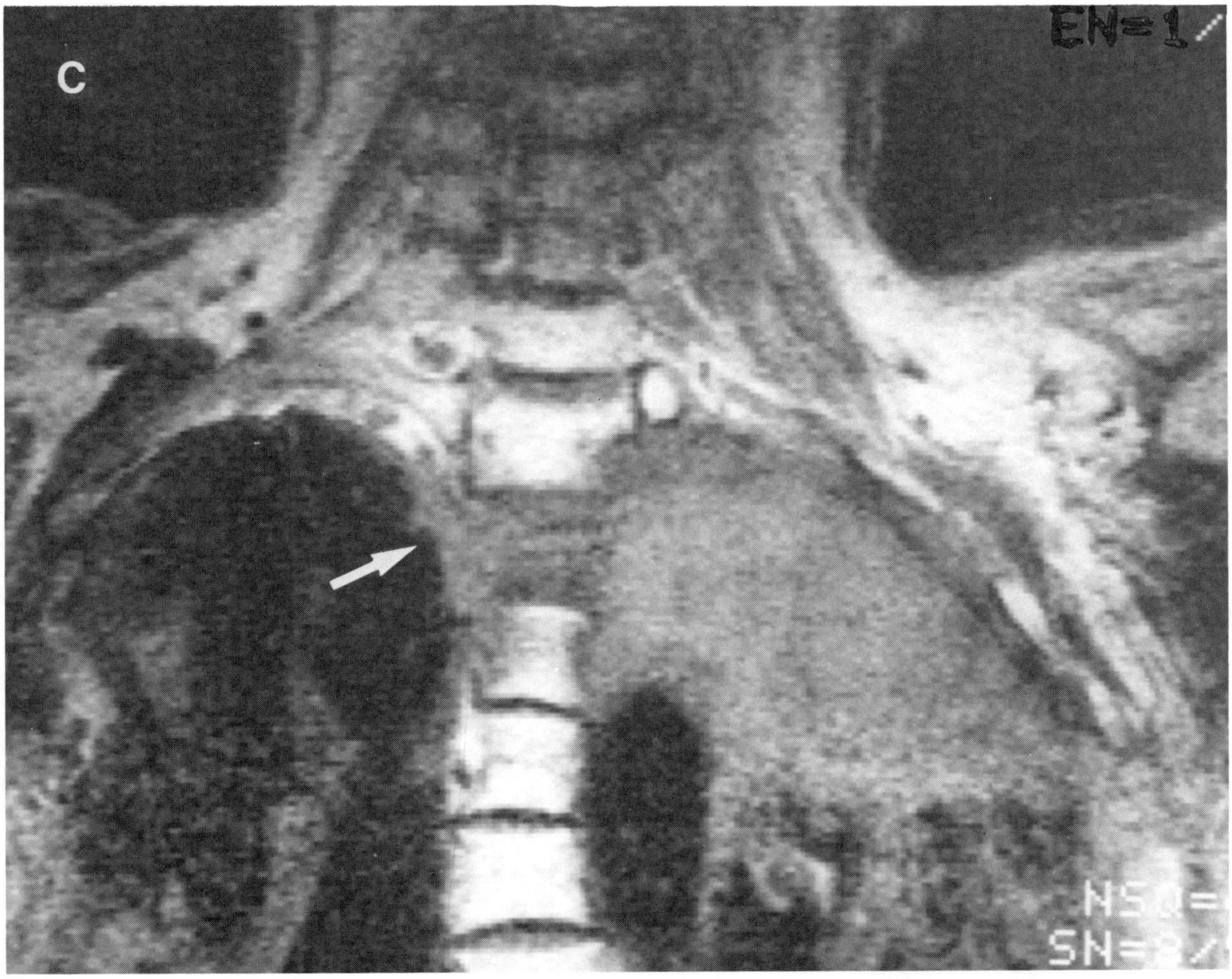

MRI OF THE MEDIASTINUM FOLLOWING PNEUMONECTOMY

Following pneumonectomy complete obliteration of the post-pneumonectomy space due to fluid collection occurs. In about 40% of the patients, the obliteration is caused by relocated mediastinal structures, the heart and great vessels rotating or shifting towards the affected side. It is a major diagnostic problem to identify tumor recurrences within the fluid filled post-pneumonectomy space. Tumor recurrences may also occur as enlarged lymph nodes in the mediastinum, which may only be separated with great difficulty from the distorted and displaced great vessels and heart.

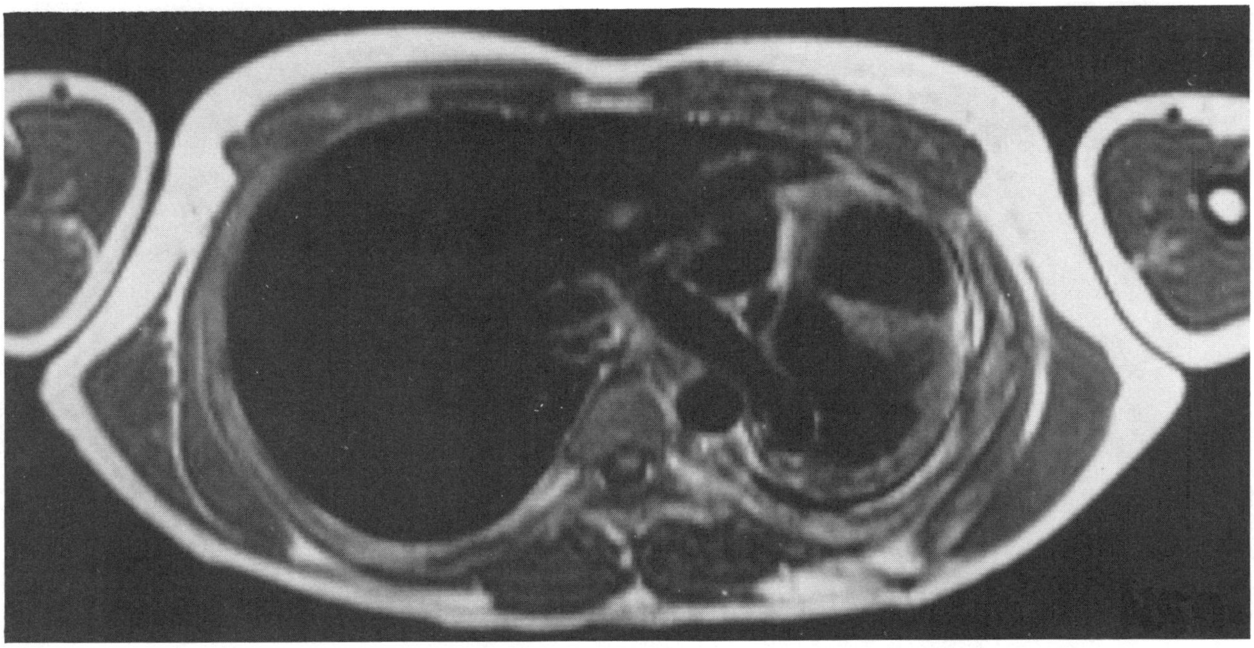

Figure 5.20. Transverse MR image with cardiac gating in a post-pneumonectomy patient shows complete shifting and rotation of the cardiovascular structures towards the left. Note that all the vascular compartments can be well individualized.

On conventional x-ray films, the post-pneumonectomy hemithorax is entirely opaque and recurrent disease cannot be detected unless it is so advanced that mediastinal shift occurs. Computed tomography provides a relatively useful diagnostic tool to recognize recurrent tumors at a much earlier stage as it allows cross-sectional imaging of the thorax. MRI is an additional and important diagnostic technique complementing the capabilities of CT scanning in this area. The main advantage of MRI over CT resides in the fact that the broncho-vascular structures are visualized with superb detail so that more subtle changes may be recognized on MRI slices (Figure 5.20). Frequent post-operative complications such as formation of intravascular emboli or empyema may readily be shown by MRI. The main bronchus stump may be very well visualized by MR images, mainly on coronal sections (Figure 5.21), which allows detection of tumor recurrence around the bronchus stump at a relatively early stage. It is hoped that MRI will provide a significant improvement in the diagnostic work-up of post-operative complications as well as in the early detection of tumor recurrency.

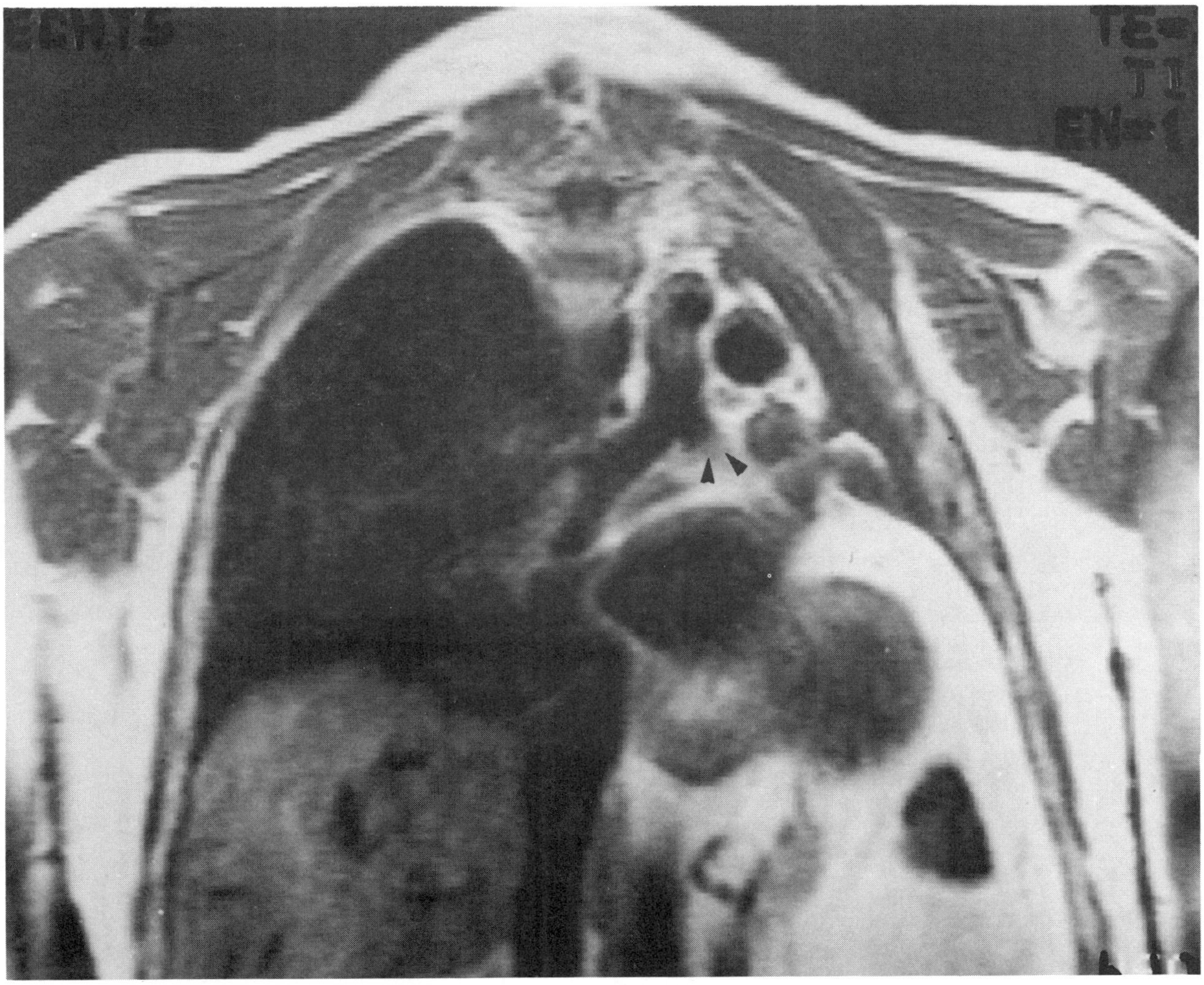

Figure 5.21. Coronal MRI section shows cardiovascular shift towards the left and elevation of the left hemidiaphragm. Left bronchus stump clearly visualized, no tumor could be seen within the surrounding fatty tissue (arrowhead).

CONCLUSIONS

Recognition of normal and abnormal mediastinal anatomy is possible with MR imaging and CT scanning. The major problem with both imaging modalities remains in the fact that abnormal morphological findings cannot be translated into histopathology. Distinction between benign and malignant disease on the basis of the imaged anatomy is not possible by MRI. Tissue characterization using T_1 and T_2 measurements remains unreliable on the present state of the art MRI machines due to the overlap of T_1 and T_2 relaxation time values in various pathological conditions. Due to long examination times, the inherent spatial resolution of MRI units still remains inferior to the spatial resolution of CT scans. This loss of spatial resolution is nevertheless partially compensated by the very high soft tissue contrast provided by MRI in the study of the mediastinum. Delineation of vessels from solid mediastinal masses and lymphadenopathy can be achieved without the need of intravenous contrast material. For this reason, we believe that MRI is able to play a major role in the TNM staging of bronchogenic carcinoma as well as in the early detection of postoperative complications. By the comparative study of T_1 and T_2 weighted MR images some indications as to the nature of mass lesions may be derived. Tumor recurrency may be recognized at an earlier stage using MRI due to its inherent high contrast sensitivity and to the three-dimensional imaging technique. An additional disadvantage of MRI was the lack of demonstrating calcifications within mediastinal masses which may be helpful in the differential diagnosis. Although there clearly remains a need to assess further the relative merit of MR imaging in the study of mediastinal pathology on larger patient populations, it can be stated that MRI adds an important diagnostic tool to the diagnostic work-up of mediastinal pathology.

REFERENCES

1. Webb WR: Magnetic resonance imaging of the chest. In: *Magnetic Resonance Annual 1986*, Kressel HY (Ed.). New York: Raven Press, 1986.

2. Epstein DM, Kressel H, Gefter H, Axel L, Thickman D, Aronchick J, Miller W: MR imaging of the mediastinum: a retrospective comparison with computed tomography. *J Comput Assist Tomogr*, *8:*670-676, 1984.

3. Fraser RG, Paré JAP: *Diagnosis of Diseases of the Chest.* Philadelphia: W.B. Saunders Co., 1979.

4. Heitzman ER: *The Mediastinum.* Radiologic correlations with anatomy and pathology. St. Louis: C.V. Mosby Co., 1977.

5. Schinz HR, Baensch WE, Frommhold W, Glauner R, Uehlinger E, Wellauer J: *Lehrbuch der Röntgendiagnostik*, Vol 4(2). Stuttgart: Georg Thieme Verlag, 1973.

6. Warnick R. Williams PL: *Gray's Anatomy*, 35th ed. Philadelphia: W.B. Saunders, Co., 1973.

7. Aronberg DJ, Glazer HS, Sagel SS: MRI and CT of the mediastinum: comparisons, controversies, and pitfalls. *Radiol Clin N Am*, *23:*439-448, 1985.

8. Gamsu G, Stark DD, Webb WR, Moore EH, Sheldon PE: Magnetic resonance imaging of benign mediastinal masses. *Radiology*, *151:*709-713, 1984.

9. Kundel HL, Kressel HY, Epstein DM: The potential role of NMR imaging in thorax disease. *Radiol Clin N Am*, *21:*801-808, 1983.

10. Sperber M: Mediastinal and hilar abnormalities. In: *Computerized Tomography of the Lung - Normal Anatomy and Most Common Disorders*, Sperber M (Ed.). New York: Futura Publishing Co., 1984.

11. McKurdo KK, de Geer G, Webb WR, Gamsu G: Normal and occluded mediastinal veins: MR imaging. *Radiology*, *159:*33-38, 1986.

12. Mills CM, Brant-Zawadzki M, Crooks LE, Kaufman L, Sheldon P, Norman D, Bank W, Newton TH: Nuclear magnetic resonance: principles of blood flow imaging. *AJNR*, *4:*1161-1166, 1983.

13. Walter E, Hübner KH: Computertomographische Charakteristika raumfordernder Prozesse im vorderen Mediastinum und ihre Differentialdiagnose. *Fortschr Rontgenstr*, *133:*391-400, 1980.

14. Sagel SS, Aronberg DJ: Thoracic anatomy and mediastinum. In: *Computed Body Tomography*, Lee JK, Sagel SS, Stanley RJ (Eds.). New York: Raven Press, 1983.

15. Dooms GC, Hricak H, Moseley ME, Bottles K, Fisher M, Higgins CB: Characterization of lymphadenopathy by magnetic resonance relaxation times: preliminary results. *Radiology*, *155:*691-697, 1985.

16. Heelan RT, Martini N, Westcott J, *et al.*: Carcinomatous involvement of the hilum and mediastinum: computed tomographic and magnetic resonance evaluation. *Radiology*, *156:*111-115, 1985.

17. Davies PL, Kaufman L, Crooks LE: Tissue characterization. In: *Clinical Magnetic Resonance Imaging*, Margulis AR, Higgins CB, Kaufman L, Crooks LE (Eds.). San Francisco: UCSF Radiology Research and Education Foundation, 1983.

18. Webb WR, Moore EH: Differentiation of volume averaging and mass on magnetic resonance images of the mediastinum. *Radiology*, *155:*413-416, 1985.

19. Johnston DL, Liu P, Wismer GL, *et al.*: Magnetic resonance imaging: present and future applications. *Can Med Asst J*, *132:*765-777, 1985.

20. Levitt RG, Glazer HS, Roper CL, Lee JKT, Murphy, WA: Magnetic resonance imaging of mediastinal and hilar masses: comparison with CT. *AJR*, *145:*9-14, 1985.

21. Edelman RR, Shoukimas GM, Stark DD, *et al.*: High-resolution surface coil imaging of lumbar disk disease. *AJNR*, *6:*479-485, 1985.

Notes

6

Hilar Abnormalities

Consecutive transaxial MR sections through the thorax allow the visualization of hilar components in a manner which is similar to CT scans. However, some significant differences exist between the spatial resolution of the two modalities and, as a result, the ability to visualize pathological changes varies from modality to modality.

In general, the diagnostic criteria which have been proposed for the interpretation of CT sections of pulmonary hila are applicable also in the study of MR images. These include the finding of a localized or generalized abnormal hilar contour, identification of discrete hilar masses, obstruction or displacement of the bronchi, and obstruction of vascular shadows.

In normal subjects, hilar structures routinely identified on spin-echo MR images are the vessels and the bronchi whose walls are emitting a similar signal. Their distinction may pose a problem when hilar transverse anatomy is not fully understood. In addition to that, the nature of hilar soft tissues which give an intermediate signal intensity is often difficult to ascertain.

Depending on the centering of the scan series and the number of MR scans performed, various hilar levels are visualized: the right upper lobe bronchus (sometimes with its anterior and posterior segmental branches); the trunchus anterior; the intermediate bronchus; the right middle lobe bronchus and parts of the basal segmental bronchi and vessels; as well as similar structures on the left, including the left upper and lower lobe bronchi and the left main pulmonary artery (Figure 3.3 to 3.7).

When it comes to identifying pathological changes in the hilar area, plain chest radiographs are of limited use. Hilar nodes can only be visualized when they are enlarged, and in many cases glandular enlargement has to be substantial before it can be recognized. For that reason, conventional tomography, including the 55 posterior oblique projections, has been considered for many years the procedure of choice to accurately localize hilar lymph nodes in relation to vessels and bronchi and assess the effects of glandular enlargement on adjacent structures (7).

The advent of computed tomography has added substantial data to the information obtained from conventional radiographic studies (8, 9). However, on CT scans of the pulmonary hila, differentiation between an abnormal soft tissue mass and normal vasculature is usually required. This is often achieved by the administration of a large bolus of contrast which results in vascular opacification. In some cases, however, a reliable distinction between a mass and a vascular structure is not possible using contrast-enhanced CT.

Studies which compared the efficacy of MRI versus CT in the evaluation of the pulmonary hilum (1-4) have clearly shown the superiority of MRI in diagnosing a hilar mass in cases in which administration of contrast during the CT study was not possible or proved to be inefficient. In addition, several reports mentioned small hilar lesions which were not convincingly visualized on CT scans, but which were detected while using MR imaging.

Unless roentgenograms of the chest made at an earlier date are available for comparison, the evaluation of enlargement of the pulmonary hilum is usually difficult. In fact, MRI is called to participate in the solving of one of the most common diagnostic dilemmas encountered in daily practice — the study of an enlarged or questionably prominent hilum and the differentiation between enlarged hilar lymph nodes, a prominent central pulmonary artery and a tumoral mass.

Due to the lack of signal from the air in the bronchial tree and flowing blood in pulmonary arteries and veins, magnetic resonance imaging, rather than CT, seems to provide more accuracy in the study of the close relationship that exists between visible bronchi, pulmonary artery branches and hilar lymph nodes.

A problem arises however on spin-echo MR images when small collections of soft tissue are visible at various hilar levels. Webb and colleagues (3) have warned against the confusion of these collections with enlarged nodes (more than 1 cm in diameter). Three specific locations have been mentioned: 1) at the bifurcation of the right pulmonary artery, 2) at the origin of the middle lobe bronchus, and 3) on the left, at the level of the left upper lobe bronchus (Figure 6.1). Collections of soft tissues can be identified also in several other hilar locations. They seem to remain in the limits of 3-5 mm and even if they represent lymph nodes, they can be considered to be of normal size.

Although inherent cardiac and respiratory movements in most patients do impair the spatial resolution of MR images of the hilum, satisfactory studies can be performed without cardiac or respiratory gating, while patients are requested to breathe lightly and avoid motion. Still, cardiac gating gives the best results in the evaluation of abnormalities located in the cardiac vicinity.

Lungs are low intensity signal structures on MRI, therefore, pathological changes in the lungs usually appear as high signal intensity areas within various gradations of grey-white levels. This

Figure 6.1 A. The bronchus intermedius (BI) is visible on the right, with the right pulmonary artery (A) anterior to it. A soft tissue collection (arrows) is visible lateral to the right pulmonary artery and anterior and lateral to the bronchus. On the left, the upper portion of the left upper lobe bronchus (UL) is visible with the left superior pulmonary vein (V) anteriorly and the descending pulmonary artery (A) posteriorly.

Figure 6.1 (A,B,C) used with permission from reference 3.

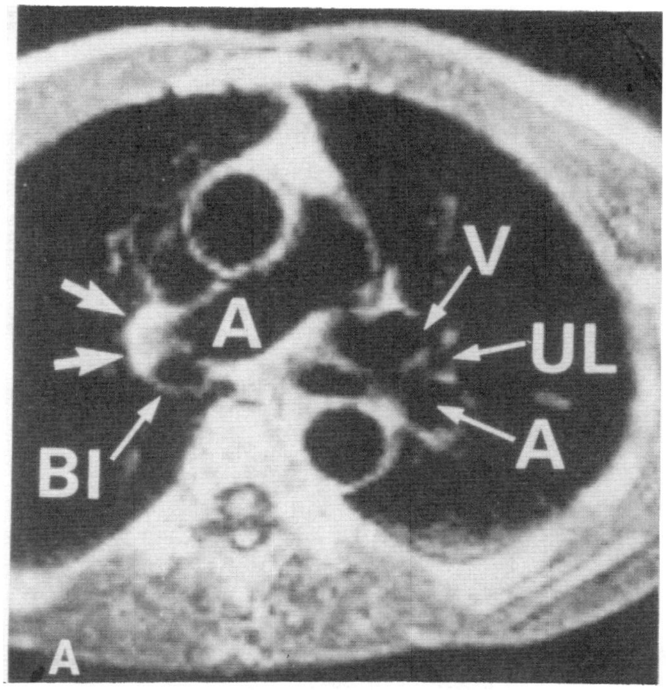

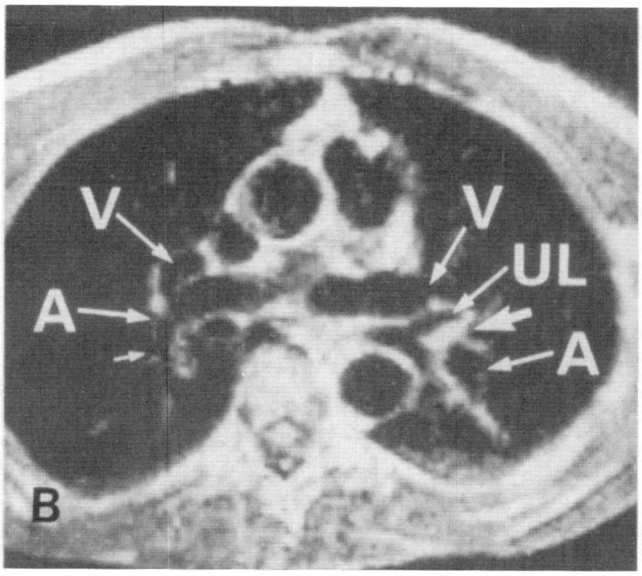

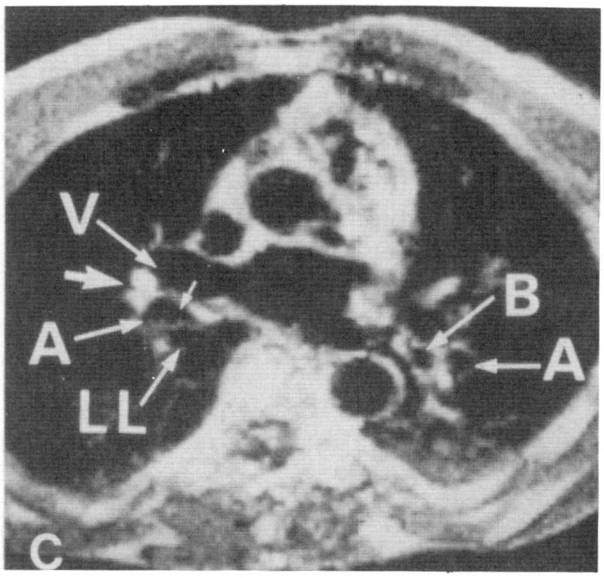

Figure 6.1 B. The right descending pulmonary artery (A) passes anteriorly and laterally to the bronchus intermedius and gives rise to arterial branches supplying the superior segment of the lower lobe (small arrow). A right superior pulmonary vein branch (V) occupies the anterior hilum. On the left, the lower portion of the left upper lobe bronchus (UL) is clearly seen with the superior pulmonary vein (V) anterior to it. A normal layer of tissue (arrow) separates the upper lobe bronchus and the descending pulmonary artery (A), incompletely seen in this patient.

Figure 6.1 C. The right middle lobe bronchus anteriorly (small arrow), the lower lobe bronchus (LL) posteriorly, and the descending pulmonary artery (A) laterally cannot be clearly distinguished. A tissue collection (large arrow) occupies the lateral hilum, in relation to the middle lobe bronchus and pulmonary artery. The superior pulmonary vein (V) is anterior. On the left, the lower lobe bronchus (B) pulmonary artery (A), and small amounts of soft tissue are visible.

explains why in the study of pulmonary pathology it is important to use T_2 weighted images with long TR values (e.g., TR 1500, TE 30) because of the improved signal to noise ratio and the relatively increased signal intensity of most masses. T_2 weighted images are also of value in differentiating higher intensity parenchymal consolidation from lower intensity centrally located lesions.

In the mediastinum, T_1 weighted images with a short TR (e.g., TR 500, TE 30) are usually sufficient because the relatively low signal intensity lesions can easily be separated from the high signal intensity mediastinal fat. This type of spin-echo imaging will provide the best contrast between a hilar mass and the adjacent mediastinal fat and will also allow the best visualization of its mediastinal extension (Figure 6.2). However, as spin-echo images obtained with a long TR seem to provide the best spatial resolution and those obtained with short TR the best constrast, in some cases it may be necessary to use pulse sequences with both long and short TRs in order to fulfill these requirements.

The anatomic proximity of the mediastinum has a great impact on the pulmonary hila. Numerous pathological processes concomitantly involve both structures, for example, a mediastinal lymphomatous mass will frequently be associated with the presence of enlarged hilar lymph nodes. In fact, most of the causes of hilar lymphadenopathy are the same as for mediastinal lymph node enlargement. Symmetrical adenopathy usually suggests the presence of sarcoidosis, and asymmetrical disease is frequently a sign of malignant lymphoma, metastatic disease or inflammatory changes.

→

Figure 6.2. A, B, C, and D. Spin echo MR images taken at various thoracic levels and performed while using a T_1-weighted pulse sequence (TR 300 or 500 msec, TE 30 or 32 msec) provide a significant difference in signal intensity between the high signal intensity normal mediastinal or hilar fat (white arrows) and intermediate signal intensity abnormal soft tissue hilar and mediastinal masses.

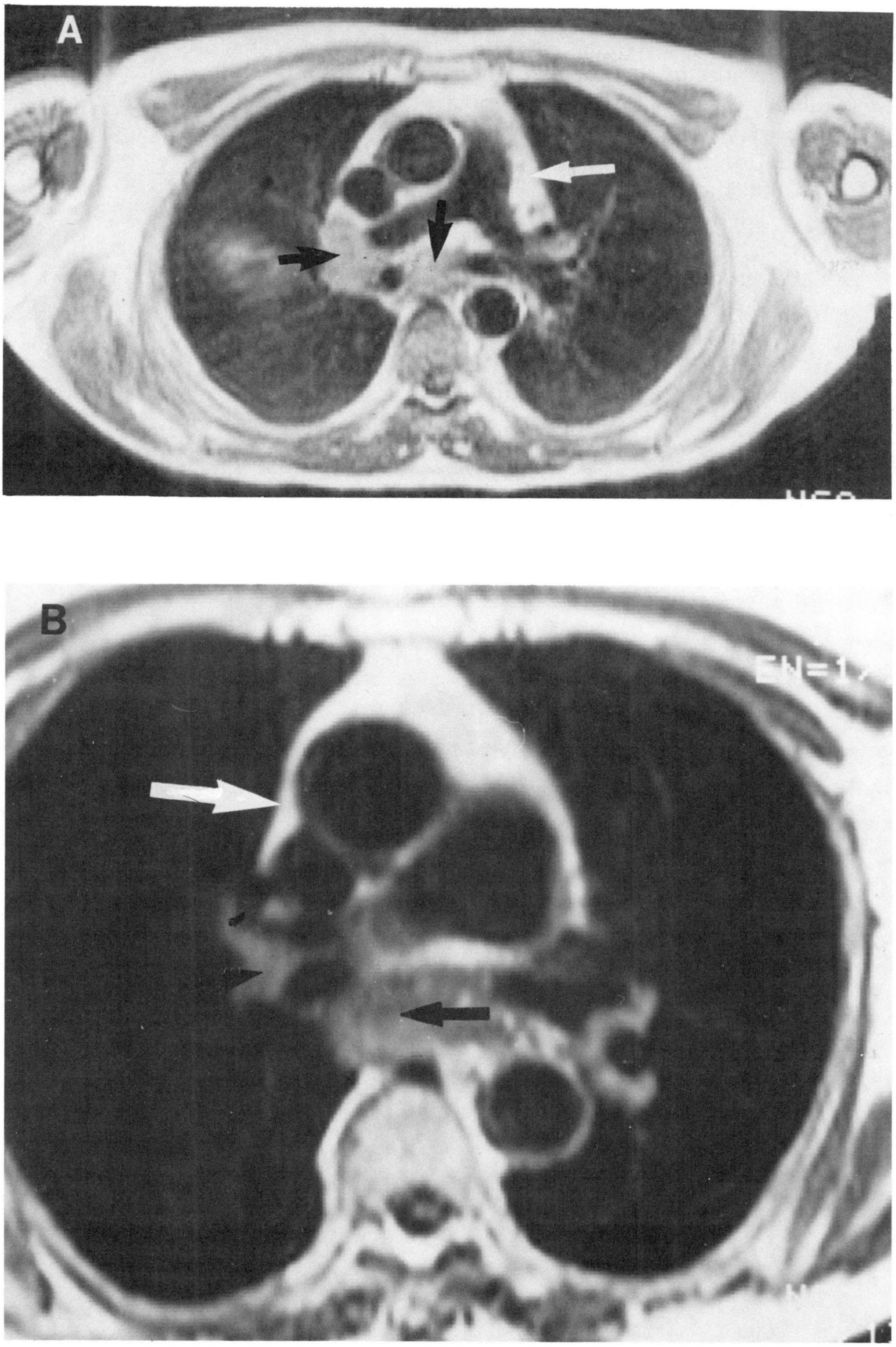
A
B

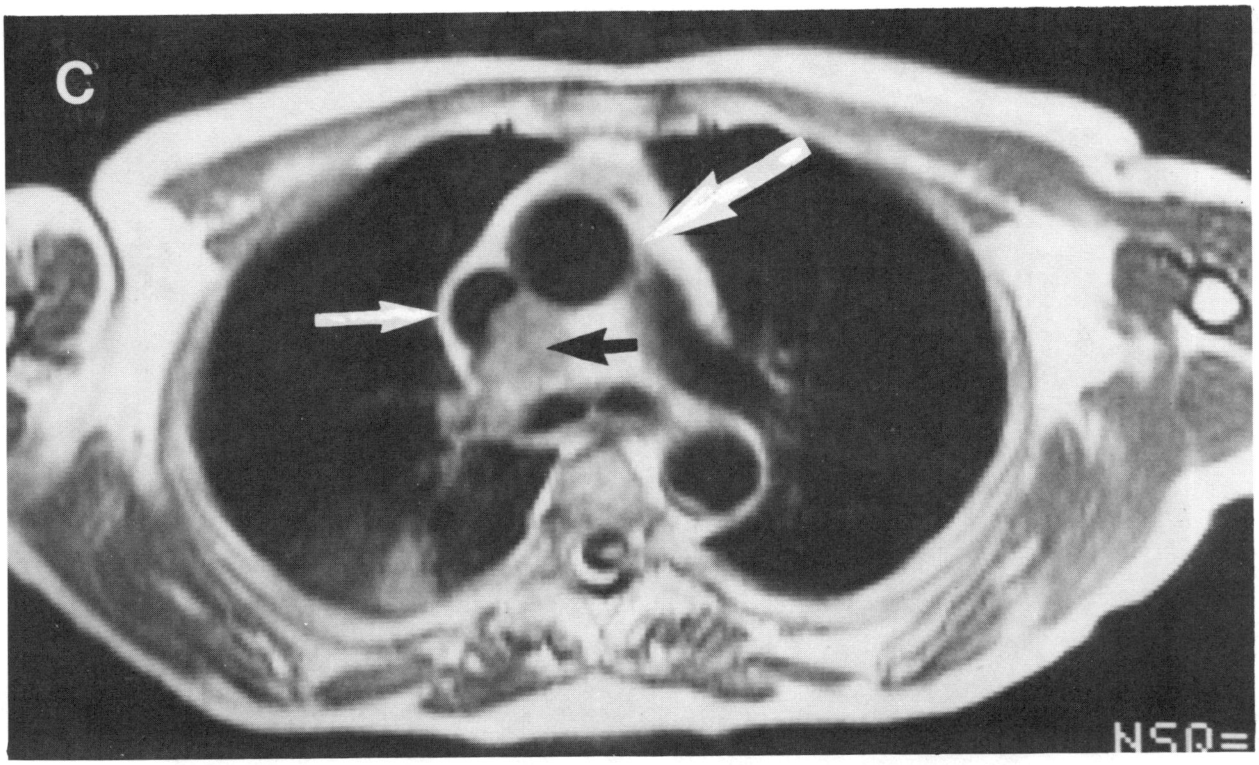
C
NSQ=

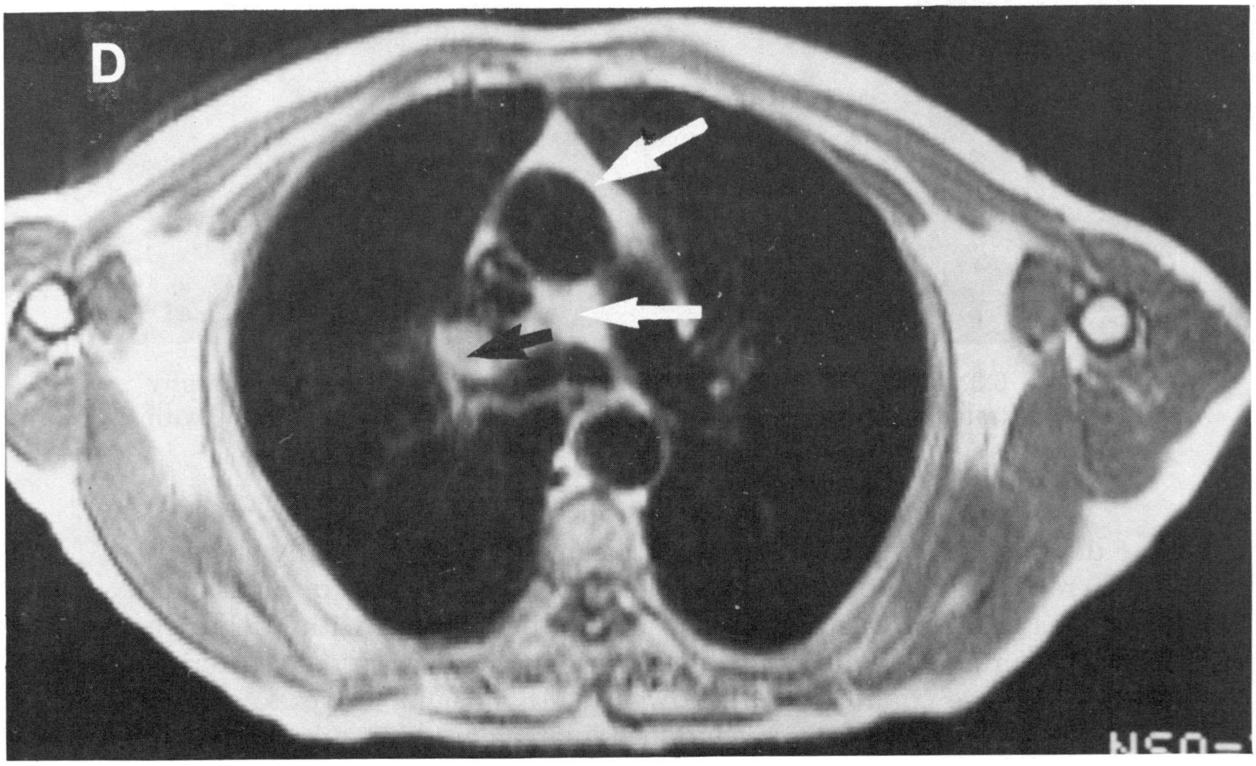
D

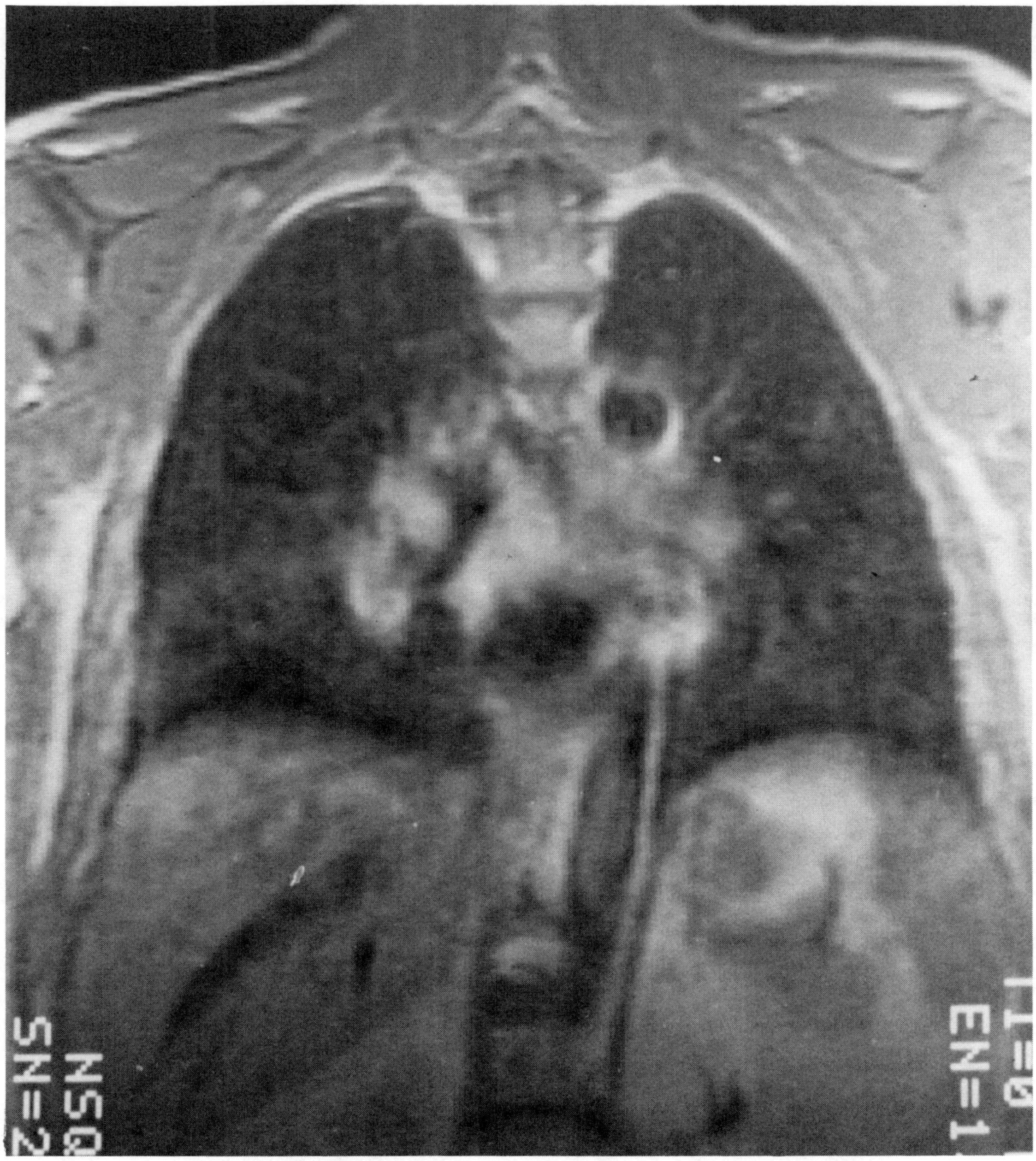

Figure 6.3. Prominent hilar and mediastinal glandular enlargement clearly demonstrated on coronal spin-echo MR image (500/30), in a patient with sarcoidosis.

Enlargement and calcification are major signs of lymphadenopathy. Lymph node calcification which is commonly encountered in granulomatous disorders of the lungs, in occupational disease, or in fungus infections cannot be detected with MRI since calcium gives no MR signal. When performed in patients suffering from these conditions (3), however, MR imaging proves to clearly visualize the extent of glandular enlargement and its relation to the adjacent vascular structures and bronchi (Figure 6.3).

Bronchogenic carcinoma presenting as a hilar lesion will usually appear as an irregular, ill-defined mass. The use of sagittal and coronal views in MR imaging of the chest permits the visualization of longer segments of intrapulmonary bronchi and therefore bronchial narrowing present in patients with lung cancer is commonly demonstrated with MRI (Figures 6.4, 6.5, and 6.6).

It has been mentioned that in MR images of the thorax in normal subjects, the major bronchi are usually well visualized (the right and left main bronchi, the right and left upper lobe bronchi and bronchus intermedius). Small bronchi are not well seen with MRI and it seems that CT, with its better spatial resolution, is superior to MRI in this area.

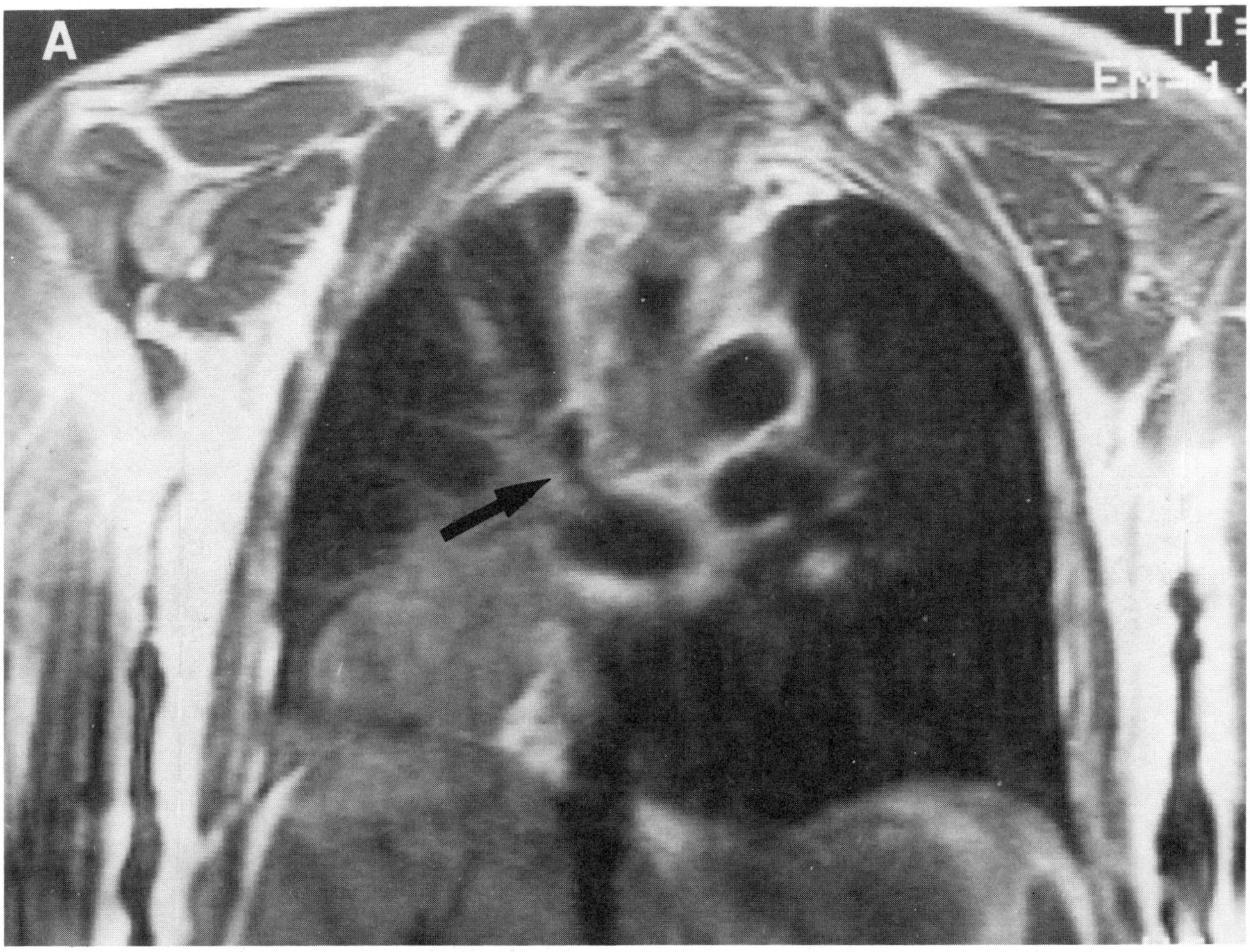

Figure 6.4 (A,B,C). Advanced bronchogenic carcinoma demonstrated on several MRI coronal cuts to prominently invade the right hilar and mediastinal areas and obstruct major bronchial and vascular structures (arrows).

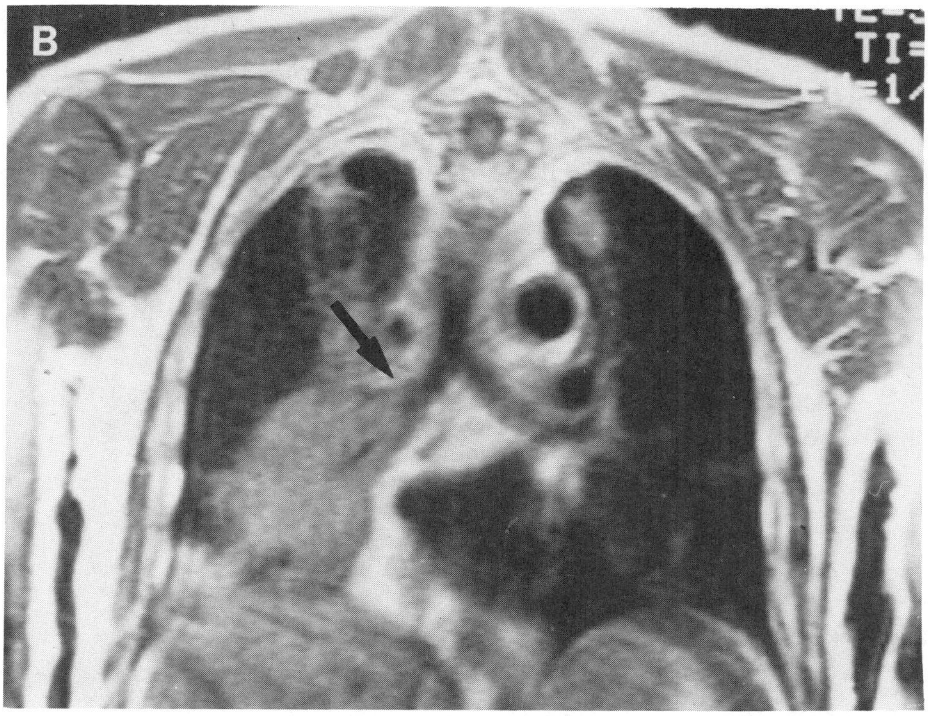
B
TI=

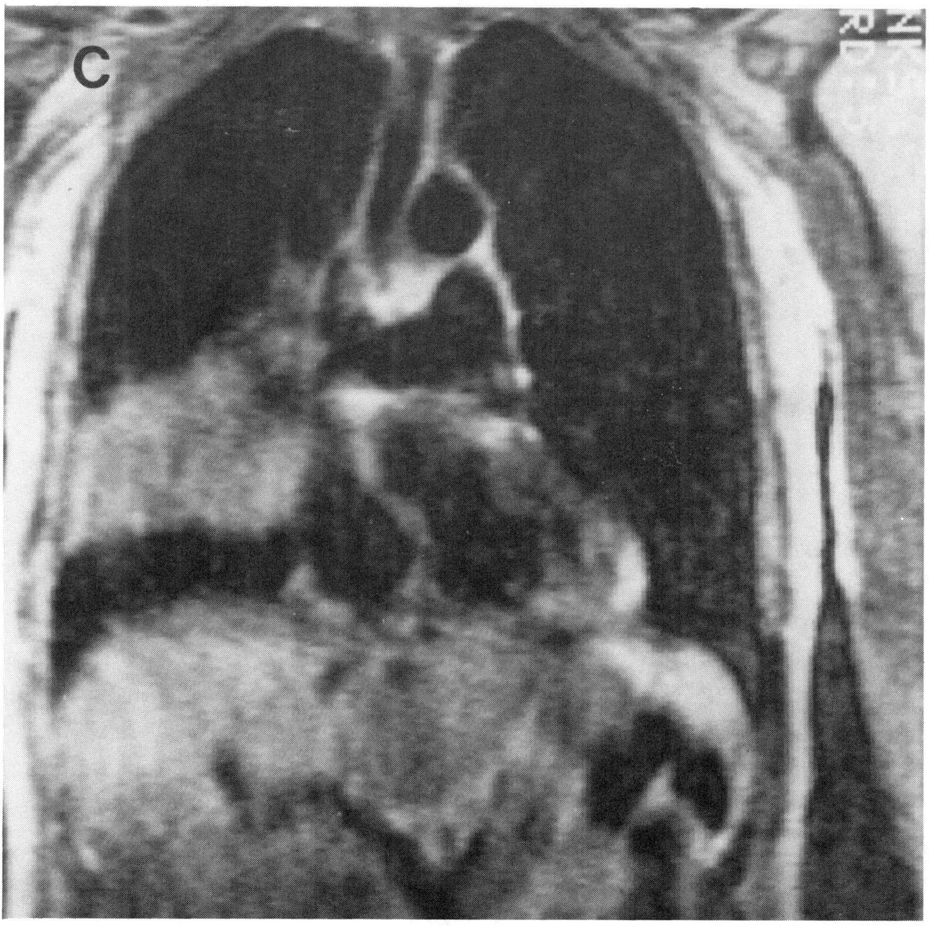
C

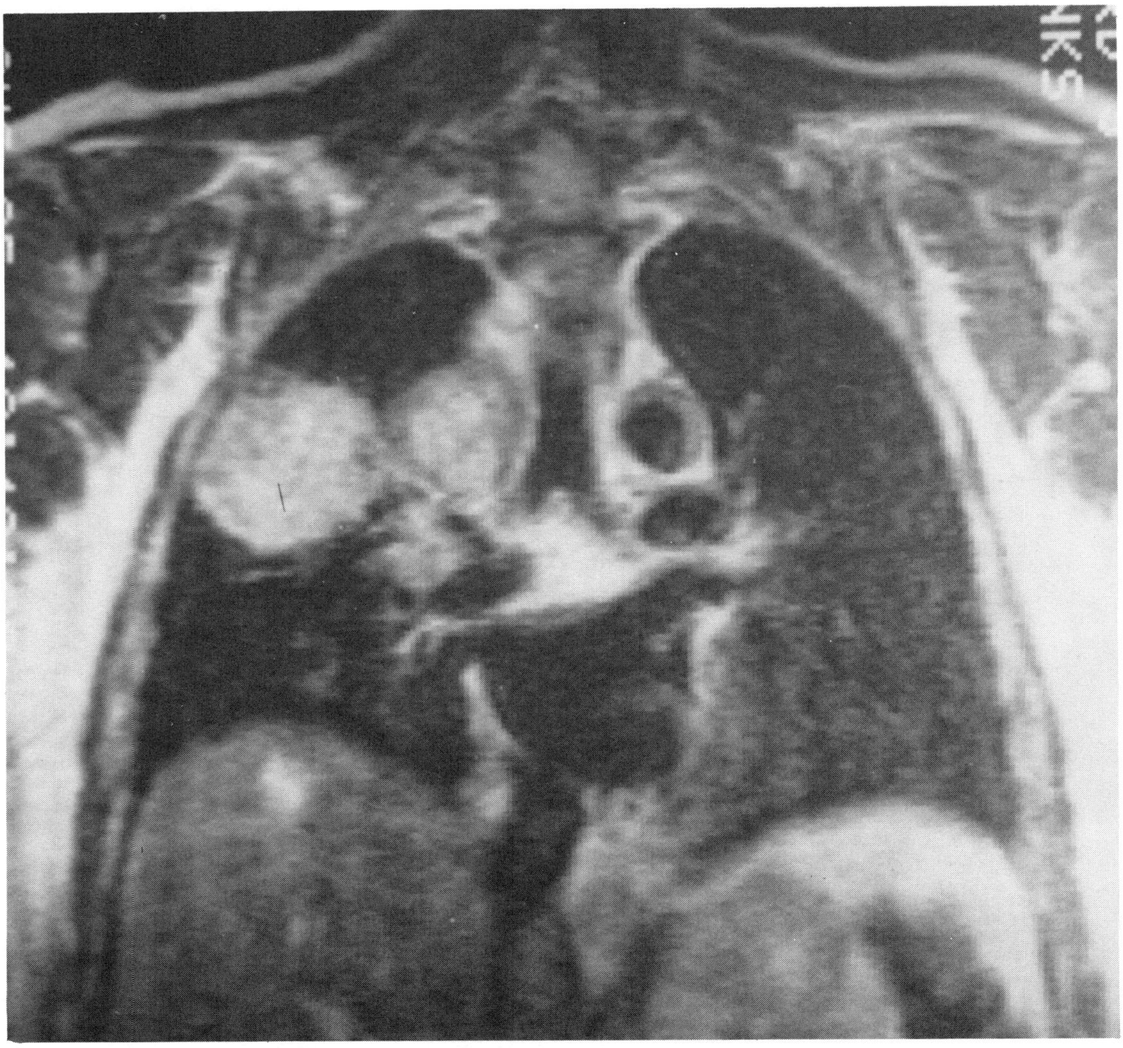

Figure 6.5. Large cell, well differentiated pulmonary carcinoma with mediastinal and hilar metastases, clearly visualized on spin-echo images (500/32).

Several other pitfalls in MRI evaluation of the hilum were identified when examining patients with bronchogenic carcinoma. The major problem was the inability of MRI to detect scattered calcifications in enlarged lymph nodes due to 1) old granulomatous disease, and 2) the lack of distinction between small adjacent lymph glands which may appear as single enlarged masses due to the limited spatial resolution of MR images (10). The same study has found MRI and CT comparable in their results in five of eleven cases with other mediastinal and hilar lesions, except for bronchogenic carcinoma (including Hodgkin's disease) and granulomatous infections.

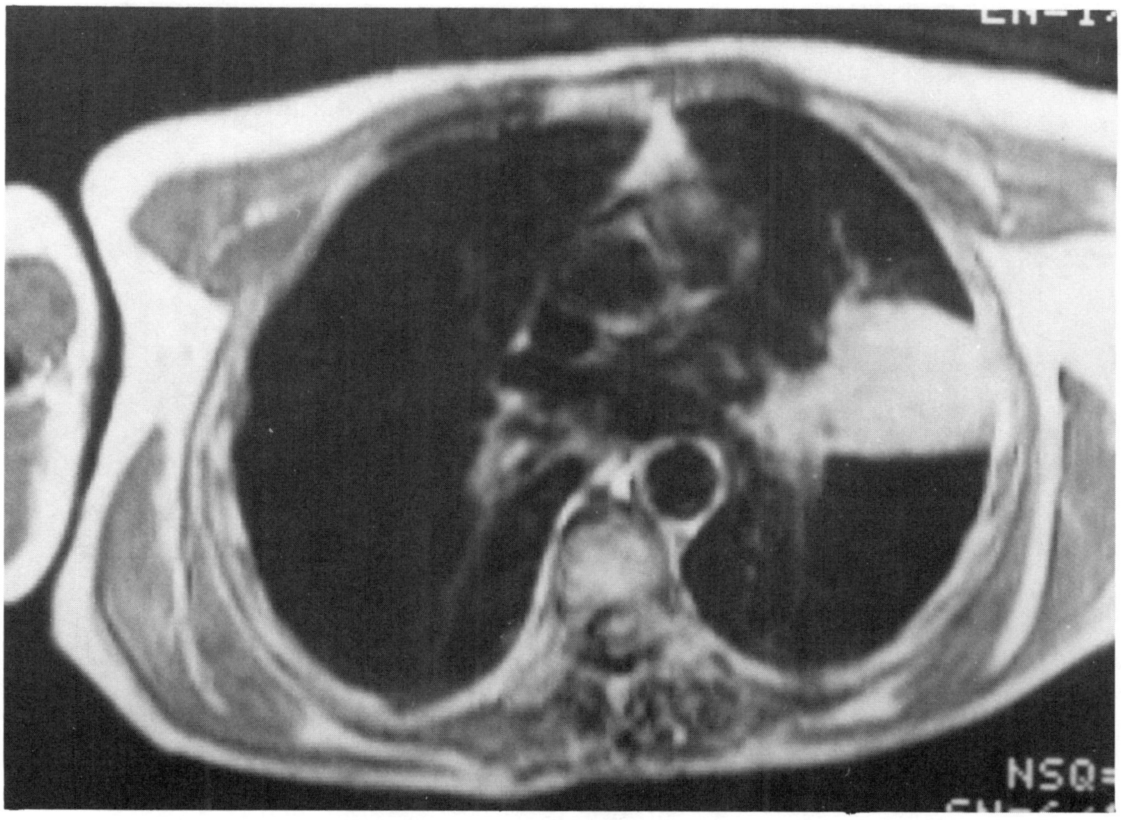

Figure 6.6. Bronchogenic carcinoma shown as a high signal intensity area on TR 1000 msec, TE 32 msec MR image, with the clear demonstration of left mediastinal and hilar invasion.

In a study by Glazer, *et al.* (11), the pulmonary hilum has been prospectively evaluated in 35 patients with lung cancer, using magnetic resonance imaging, dynamic computed tomography and 55° posterior oblique tomography. For the identification of hilar adenopathy, the authors used criteria suggested by previous investigations (3) which include recognition of enlarged hilar lymph nodes as regions of increased signal density larger than 10 mm in diameter. Results of the study basically emphasize the lack of specificy of dynamic CT and MRI which are both able to routinely detect nodes of 10 mm or more in diameter, while oblique tomography can visualize much larger nodes (exceeding 20 mm in diameter). No significant differences were demonstrated between the three imaging modalities in the overall accuracy of hilar evaluation (Table 6.1).

TABLE 1
COMPARATIVE RADIOLOGIC DATA FOR ASSESSMENT OF HILAR METASTASIS IN LUNG CANCER

	55° Oblique Tomography	*Imaging Method* *Dynamic CT*	*MRI*
No. of patients	19	19	19
False positive	3	5	5
False negative	2	1	0
True positive	7	8	9
True negative	7	5	5
Sensitivity	7/9(78%)	8/9(89%)	9/9(100%)
Specificity	7/10(70%)	5/10(50%)	5/10(50%)
Accuracy	14/19(74%)	13/19(68%)	14/19(74%)

(From Ref. 11, with permission)

The excellent contrast resolution offered by MRI raised the hope that this new imaging modality would be able to specifically characterize diseases within lymph nodes and differentiate between benign and malignant processes.

Calculated magnetic resonance relaxation times, T_1 and T_2, derived either from spectroscopy data (5) or MR images (5, 10) failed to allow recognition of specific processes based on these MRI parameters. Comparison of measurements obtained from enlarged lymph nodes present in a large variety of pathological conditions including inflammation, tuberculosis, sarcoidosis and non specific enlargement, the same as lymphoma and metastatic carcinoma, showed a clear overlap of the T_1 and T_2 values between normal and malignant lymph nodes.

Some of the suggested reasons for this overlap seem to be related to the great variations in the water content of lymph nodes, a factor on which T_1 and T_2 measurements are mostly dependent (5, 11). According to one report (5), spectroscopic analysis revealed T_1 and T_2 increased values of nodes involved by neoplasm compared to normal specimens and T_2 relaxation times which were greater for acute inflammatory nodes than for nodes involved by granulomatous disease or malignancy. Such findings could not be confirmed by other investigators and whether T_1 and T_2 relaxation times can provide reliable information for the specific characterization of lymphadenopathy remains uncertain.

REFERENCES

1. Cohen AM, Creviston S, Li Puma JP, *et al.*: NMR evaluation of hilar and mediastinal lymphadenopathy. *Radiology, 148:*737-742, 1983.

2. Cohen AM, Creviston S, Li Puma JP, *et al.*: Nuclear magnetic resonance imaging of the mediastinum and hili: Early impression of its efficacy. *AJR, 141:*1163-1169, 1983.

3. Webb WR, Gamsu G, Stark DD, Moore EH: Magnetic resonance imaging of the normal and abnormal pulmonary hila. *Radiology, 152:*89-94, 1984.

4. Gamsu G, Webb WR, Sheldon P, *et al.*: Nuclear magnetic resonance imaging of the thorax. *Radiology, 147:*473-480, 1983.

5. Dooms GC, Hricak H, Moseley ME, *et al.*: Characterization of lymphadenopathy by magnetic resonance relaxation times: Preliminary results. *Radiology, 155:*691-697, 1985.

6. Heelan RT, Martini N, Westcott JW, *et al.*: Carcinomatous involvement of the hilum and mediastinum: Computed tomographic and magnetic resonance evaluation. *Radiology, 156:*111-115, 1985.

7. Favez G, Willa C Heizer F: Posterior oblique tomography at an angle of 55 in chest roentgenology. *Am J Roentgenol Radium Ther Nucl Med, 120:* 907-915, 1974.

8. Shevland JE, Chiu LC, Shapiro RL, *et al.*: The role of conventional tomography and computed tomography in assessing the resectability of primary lung cancer. A preliminary report. *CT, 2:*1-10, 1978.

9. Mintzer RA, Malave SR, Neiman HL, *et al.*: Computed vs conventinal tomography in the evaluation of primary and secondary pulmonary neoplasms. *Radiology, 132:*653-659, 1979.

10. Levitt RG, Glazer HS, Roper CL, *et al.*: Magnetic resonance imaging of mediastinal and hilar masses: Comparison with CT. *AJR, 145:*9-14, 1985.

11. Glazer GM, Gross BH, Aisen AM, *et al.*: Imaging of the pulmonary hilum: A prospective comparative study in patients with lung cancer. *AJR, 145:*245-248, 1985.

Notes

7

Pulmonary Nodules Including Bronchogenic Carcinoma

The pulmonary nodule is a common presentation of lung cancer, the same as benign pulmonary lesions. Its radiological evaluation is, in most cases, a challenging process which includes the performing of multiple radiological investigations with the goal of establishing non-histological criteria for benignity or malignancy.

Qualitative characteristics of the discovered lesion such as size, shape, appearance of borders, homogeneity and amount or distribution of calcifications are taken into consideration on radiological images in an attempt to provide an accurate diagnosis and prevent unnecessary invasive procedures.

Serial conventional radiographs may allow one to follow and assess the various changes which a particular lesion undergoes over a period of time. Also, the use of low-kvp spot radiographs usually permit the visualization of calcification within a pulmonary nodule.

While the finding of centrally located, coarse calcifications practically determines the diagnosis of a benign process, the presence of asymmetrical, eccentric calcifications raises a high suspicion of a nodule being malignant (1, 2). In this case, conventional radiography should be supplemented by conventional or computed tomography (CT).

It has to be mentioned, however, that despite the extensive use of CT in the preoperative evaluation of solitary pulmonary nodules, the accuracy of CT quantitative measurements has been disappointing, as no universal values could be established for detection of calcifications in pulmonary nodules. Additionally, CT has been found to have several other limitations in the studies of thoracic masses, including its inability to establish whether a benign or malignant process is the primary cause for an area of pulmonary consolidation or atelectasis. Hilar pathology also seems to be better imaged by conventional tomography in the antero-posterior and 55° oblique positions.

With the advent of MRI, studies performed in order to establish its value in the detection of pulmonary nodules and the staging of bronchogenic carcinoma have compared the new modality with the previously existent techniques (6-12). Since the best treatment for bronchogenic carcinona in an asymptomatic patient remains the resection of localized tumor, MRI has been called to participate in the evaluation of patients with suspected lung cancer with the aim of obtaining a diagnosis and detecting metastatic dissemination, while assessing the patient's ability to undergo a pulmonary resection if necessary. The resectability of a primary lesion can accurately be evaluated with the use of MRI, by demonstrating the presence and location (or absence) of mediastinal node enlargement or by revealing direct invasion of intrathoracic structures.

In studies by Webb, Martini, and their respective groups, the value of magnetic resonance in the staging of bronchogenic carcinoma has been compared to that of conventional and computed tomography and the results correlated with pathological findings (8, 9, 11). In the study by Webb, *et al.* (8), in a series of 33 patients, MRI seemed to clearly demonstrate the presence of mediastinal lymph nodes, providing, however, information comparable to that obtained from CT scans. Both modalities classified nodes as being normal when smaller than 1.0 cm, suspicious when between 1.0-1.5 cm and abnormal when larger than 1.5 cm.

For the identification of mediastinal adenopathy by CT the use of contrast material injection is mandatory in order to enhance and identify vascular structures. On spin echo MR images, however, normal and abnormal mediastinal lymph nodes can be easily distinguished from surrounding tissues by their differences in T_1 relaxation time values. On MR images obtained with short TR values (ex. 0.5 msec), normal and abnormal lymph nodes appear to be less intense than fat and well separated from the low signal intensity vascular and bronchial lumen (Figure 7.1). Some diagnostic problems may arise on T_2 weighted images (TR 1.5-2.0 msec), when the intensity of the nodes increases and they may be more difficult to identify. Also, due to the poorer spatial resolution of MRI, discrete neighboring lymph nodes may appear on MR images as a large single and suspicious mass.

Although the authors have performed T_1 and T_2 value measurements, the same as in previous reports (13, 14, 15), no clear differences could be found between benign and malignant lesions where the measurements were concerned. Also, comparison between the MR characteristics of the primary pulmonary mass and the discovered lymphadenopathy did not permit the distinction between involved and uninvolved lymph nodes.

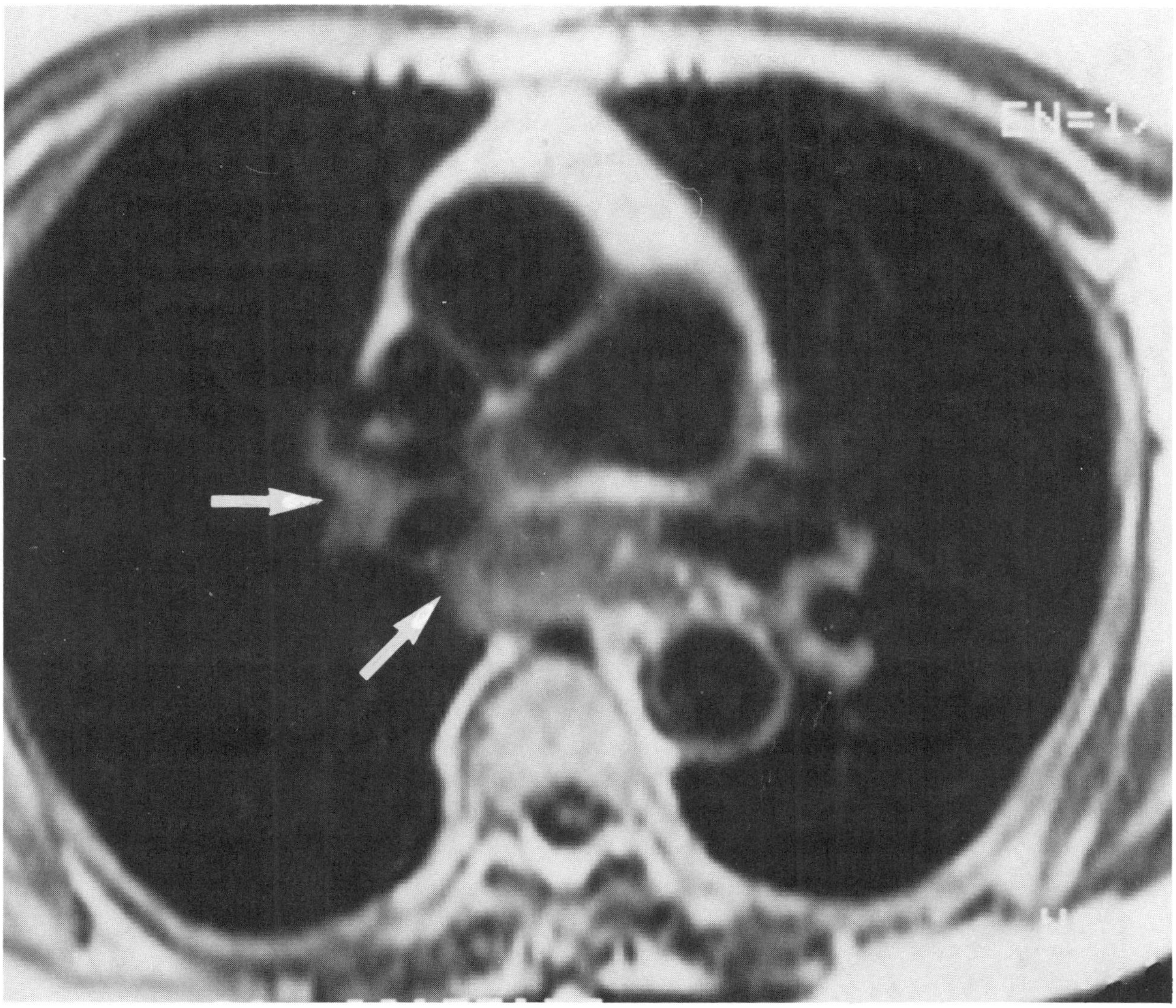

Figure 7.1. Intermediate signal intensity metastatic masses (arrows) are visible on this axial MR image of the thorax, in a patient with bronchogenic carcinoma (TR 500 msec, TE 30 msec), well separated from the vascular and bronchial structures.

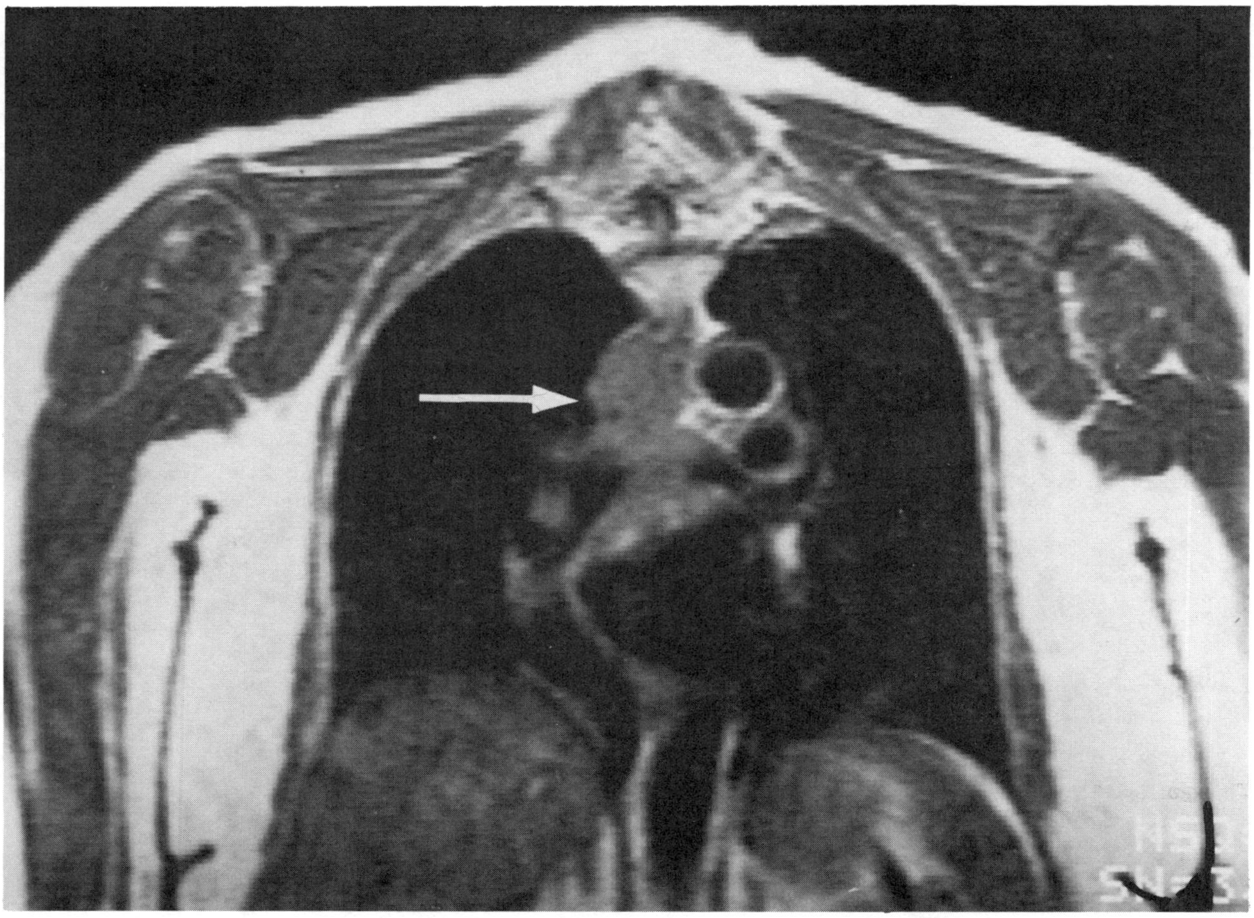

Figure 7.2. Extensive right metastatic mediastinal mass (arrow) clearly demonstrated on an MR image obtained with a short TR (600 msec) and a TE of 32 msec.

Our personal experience also demonstrates that MRI easily diagnoses tumoral extension to the mediastinum by clearly separating the intermediate signal intensity tumor from the low signal intensity vascular structures such as the superior vena cava or the pulmonary arteries and the high signal intensity fat (18) (Figures 7.2, 7.3, 7.4, 7.5).

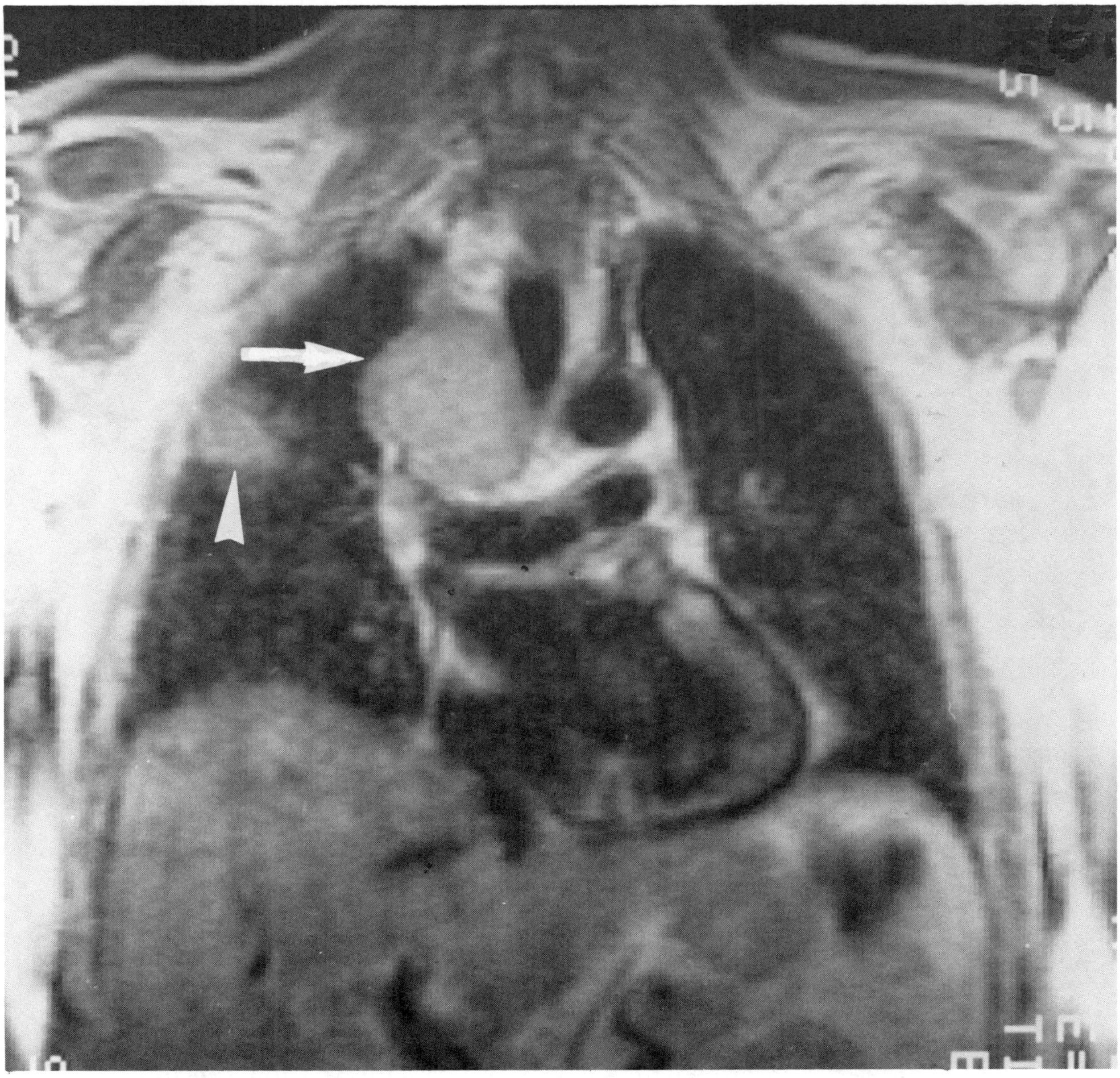

Figure 7.3. MR image obtained with a TR of 500 msec and a TE of 32 msec. Large metastatic lesion (arrow) from a primary bronchogenic carcinoma (arrow head), demonstrated in the area of the superior vena cava and producing the patient's superior vena cava syndrome.

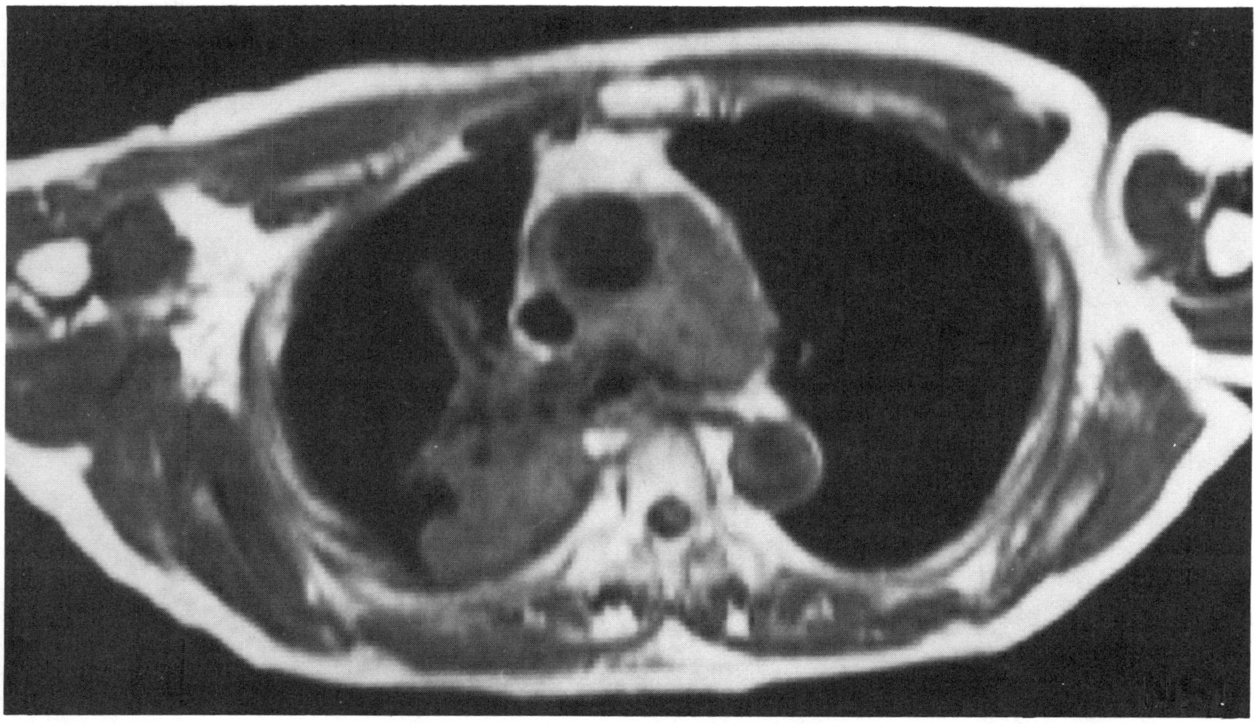

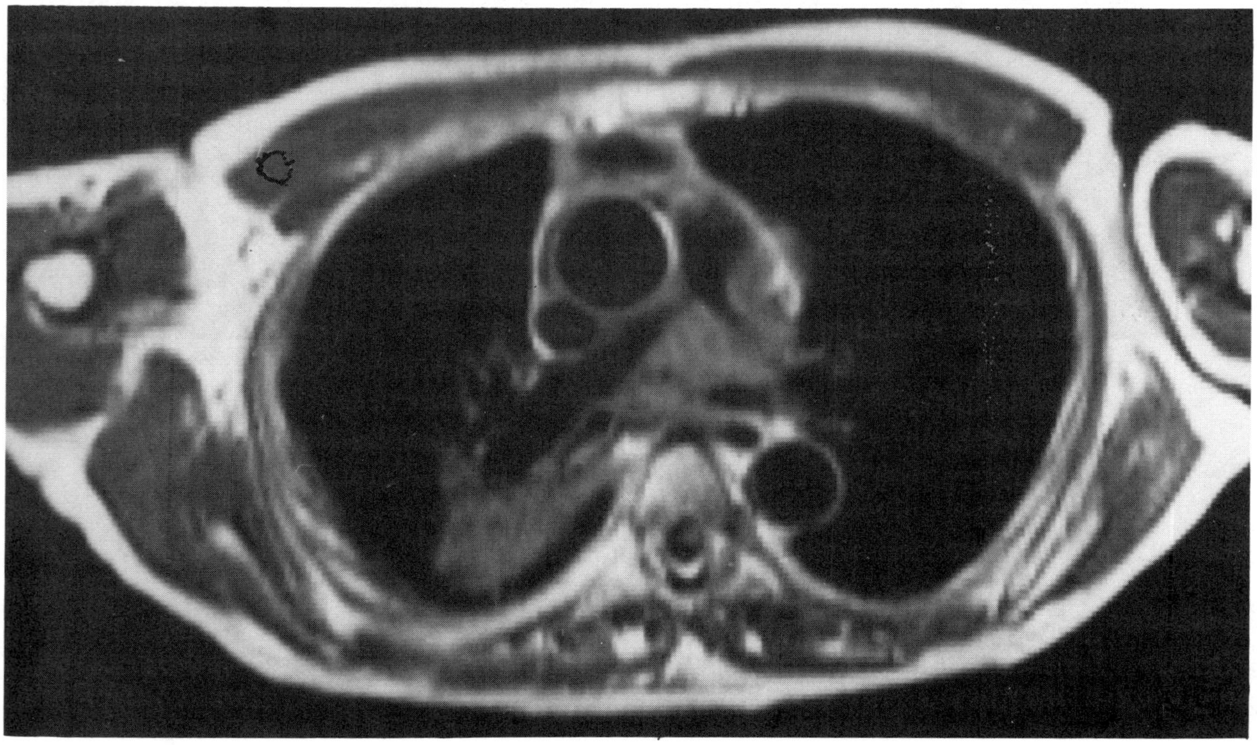

Figures 7.4 and 7.5. Prominent mediastinal involvement in a patient with bronchogenic carcinoma visualized as intermediate signal intensity masses on T_1 weighted images.

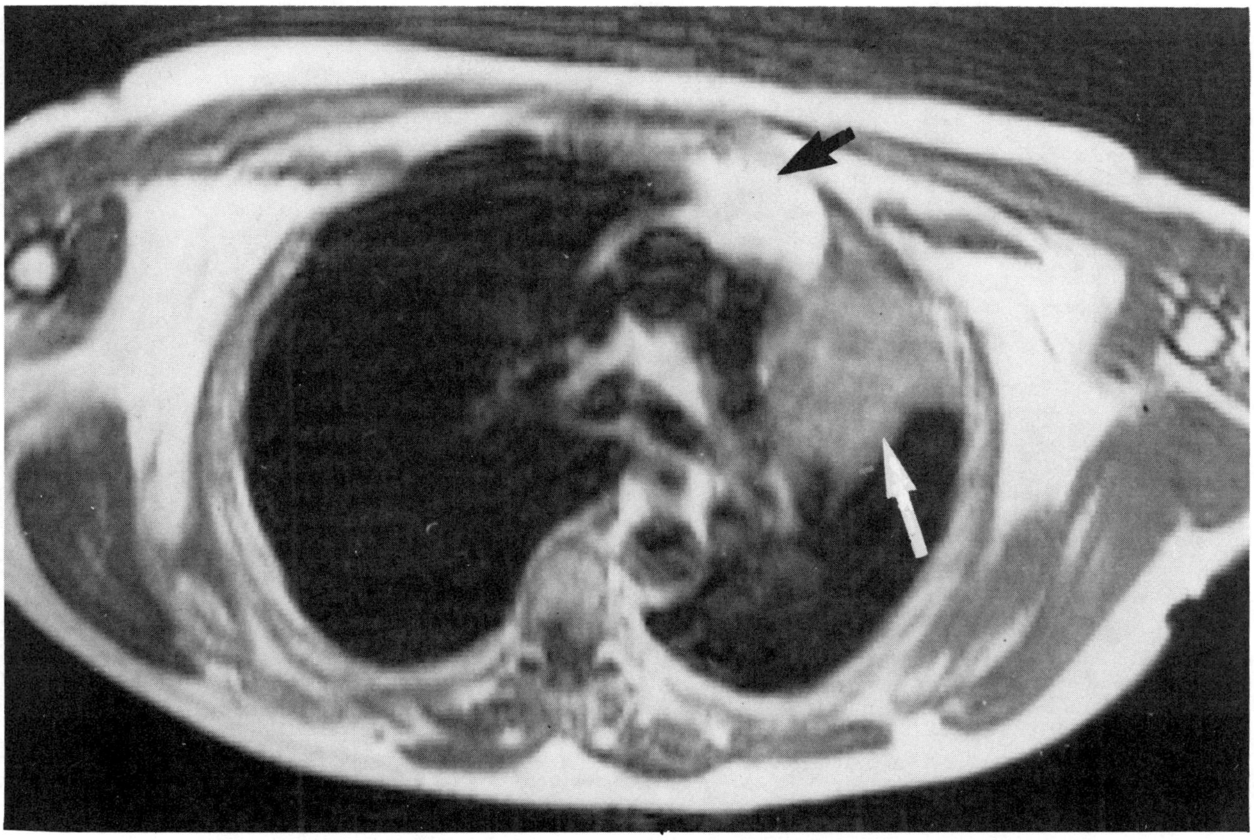

Figure 7.6. Left pulmonary mass with an atelectatic component (white arrow), clearly identified and separated from the mediastinal fat (black arrow) (TR 500 msec, TE 32 msec).

In a study by Martini, *et al.* (11), mediastinal lymph node dissection or sampling has been performed and correlated with preoperative studies in 34 patients with surgically confirmed carcinoma of the lung. Both CT and MRI have been found to be highly accurate in assessing the presence of mediastinal adenopathy with a sensitivity rate of 87%. Direct extension into the mediastinum adjacent to a pulmonary mass is easily distinguished from fat with MR when using short TR images (Figures 7.6, 7.7). However, in the above comparitive study neither CT nor MRI correlated well with surgical findings, when the sensitivity rate for CT was 55% and 64% for MR.

An additional important area to be evaluated as a criterion for operability of a primary lung lesion is the pulmonary hilum, when MRI is required to assist in the identification of hilar masses and bronchial abnormalities. In a study by Glazer, *et al.* (9), hilar adenopathy was diagnosed on MR images when a region of increased signal intensity was observed that was larger than 10 mm in diameter, as suggested in a previous report by Webb, *et al.*

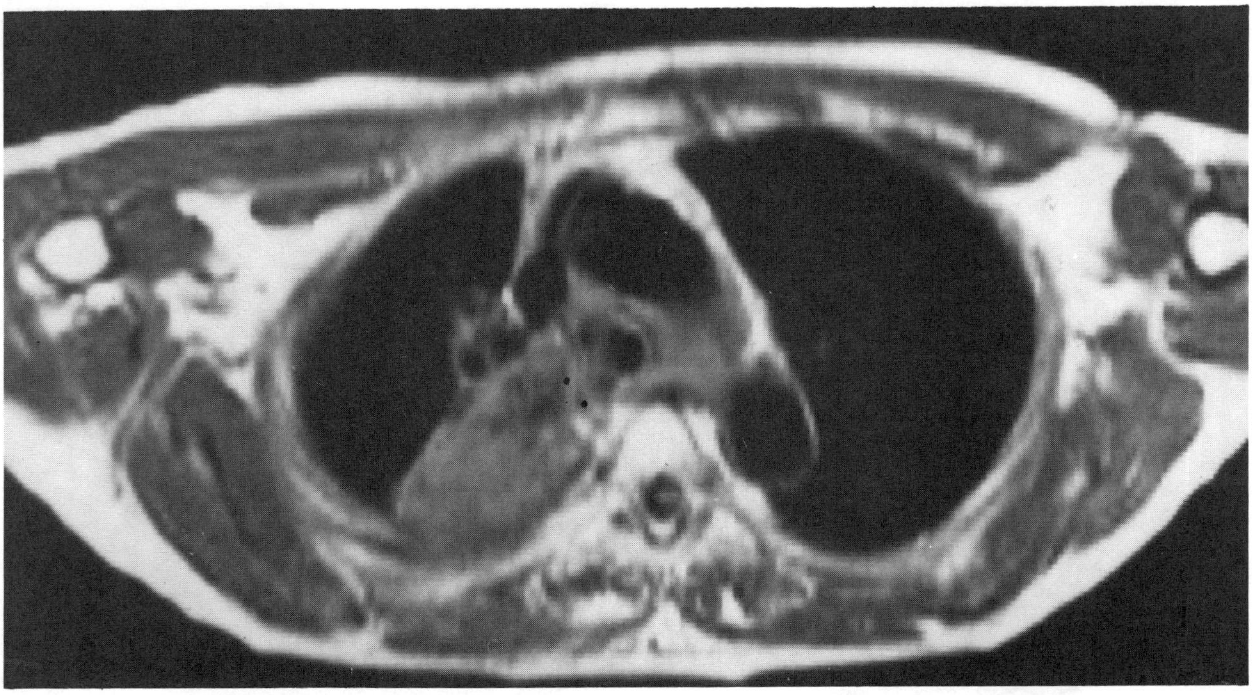

Figure 7.7. Direct mediastinal invasion from a right sided pulmonary mass well diagnosed on MR images taken with a short TR (500 msec).

(7). MR images were compared with dynamic CT and oblique tomography, when MRI and dynamic CT were found to be highly sensitive but relatively non-specific in diagnosing hilar metastasis. Oblique tomography had had fair sensitivity and specificity while detecting nodes exceeding 20 mm in mean diameter. The low specificity of MR and dynamic CT in the above study was due to the detection of benign hilar nodes of moderate size (10-16 mm).

It seems that hilar masses or enlarged hilar nodes are more sharply defined and more clearly visualized on MR images when they contrast with the adjacent low signal intensity lung, bronchi and hilar vessels. On the contrary, bronchial abnormalities are better demonstrated on CT, mainly because of the better spatial resolution of this modality. Lobar and segmental bronchi are not entirely demonstrated on MR images and one has to be cautious about diagnosing a nonvisualized small bronchus on MR as pathological.

Bronchogenic carcinoma often presents with distal pulmonary collapse. Seventeen such patients have been studied by Tobler, *et al.* (12), when magnetic resonance imaging was compared to computed tomography in the ability to identify a contour abnormality secondary to tumor presence, to discover bronchial obstruction and separate proximal tumor from distal collapse. CT and MRI were found to be equal in their capacity to

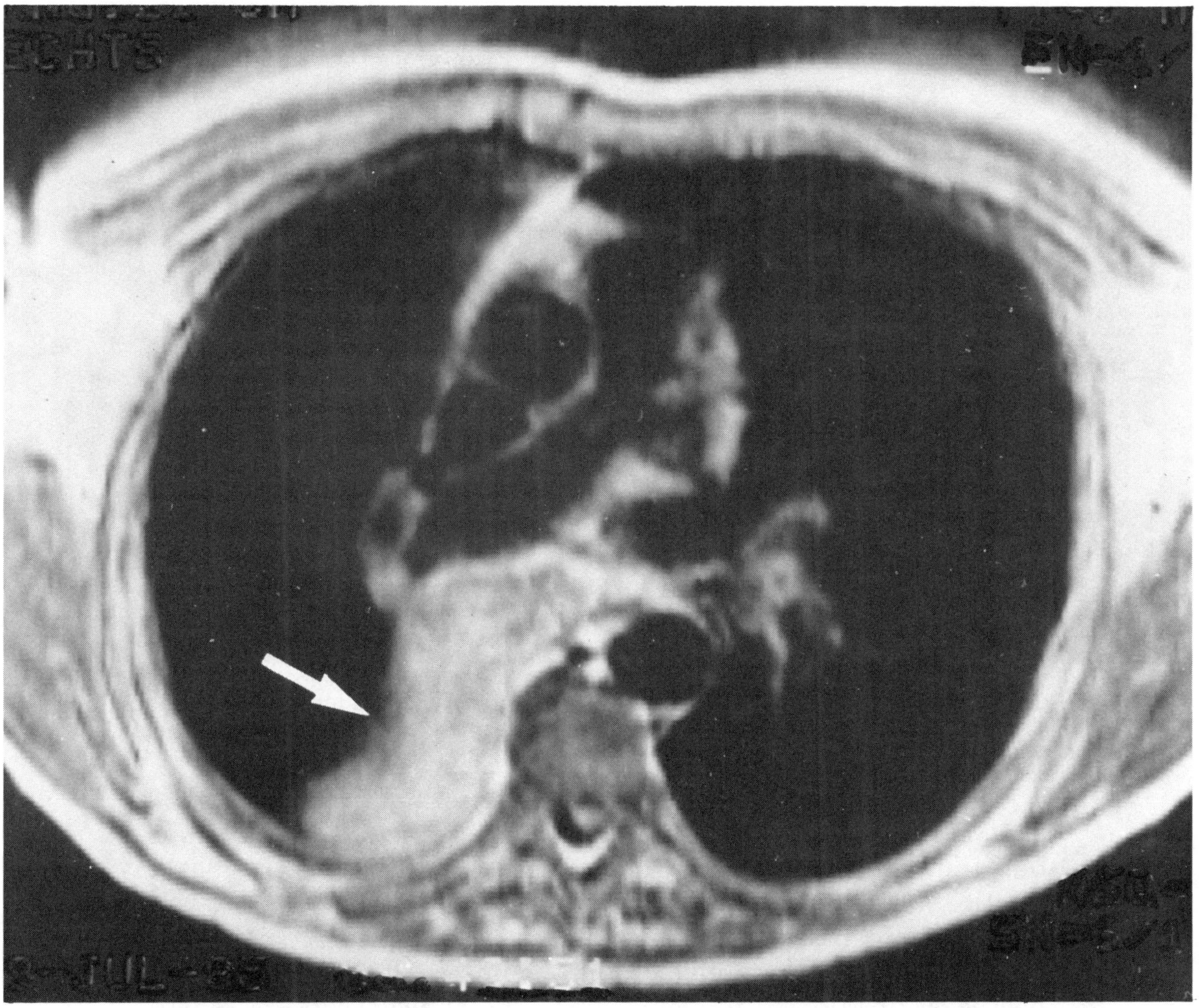

Figure 7.8. Right lower lobe tumoral process (arrow) involving the posterior mediastinum, impossible to differentiate on MR images from collapsed lung parenchyma, based on signal intensities (TR 500 msec, TE 32 msec).

visualize a contour abnormality (70% of cases). Because of the poor spatial resolution of MRI, bronchial narrowing could be identified only in 7 patients out of 17, while CT succeeded in demonstrating bronchial narrowing as a secondary sign of bronchogenic carcinoma in 15 out of 16 cases.

While attempting to separate the tumoral mass from collapsed lung parenchyma, CT with bolus injection of contrast was able to make such a differentiation. Although T_2 weighted images seemed to enable separation of the two entities by signal intensities, MRI showed a poorer ability to distinguish between tumor and collapse, mainly due to heterogeneity in the signal intensity of tumors, as shown by measuring the relative intensity of a different group of 15 tumors (Figures 7.8, 7.9, 7.10, 7.11).

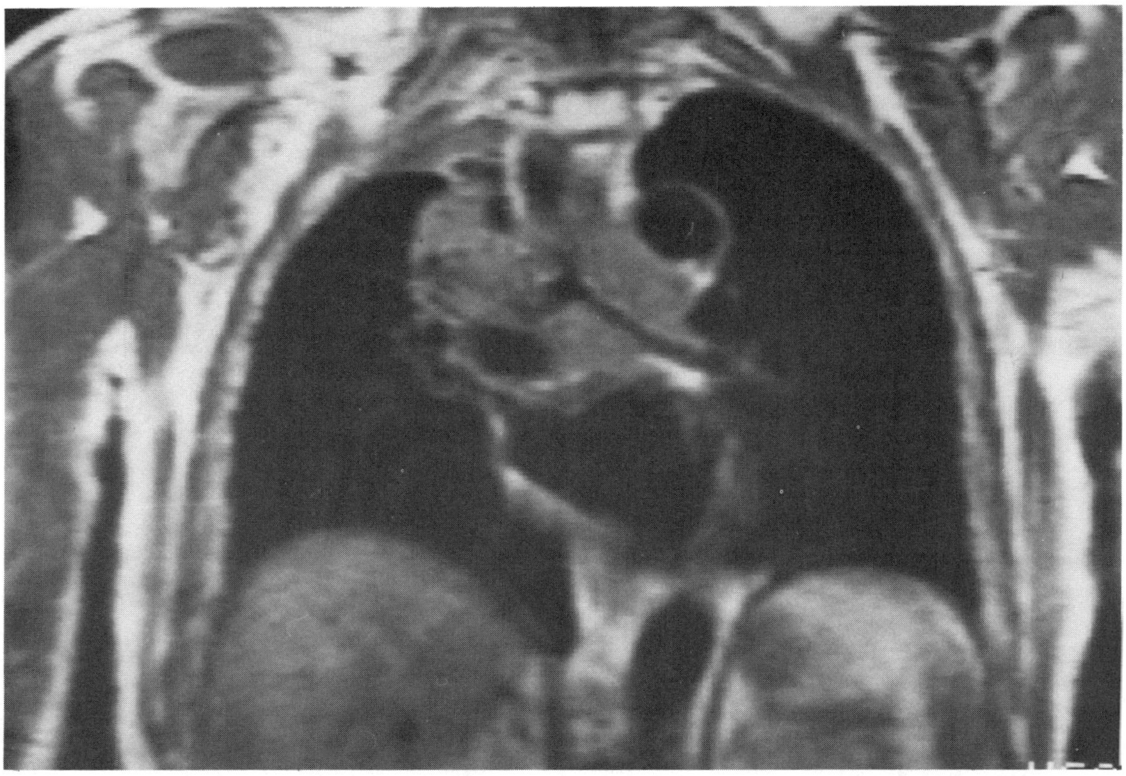

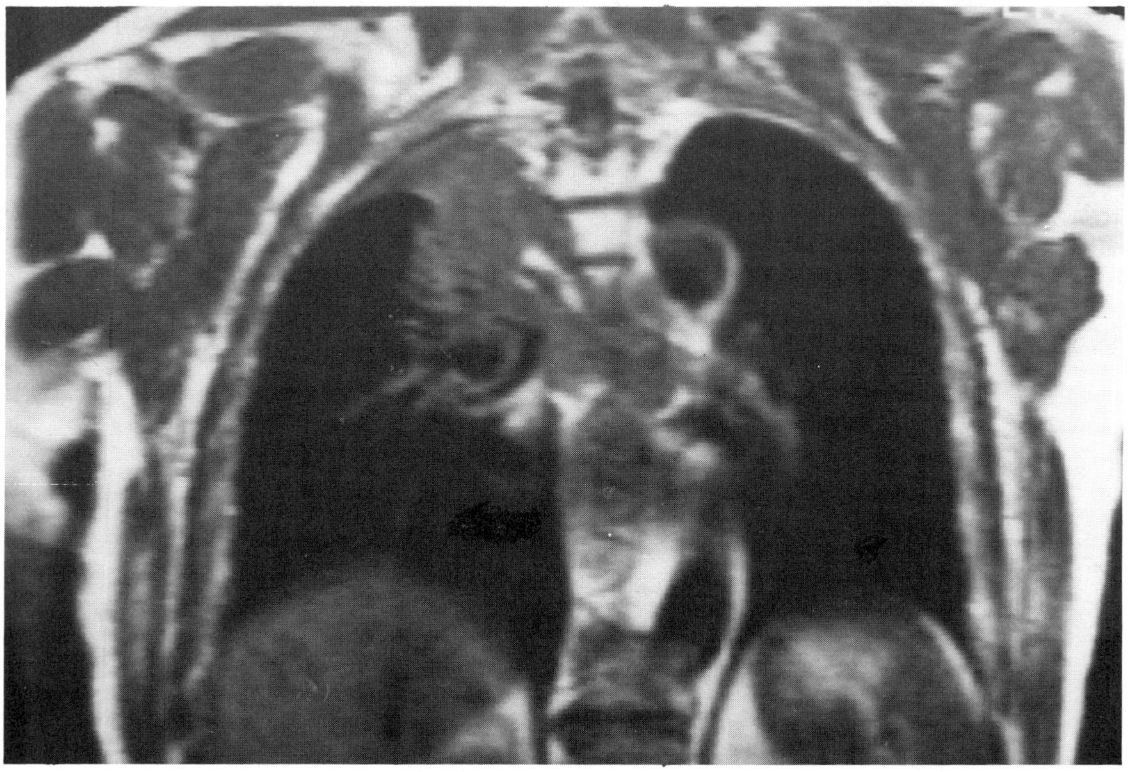

Figures 7.9, 7.10, and 7.11. Consecutive MR images obtained with a TR of 600 msec clearly visualize a tumoral mass in the right upper lung area extensively invading the mediastinum.

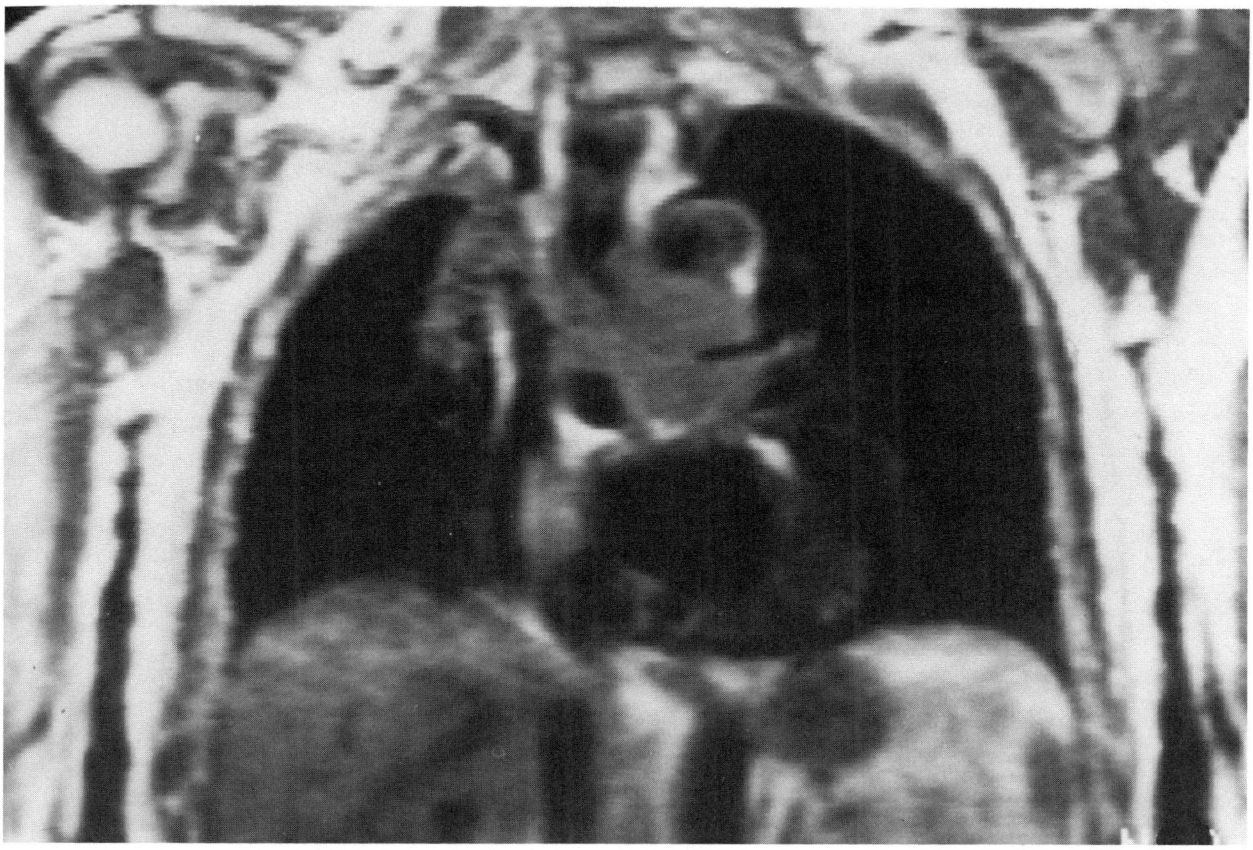

Pleural fluid collection is a common finding in patients with bronchogenic carcinoma. With MR, fluid collections are better visualized on images obtained with long TR and TE values (2,O sec, 50 msec) (Figures 7.12, 7.13). Bronchial carcinoma is often associated with distant metastatic spread. While MRI is unable to demonstrate bone destruction due to lack of signal from calcified tissues, it can, however, accurately visualize adrenal or liver metastases. If there are no time limitations, MR images of the upper abdomen should be included in the MR study of patients with lung cancer.

An exciting area in which MR may prove to be a valuable diagnostic technique is the study of the post-pneumonectomy chest. MR images may provide useful information concerning the immediate and long term pathological changes. In patients who underwent pneumonectomy for a lung cancer, MR images demonstrate variable degrees of fluid collection, pleural thickening and mediastinal shift and rotation (Figures 7.14, 7.15, 7.16). Recurrent tumor may appear as an area of high signal intensity which can be differentiated from the intermediate signal intensity fibrotic changes (see also Chapter 5).

The differences between CT and MR imaging are also emphasized in studies which attempt to assess the ability of MR in detecting single and multiple lung nodules. Computed tomography has been demonstrated to be a highly sensitive modality in the diagnosis of pulmonary nodules (16, 17). Most pulmonary nodules larger than 3 mm in diameter are visible on CT scans. However, nodules detected by this method in a patient with a known malignant lesion do not necessarily represent metastases and no reliable method has been found to enable the distinction between benign and malignant pulmonary nodules. Additionally, on CT scans, even with contrast enhancement, nodules adjacent to blood vessels may be difficult to discover.

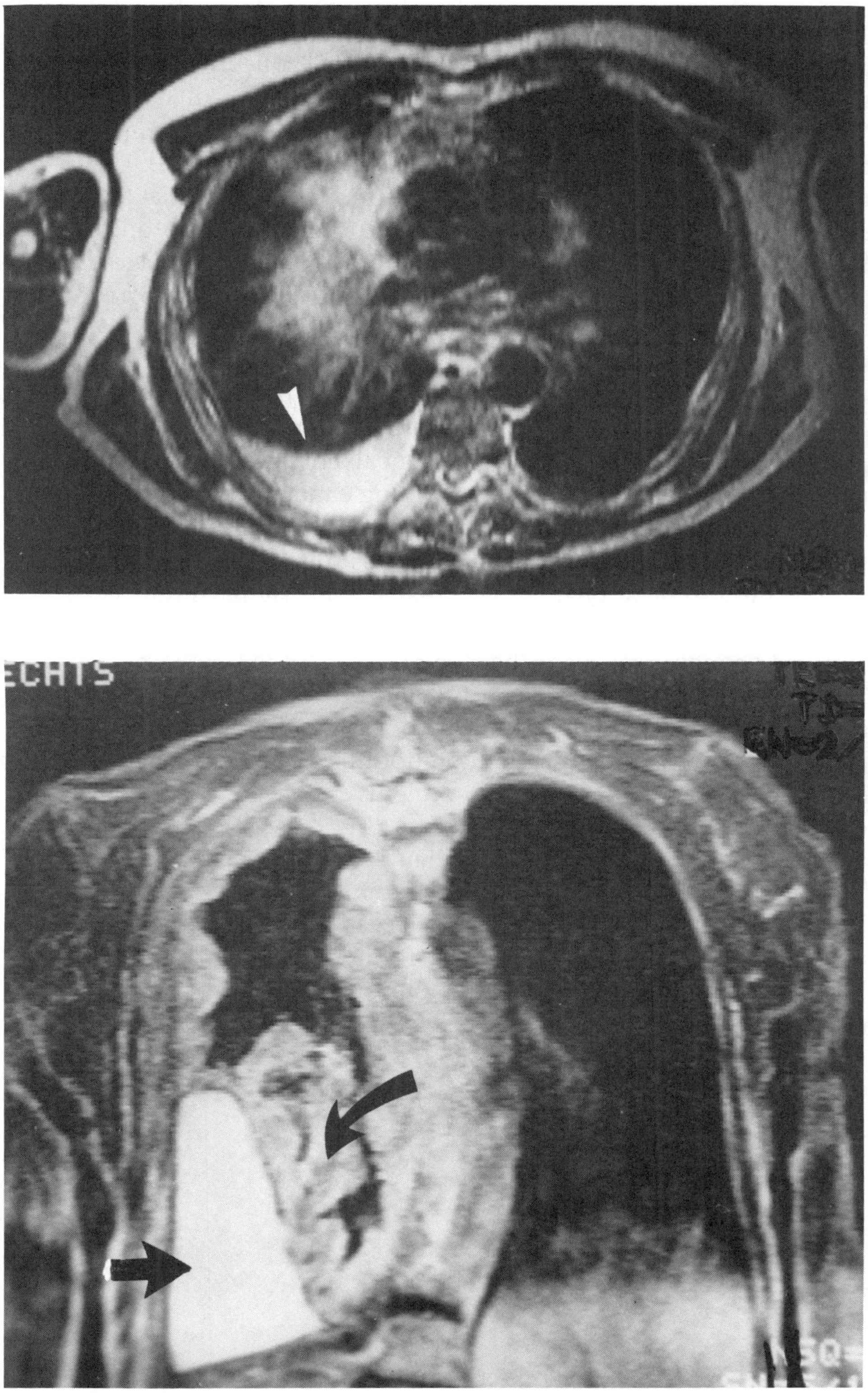

Figures 7.12 and 7.13. In a mesothelioma patient, MR images obtained with long TR and TE (3000 msec, 32 msec) permit a good separation between the high signal intensity pleural effusion (arrow) and the extensive pleural involvement (curved arrow).

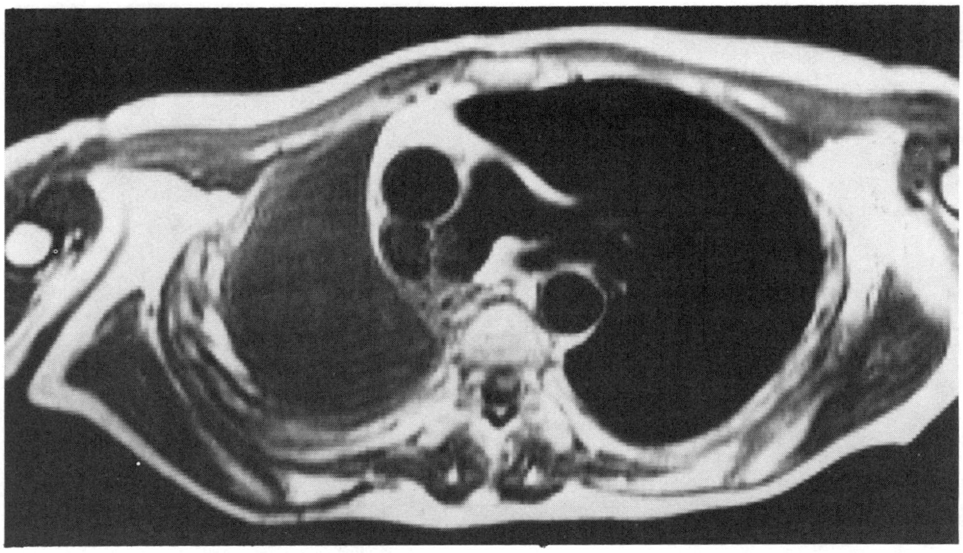

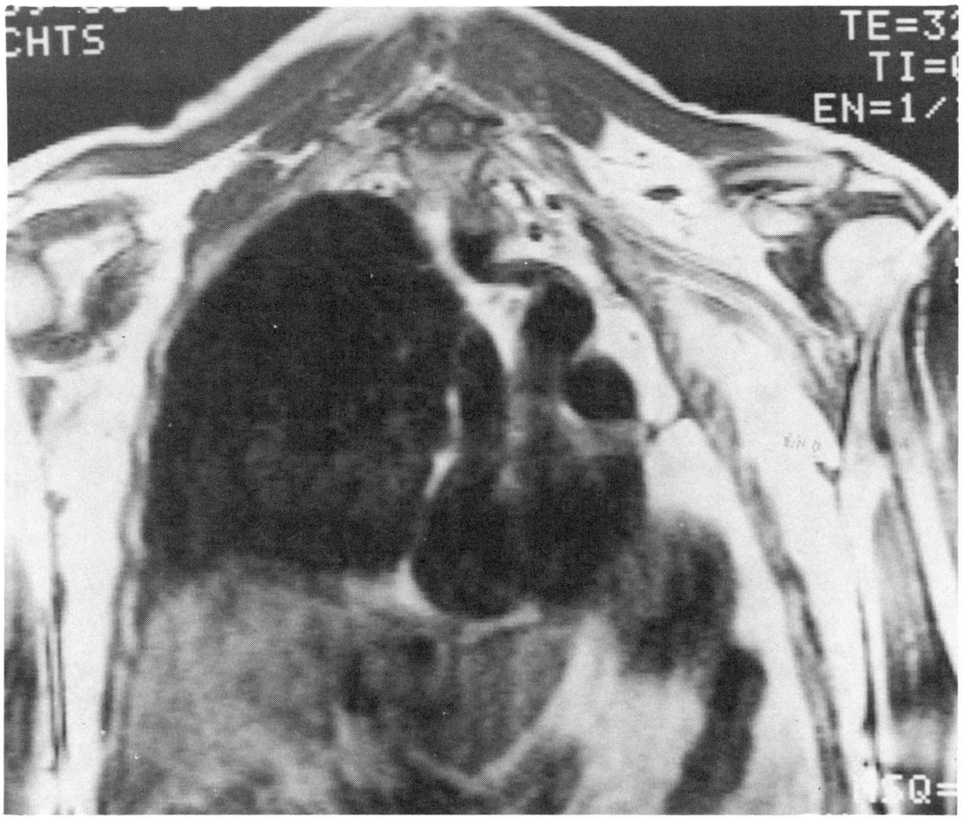

Figures 7.14, 7.15, and 7.16. Sagittal and coronal MR images performed in patients which underwent pneumonectomy for lung cancer, demonstrate variable degrees of mediastinal shift, easily separating the contents of the post-pneumonectomy hemithorax from fat and vascular structures.

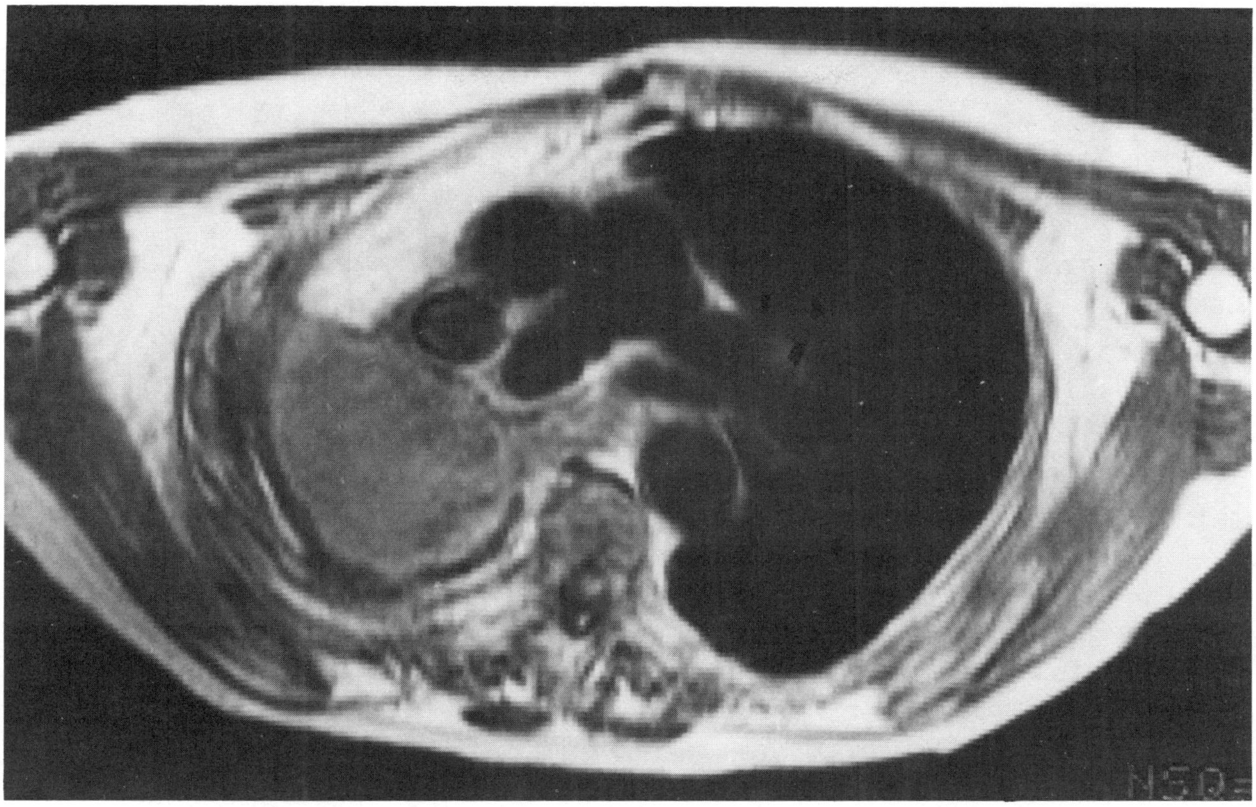

MRI, on the contrary, is easily able to differentiate between the high signal intensity of a pulmonary nodule and the low signal intensity of blood vessels and lung parenchyma (Figures 7.17, 7.18, 7.19). Limitations of this modality include its reduced spatial resolution, particularly in the subpleural and diaphragmatic areas where often metastatic nodules are located. Also, because of the low signal-to-noise ratio of the normal lung parenchyma and nonvisualization of most segmental bronchi or normal fissures, it is difficult to establish the exact location of a nodule on MR images.

In a study performed by Müller, *et al.* (10), 25 patients with pulmonary nodules were examined by CT and MRI. Neither modality discovered lesions which were less than 1.5 cm in diameter. On MR images, long repetition times (2.0 sec) were beneficial in demonstrating pulmonary nodules, especially those close to blood vessels. CT, with its superior spatial resolution, enbled better detection of nodules close to the diaphragm, the pleura or each other.

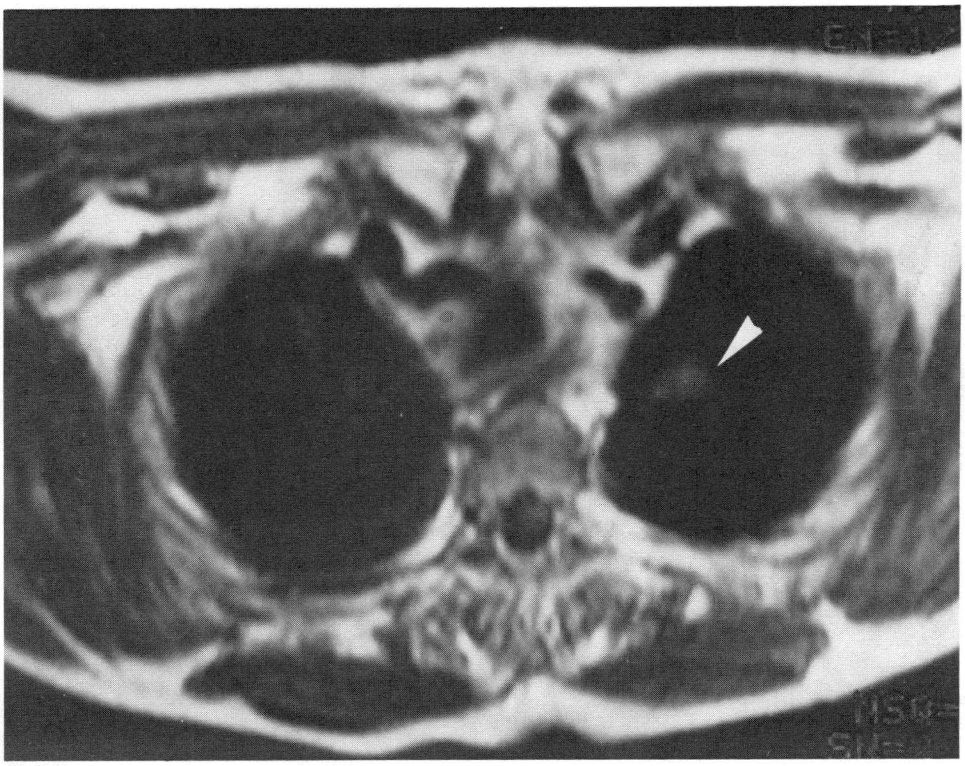

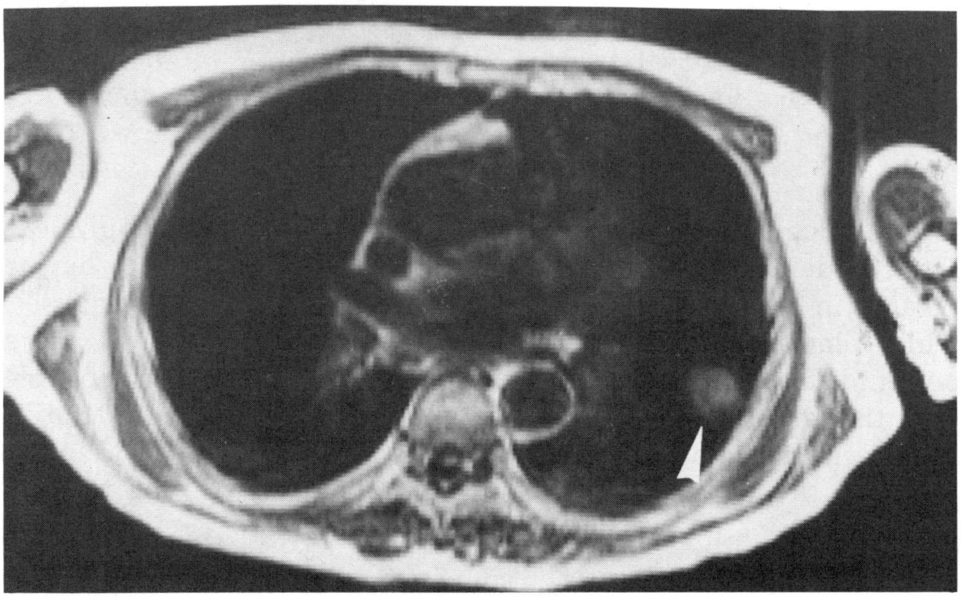

Figures 7.17 and 7.18. Solitary pulmonary nodules identified as intermediate signal intensity lesions, well differentiated from the low signal intensity lung parenchyma (TR 600 msec, TE 32 msec).

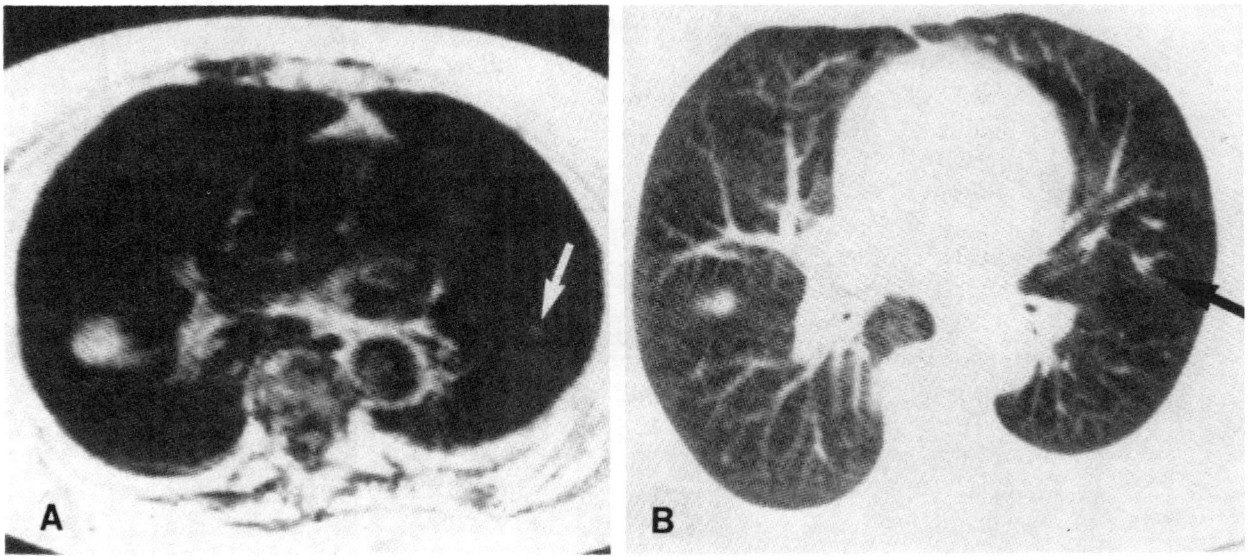

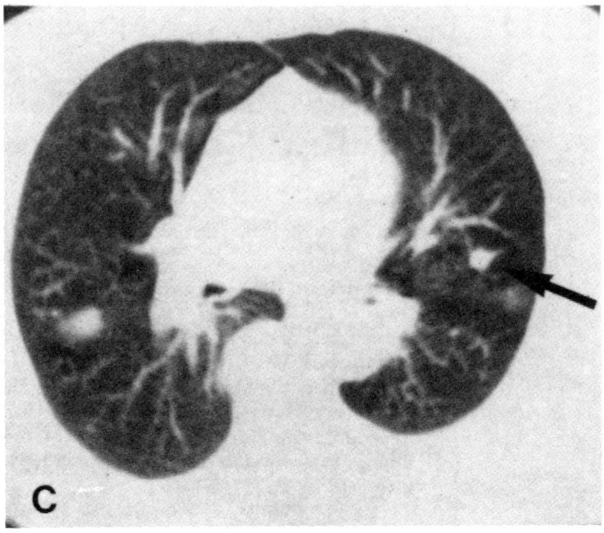

Figure 7.19

A) With MR, a small nodule is noted on the left side (arrow). A larger nodule is present in the right lung.

B) Left nodule was thought to represent a vessel on the CT scan (arrow). Right nodule is clearly seen, although it appears smaller. The reason for this discrepancy in size is not known.

C) A repeat CT scan obtained 3 months later clearly shows the left nodule, which has grown in the interval (arrow).

(From reference 10 with permission.)

As demonstrated, MR imaging can be considered equivalent to CT in demonstrating most of the intrathoracic pathology having a value in the initial diagnosis and staging of pulmonary masses. While hilar adenopathy seems to be better shown with MR and a better distinction of peripheral nodules from vessels is possible with this modality, there is a need for more extensive comparative studies in order to fully appreciate the exact place of MRI in the complex preoperative assessment of patients with lung tumors.

REFERENCES

1. Rigler LG: An overview of cancer of the lung. *Semin Roentgenol*, *12:*161–164, 1977.

2. Heitzman ER: *The Lung: Radiologic-pathologic Correlations.* St. Louis, MO: CV Mosby Co., 1973.

3. Osborne DR Korobkin M, Ravin CE, Putman CE, Wolfe WG, Sealy WC, Young WG, *et al.*: Comparison of plain radiography and computed tomography in detecting intrathoracic lymph node metastases from lung carcinoma. *Radiology, 142:*157-161, 1982.

4. Lewis JW Jr., Madrazo BL, Gross S, *et al.*: The value of radiographic and computed tomography in the staging of lung carcinoma. *Ann Thor Surg, 34:*553-557, 1982.

5. Glazer GM, Francis IR, Shirazi KK, Bookstein FL, Gross BH, *et al.*: Evaluation of the pulmonary hilum: comparison of conventional radiograph, 55° posterior oblique tomography and dynamic computed tomography. *J Comput Assist Tomogr, 7:*983-989, 1983.

6. Cohen AM, Creviston S, Li Puma JP, *et al.*: NMR evaluation of hilar and mediastinal lymphadenopathy. *Radiology, 148:*739-742, 1983.

7. Webb WR, Gamsu G, Stark DD, *et al.*: Magnetic resonance imaging of the normal and abnormal pulmonary hila. *Radiology, 152:*89-94, 1984.

8. Webb WR, Jensen BG, Sollitto R, *et al.*: Bronchogenic carcinoma: staging with MR compared with staging with CT and surgery. *Radiology, 156:*117-124, 1985.

9. Glazer GM, Gross BH, Aisen AM, *et al.*: Imaging of the pulmonary hilum: a prospective comparative study in patients with lung cancer. *AJR, 145:*245-248, 1985.

10. Müller NL, Gamsu G, Webb WR: Pulmonary nodules: detection using magnetic resonance and computed tomography. *Radiology, 155:*687-690, 1985.

11. Martini N, Heelan R, Westcott R, *et al.*: Comparative merits of conventional, computed tomography and magnetic resonance imaging in assessing mediastinal involvement in surgically confirmed lung carcinoma. *J Thorac Cardiovasc Surg, 90:*639-649, 1985.

12. Tobler J, Levitt RG, Glazer HS, *et al.*: Differentiation of proximal bronchogenic carcinoma from distal consolidation or collapse by magnetic resonance imaging. Presentation at the meeting of the Soceity of Thoracic Radiology, Bal Harbor, FL, 1985.

13. Gamsu G, Webb WR, Sheldon P, *et al.*: Nuclear magnetic resonance imaging of the thorax. *Radiology, 147:*473-480, 1983.

14. Webb WR, Gamsu G, Stark DD, *et al.*: Evaluation of magnetic resonance sequences in imaging mediastinal tumors. *AJR, 143:*723-727, 1984.

15. Ross JS, O'Donovan PB, Novoa R, *et al.*: Magnetic resonance of the chest: initial experience with imaging in vivo T_1 and T_2 calculations. *Radiology, 152:*95-101, 1984.

16. Muhm JR, Brown LR, Crowe JK, *et al.*: Comparison of whole lung tomography and computed tomography for detecting pulmonary nodules. *AJR, 131:*981-984, 1978.

17. Shaner EG, Chang AE, Doppman JL, *et al.*: Comparison of computed and conventional whole body tomography in detecting pulmonary nodules: a prospective radiologic-pathologic study. *AJR, 131:*51-54, 1978.

18. Sperber M, Kaiser MC: MR imaging in pulmonary abnormalities - advantages and limitations. *Respiration,* accepted for publication.

8

Benign Pulmonary Conditions

A large variety of benign clinical conditions still require an accurate, non-invasive means of diagnosis. Attempts have been made to evaluate the potential of MRI in the discovery and determination of extent of such conditions as pulmonary embolism, abscess collections, congenital bronchial abnormalities, pulmonary airspace and interstitial diseases, and chronic lung disorders.

At the present time, there is no safe and definite method to establish the presence of a pulmonary embolism, as arteriography is a rather complicated procedure and involves a certain risk in a number of patients. MRI may contribute to this often urgent and lifesaving diagnosis by its ability to visualize the vascular anatomy of the chest without the administration of contrast materials.

On MR images there is little or no signal from the vascular lumen, which therefore appears dark and well-defined on the background of high intensity signal mediastinal fat. Cases have been described of angiographically demonstrated pulmonary emboli when patients showed an intense signal within pulmonary arteries at the level of lodged clots, while the remaining normal vascular segments presented no intraluminar signal (1, 2) (Figure 8.1). In the published cases, pulmonary emboli were relatively easily diagnosed on MR images. However, it has to be taken into consideration that possible diagnostic difficulties may be encountered due to the intraluminal signal resulting from slow vascular flow, which may be mistaken for the presence of an embolus. also, existent areas of airspace disease or atelectasis can give an intense signal, resulting in the concealment of small peripheral emboli. The same is true about the present limitations in the resolution of MRI, which is not sufficiently high to allow detection of small clots.

Several imaging modalities are usually employed in the evaluation of abscess collections including sonography, radionuclide scans and CT. MRI is adding to this area its improved soft tissue contrast and ability to visualize a lesion in multiple planes.

While studying a discovered abscess on MR images, several features of the lesion have to be taken into consideration, includ-

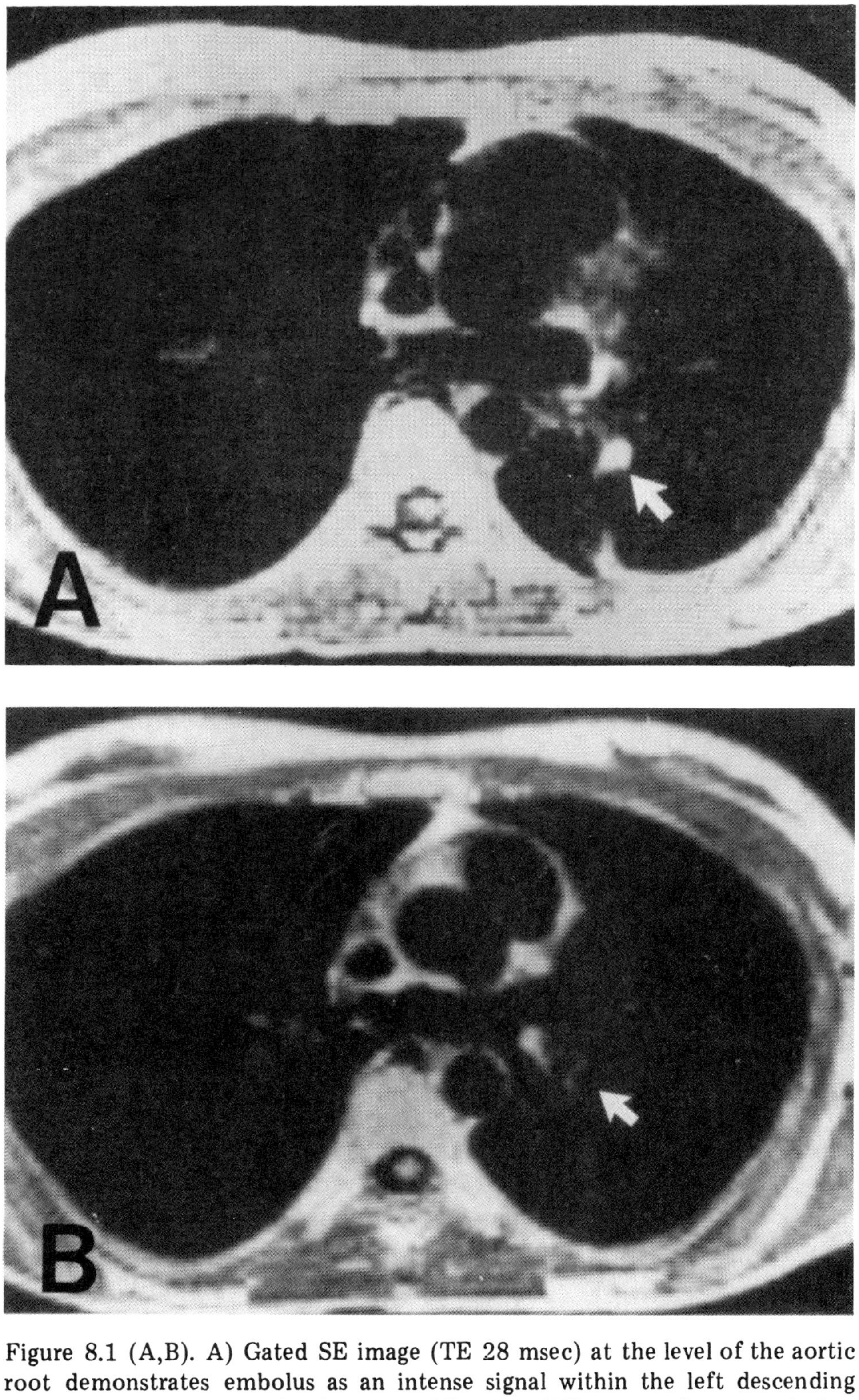

Figure 8.1 (A,B). A) Gated SE image (TE 28 msec) at the level of the aortic root demonstrates embolus as an intense signal within the left descending pulmonary artery (arrow). B) Repeat SE image (TE 28 msec) obtained after one week of anticoagulant therapy demonstrates an absence of signal in the left descending pulmonary artery (arrow), indicating lysis of the embolus (Reference 2, with permission).

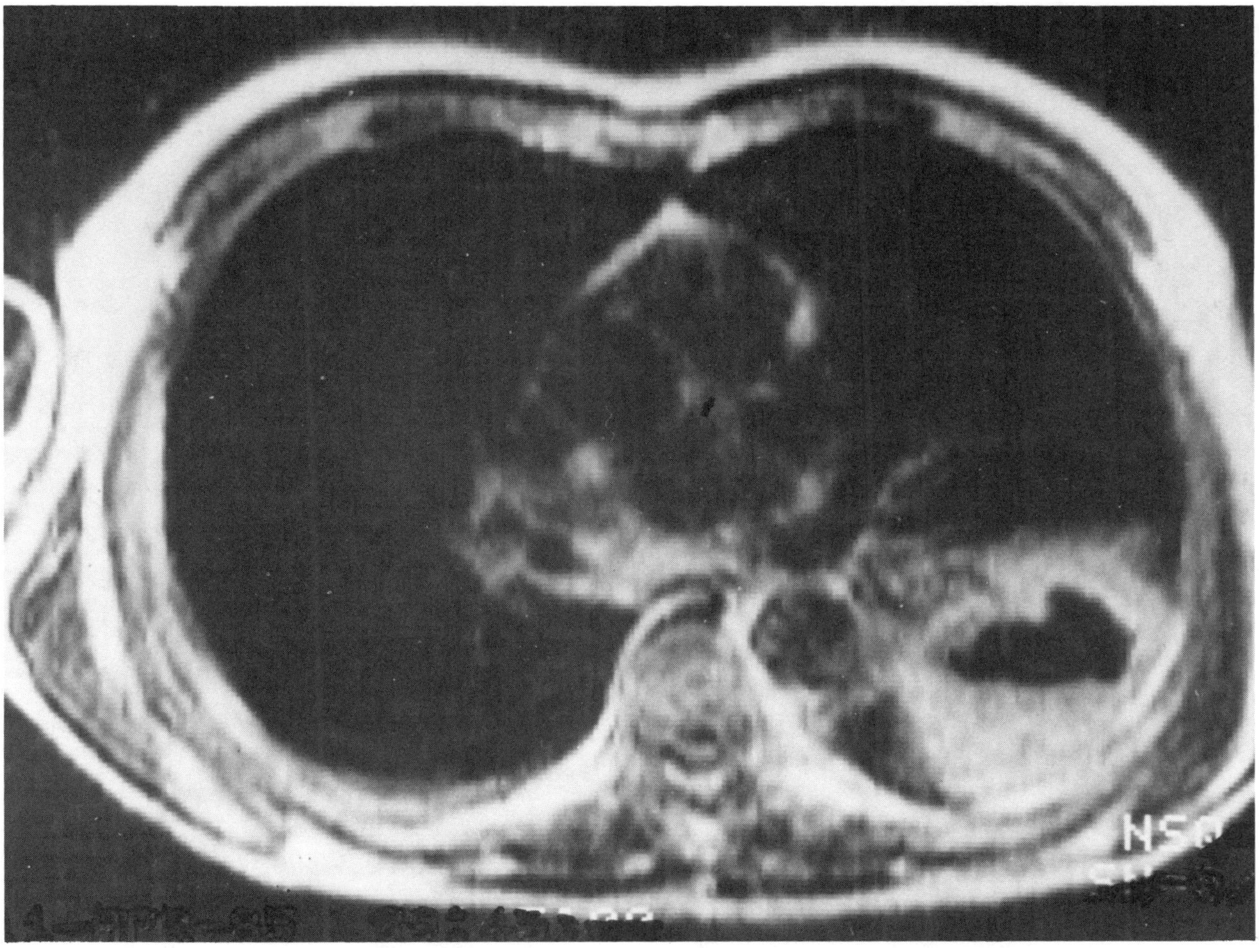

Figure 8.2. T_2 weighted image of an intrathoracic abscess, showing the high signal intensity of the lesion which has an internal air-fluid level.

ing the presence or absence of a capsule, internal gas collections, effects on adjacent structures (such as vessels, muscles and bones), and the exact extent of the lesion. When employing short repetition times (TR), thoracic as well as abdominal abscess collections present on MR a low signal intensity, either homogeneous or heterogeneous. On T_2 weighted images, these lesions seem to present a relatively higher signal intensity (3) (Figure 8.2).

Findings on MR images when compared to those on CT scans show that there is a better delineation of the extent of the inflammatory changes on surrounding tissues with MRI, as high signal intensity areas are seen on adjacent muscles, regardless of the TR or TE used to obtain the images. Also, there is no need for contrast agent injection on MRI for the visualization of the abscess capsule. On CT, if the abscess does not contain gas and does not have a low attenuation number, it is difficult to separate it from adjacent structures. Surgical clips produce known artifacts on CT images, disadvantage which is not true at the same extent with MRI. In the future, more studies are required in order to establish how sensitive and specific MRI is in differentiating between abscesses, necrotic tumors, and various fluid collections.

The normally aerated lung yields a very low signal intensity and therefore appears dark. There is an impression that emphysematos changes on MR images can be differentiated from normal lung tissue by their even lower signal intensity. Furthermore, high intensity branching structures in patients with chronic lung disease have been confirmed pathologically as representing endobronchial mucus plugs (4) (Figures 8.3, 8.4) and have been clearly differentiated on MR images from the pulmonary vessels. This finding can be of major importance, for example, in the study of children with cystic fibrosis. The lack of ionising radiation makes MRI an ideal diagnostic modality in the pediatric age group.

Congenital abnormalities such as bronchogenic cysts are clearly delineated with MRI, when the high intensity fluid content of the cyst is well visualized, the same as the accurate relationships of the lesion to the mediastinal and pulmonary structures (Figure 8.5).

There are not sufficient studies available about the use of MRI in the evaluation of pulmonary airspace diseases and the differentiation of their causes. However, some experimental studies have been performed with the goal to elucidate the potential of MRI in this area (5, 6).

In a study by Moore *et al.* (5) a phantom was constructed to simulate pulmonary airspace disease with varying degrees of residual aeration. A matrix of gelatin has been whipped with air and combined with unwhipped gelatin in different ratios, yielding varying numbers of bubbles of uniform size equally distributed in a stable matrix. Sixteen patients with a variety of disorders including pulmonary edema, pneumonia, pneumonitis, pulmonary hemorrhage, and alveolar proteinosis were studied by MRI, while means and standard deviations of T_1 and T_2 measurements were determined for each patient and for each disease process.

The mean T_1 values measured from patients with pulmonary edema, post-obstructive pneumonitis, pulmonary hemorrhage, radiation pneumonitis, and lobar pneumonia were in the same range, with the longest T_1 values recorded in patients with lobar pneumonia. Among the patients with pulmonary edema, it seems that the longest T_1 values were found in a patient with acute edema and the lowest T_1 values in cases in which edema was chronic.

In patients with alveolar proteinosis, the T_1 calculated values were the lowest when compared with all other conditions in which

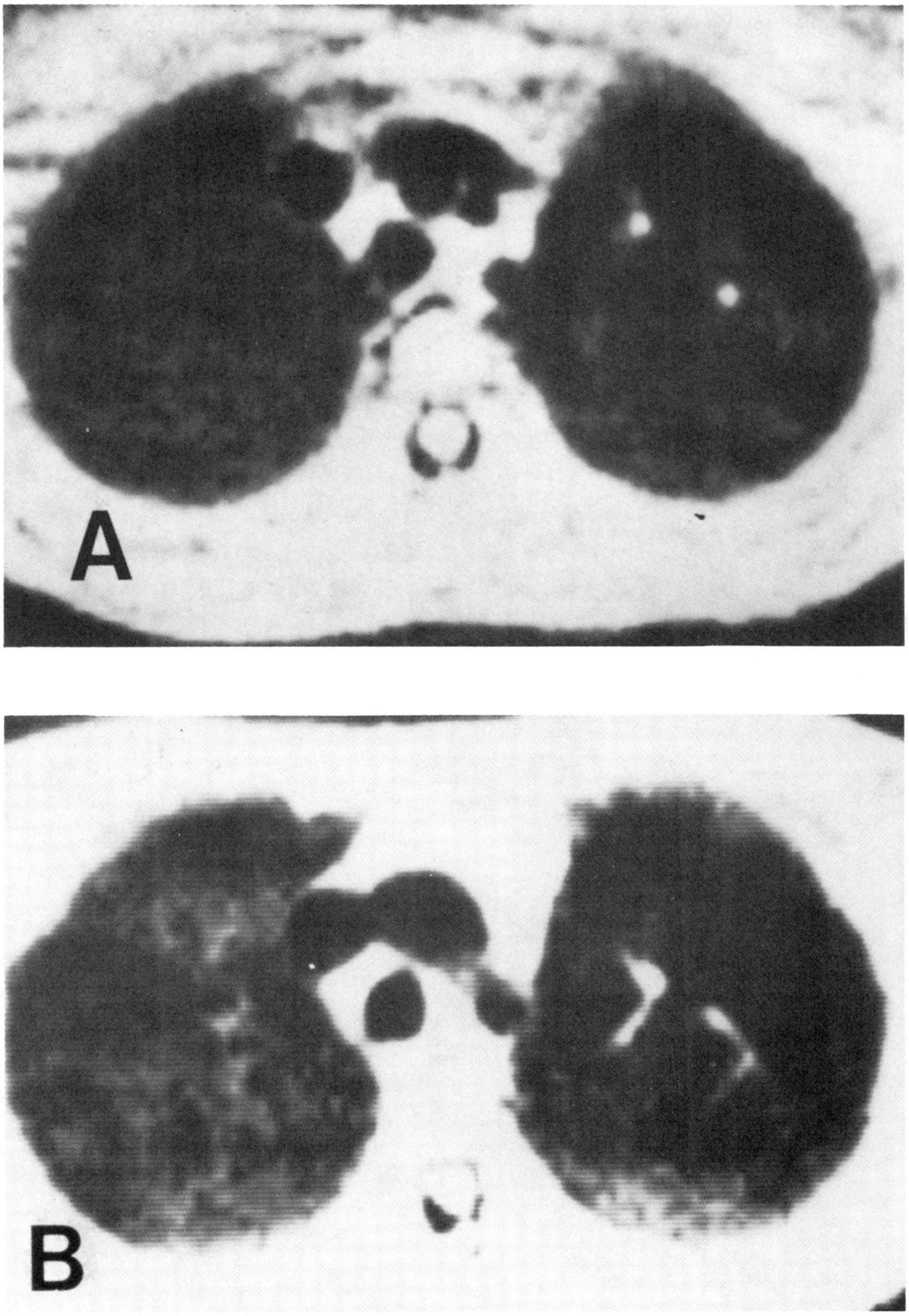

Figure 8.3 (A,B). MR cross-sectional image (TE 28 msec, TR 2.0 sec) near the thoracic apex of the same patient. The emphysema of the left upper lobe is evident as decreased intensity, compared with the normal right lung. Also seen are two small high-intensity branching structures that represent endobronchial mucus plugs. The endobronchial plugs could not be distinguished from vascular structures on CT images. A hilar bronchogenic cust with secondary emphysema and mucoid-impacted bronchi were confirmed pathologically (Reference 4, with permission).

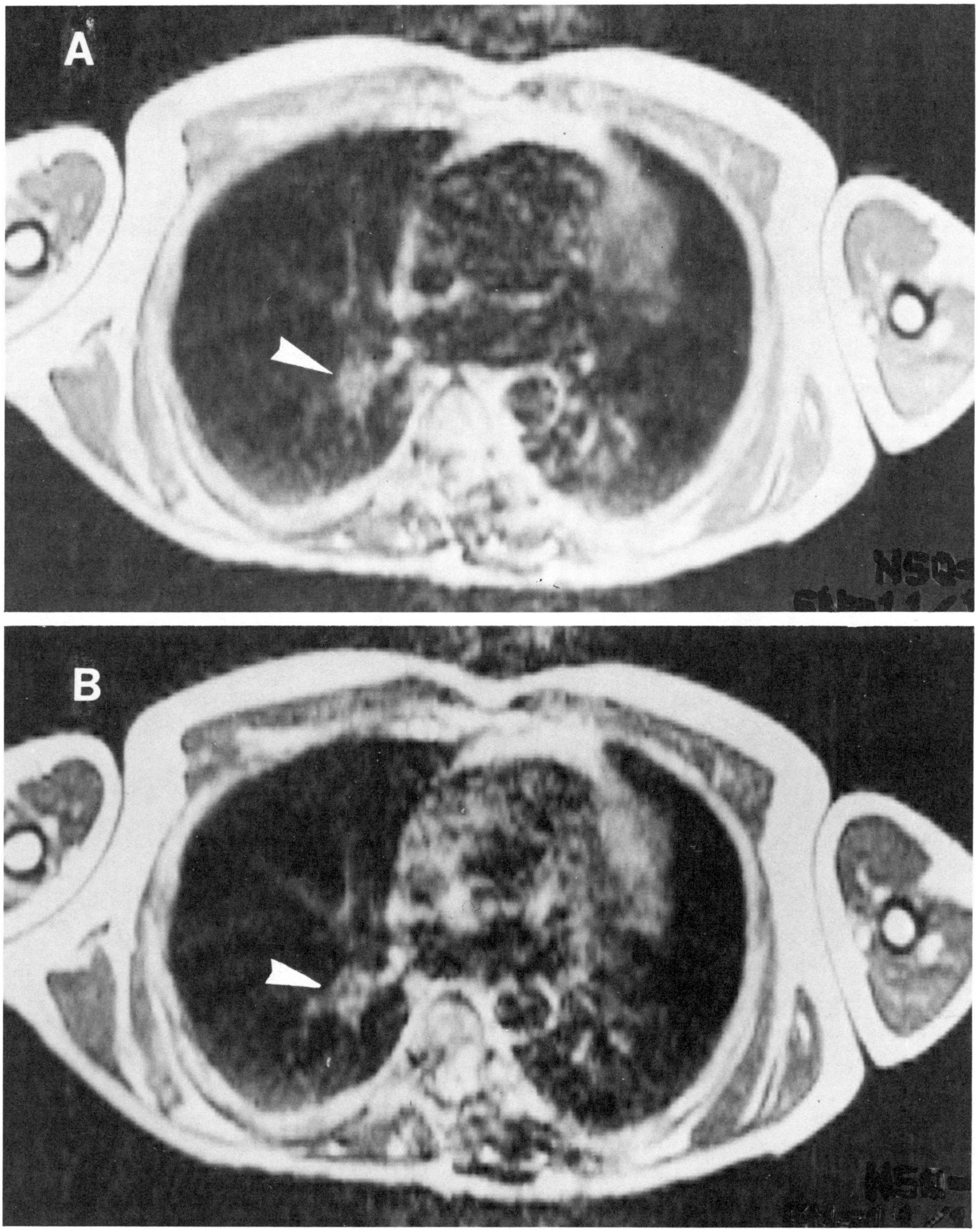

Figure 8.4 (A,B). First and second echo in a T_2 weighted image of the thorax obtained in a patient with antracosilicosis, demonstrate the increased signal intensity nodes (arrows) and the prominent interstitial markings at the hila.

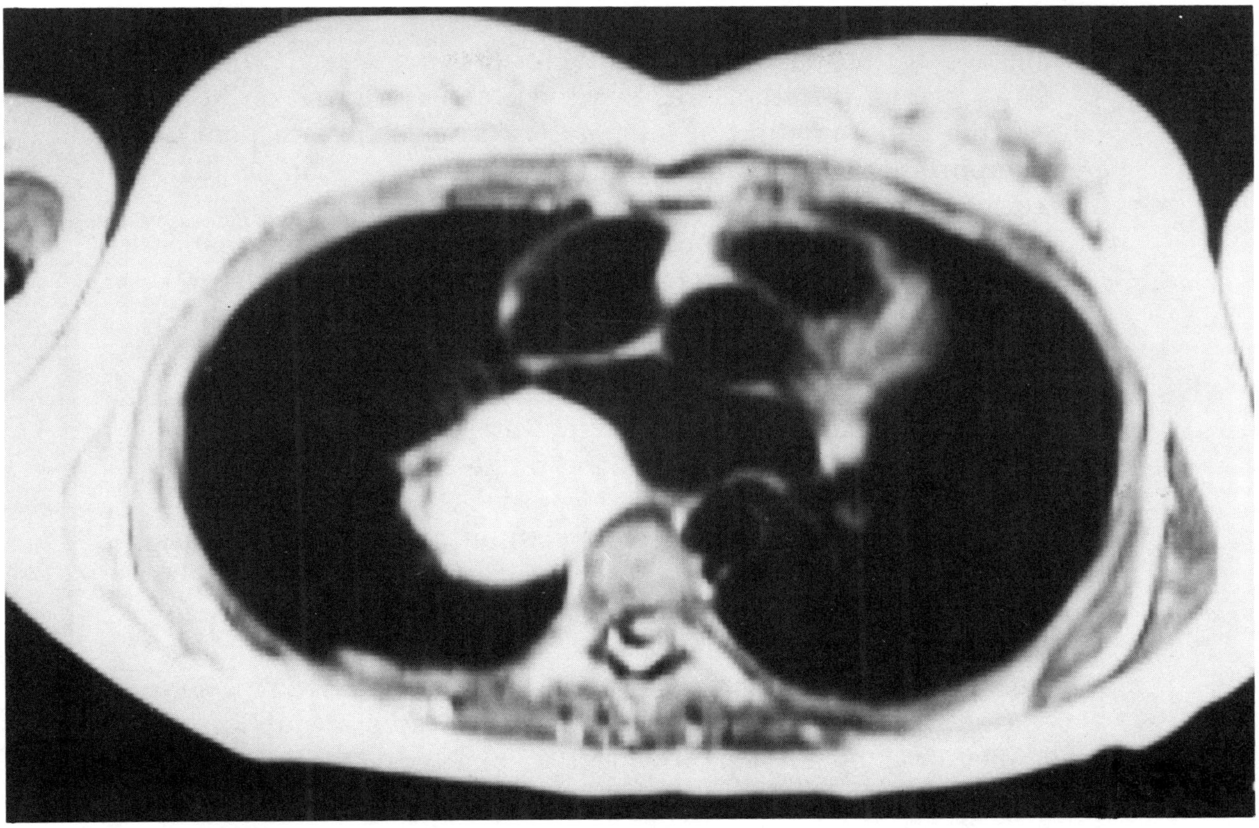

Figure 8.5. Bronchogenic cyst in which the contained fluid presents an extreme high signal intensity on T_2 weighted images.

measurements were performed. T_1 values were intermediate in patients with pneumocystic carinii pneumonia.

On the contrary, T_2 measurements were not useful in distinguishing between various airspace disorders. By using the phantom, the T_1 and T_2 values were plotted against the density of the gelatin foams and revealed that T_1 and T_2 values remained relatively constant, regardless of the degree of aeration within the tested range.

However, the effects of residual aeration cannot be accurately assessed in clinical conditions, because in disease processes the amount and type of alveolar contents changes from one phase of the disease to the other. At the present time, it is considered that these variations result from the various combinations of water, protein, cells and blood forming the alveolar content in the different clinical conditions, but there is a possibility that several other factors of same importance are involved and influence the accuracy of T_1 and T_2 measurements. When trying to identify these factors and looking forward to a possible clinical use of this method, further study is required in order to understand the real significance of the above experimental results.

An exciting different area in which MRI can prove to be of value is the determination of lung water content, measurement of great importance in the monitoring of pulmonary edema, characterized by an increase in the lung water content.

In vitro measurements of lung water by magnetic resonance have been published and the results seem to be encouraging (8, 9). The authors presented the way in which magnetic resonance can be used for the qualitative and visual determinations of the spatial distribution of lung water in animals and humans. Extremely accurate quantitative measurements of lung water content and distribution were obtained in both normal and saline-filled lungs, independent of perfusion and ventilation processes.

In a study by MacLennan, *et al.* (10), magnetic resonance has been used to show that the water content of lung tissue could be predicted accurately from the intensity of signal resulting from a 90° saturation recovery sequence. The water contained in an image section may, in this manner, be calculated by reference to 100% water standard. The total vascular and intravascular pulmonary water measured by MRI in six health volunteers was 292 gram, which is less than predicted by other indirect methods and postmortem values. Some of the explanations for this underestimation can be found in the signal reduction of 10% due to partial saturation. Also, the partial volume effect found in each tomographic technique causes the loss of lung tissue around the lung edges. By imaging in thin slices, this effect can be diminished resulting, however, in a longer examination time. Respiratory movement can also be a reason for inaccurate measurements.

A further sophistication of this method will be to succeed in distinguishing vascular from extravascular water, possibly by identifying the vascular component with appropriate contrast agents or by measurements of its flow and relaxation values. As in other areas of pulmonary diagnosis, there is a need for further development in MRI technology, together with extensive clinical studies in order to assess the full value of MRI in this field.

REFERENCES

1. Thickman D, Kressel HY, Axel L: Demonstration of pulmonary embolism by magnetic resonance imaging. *AJR, 142:*921-922, May 1984.

2. Moore EH, Gamsu G, Webb WR, Stulbarg MS: Pulmonary embolus: detection and follow-up using magnetic resonance. *Radiology, 153:*471-472, 1984.

3. Wall SD, Fisher MR, Amparo EG, *et al.*: Magnetic resonance imaging in the evaluation of abscesses. *AJR, 144:*1217-1221, 1985.

4. Brash RC, Gooding CA, Zallemand DP, *et al.*: Magnetic resonance imaging of the thorax in childhood. *Radiology, 150:*453-463, 1984.

5. Moore EH, Webb WR, Muller N, *et al.*: MRI of pulmonary airspace disease: experimental model and preliminary clinical results. *AJR, 146:* 1123-1128, 1986.

6. Skalina S, Kundel HL, Wolf G, *et al.*: The effect of pulmonary edema on proton nuclear magnetic resonance relaxation times. *Invest Radiol, 19:*7-9, 1984.

7. Huber DJ, Kobzik L, Melanson G, *et al.*: The detection of inflamation in collapsed lung by alterations in proton nuclear magnetic relaxation times. *Invest Radiol, 20:*460-464, 1985.

8. Hayes CE, Case TA, Ailon DC, *et al.*: Lung water quantitation by nuclear magnetic resonance imaging. *Science, 216:*1313-1315, 1982.

9. Cutillo AG, Morris AH, Glatter DD, *et al.*: Determination of lung water content and distribution by nuclear magnetic resonance. *J App Physiol, 57:*583-588, 1984.

10. MacLennon FM, Foster MA, Smith FW, *et al.*: Measurement of total lung water from nuclear magnetic resonance images. *Br J Radiol, 59:*553-560, 1986.

Notes

9

Pleural and Diaphragmatic Abnormalities

The chest wall is covered by a thin sheet of mesothelial cells (parietal pleura) while the lungs are similarly lined by the visceral pleura. Between both pleural layers exists a potential space that can be involved in various pathological processes:

1. Pleural effusions
2. Localized diffuse pleural thickening
3. Neoplastic disease.

The thin pleural layers can only be depicted by CT when they run axially in the slice, in which case they fill a volume element and produce adequate contrast with the adjacent structures. In general, the pleural layers of a healthy person cannot be depicted by CT. If pleural thickening occurs, these changes are visualized only in those cases in which the increase in volume or the degree of deformity in the horizontal plane is sufficient enough to be detected on axial slices. Due to inherent relatively reduced spatial resolution with the present state-of-the-art MRI devices, there is a need for quite advanced pleural pathology in order to enable visualization in an axial plane. Nevertheless, because imaging possibilities exist in the coronal and sagittal planes, relatively discreet pleural thickening may be depicted. Pleural changes usually have intermediate or high signal intensity and for this reason they can easily be separated from pulmonary structures which have extremely low signal intensity on all pulse sequences (Figure 9.1) because of their extremely low hydrogen content. This is particularly true in obese patients in which abundant extrapleural fat, showing high signal intensity on T_1 and T_2 images is lining its outer surface.

PLEURAL EFFUSIONS

Accumulations of fluid in the pleural cavity occur in a large variety of disorders and constitute, therefore, a non-specific radiological sign. The most common causes are inflammation and malig-

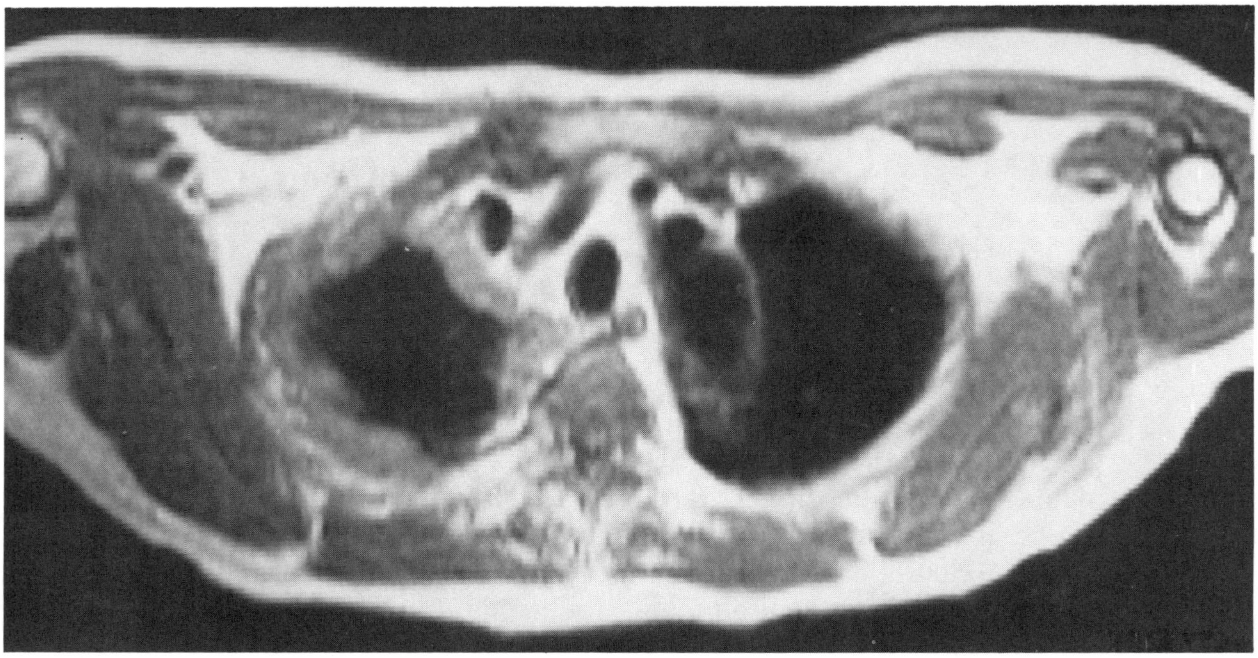

Figure 9.1. Diffuse apical pleural thickening on the right side. On T_1 weighted images these changes have intermediate signal intensity and can easily be separated from low intensity lungs.

nant infiltrations from lung disease, as well as transudation due to cardiac decompensation. Effusions may be unilateral or bilateral, but any entity that causes fluid to accumulate within both pleural spaces can also result in unilateral effusion so that no conclusion as to its etiology can be made. Thoracentesis and pleural biopsy are extremely important procedures in characterizing the nature of a pleural effusion identified radiographically. With the advent of MRI, it was hoped that it could provide a reliable diagnostic tool capable of distinguishing inflammatory from non-inflammatory effusions since there seems to be a correlation between T_1 and T_2 relaxation times of the effusion and its lipid and/or protein content (1). From experimental studies it appears that there is a significant overlap of T_1 and T_2 relaxation times of various body fluids, and that there was only a moderate correlation between protein content and T_1 and T_2 relaxation times (2).

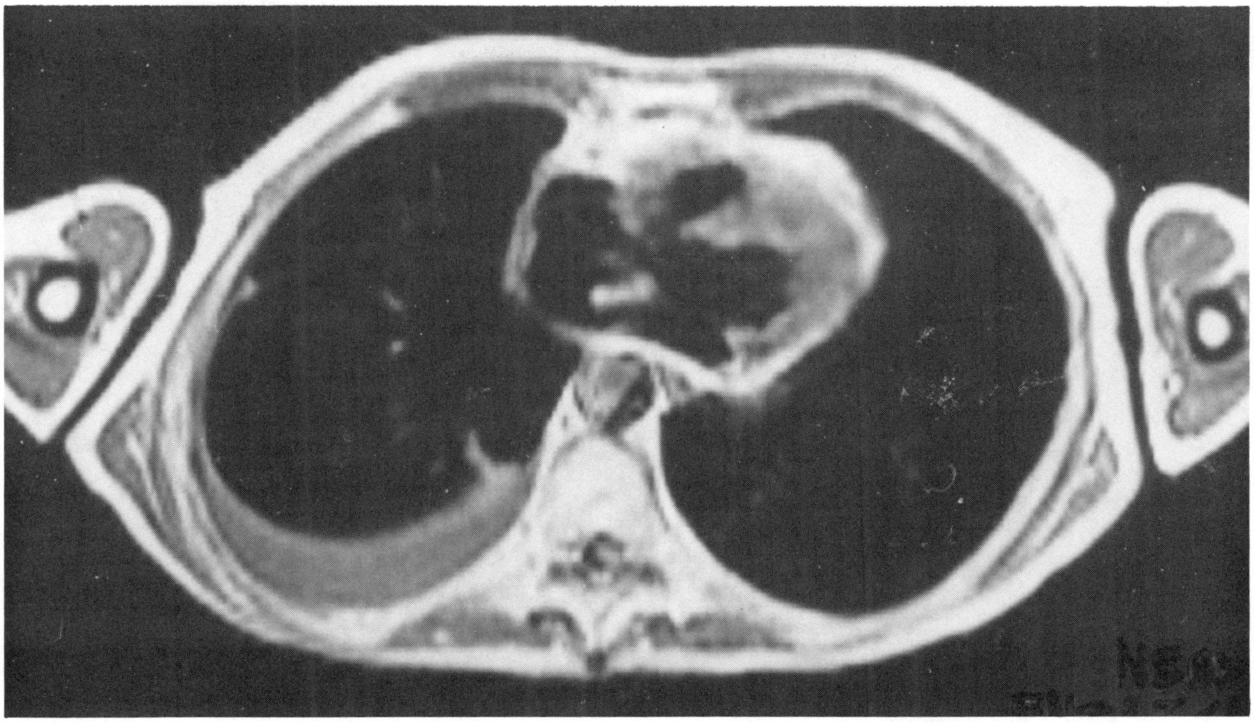

Figure 9.2. Pleural effusion showing relatively low signal intensity on T_1 image.

Blood effusions show high signal intensity on both T_1 and T_2 weighted images. Similarly, chylous or purulent pleural collections have also relatively high signal intensity with T_1 and T_2 relaxation times. In our experience, the signal intensity of pleural effusions is relatively low on T_1 weighted images in the vast majority of the cases (Figure 9.2). On T_2 weighted images the signal intensity of this pleural fluid usually increases quite significantly, but exceptions to this are seen (Figure 9.3). We believe that it is possible that these variations in signal intensity could be closely related to the age of a pleural effusion as connective tissue organization of fibrin-containing exudate may take place within relatively short time intervals.

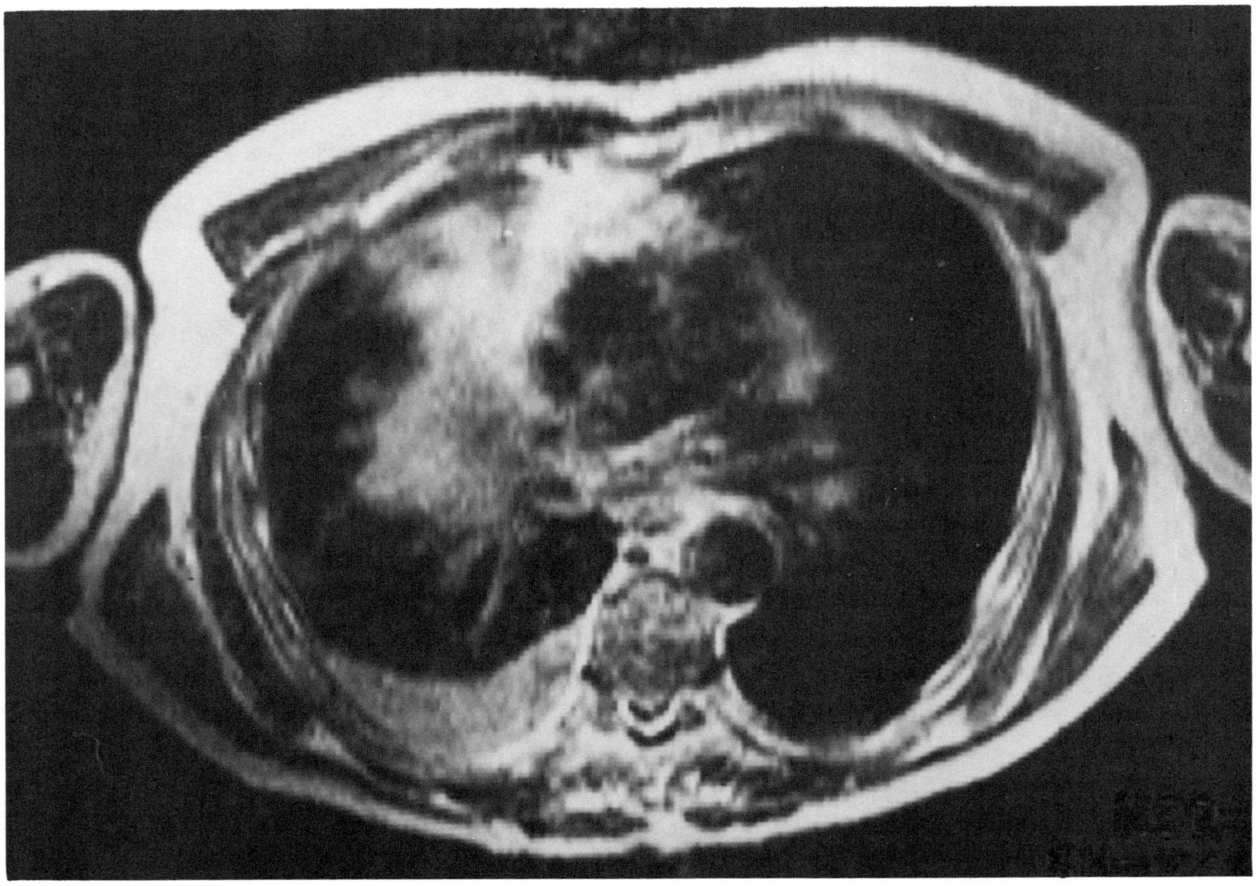

Figure 9.3. Relatively low signal intensity of right pleural effusion on T_2 image (TR 3000, TE 64 msec). Note extensive fibrosis after irradiation.

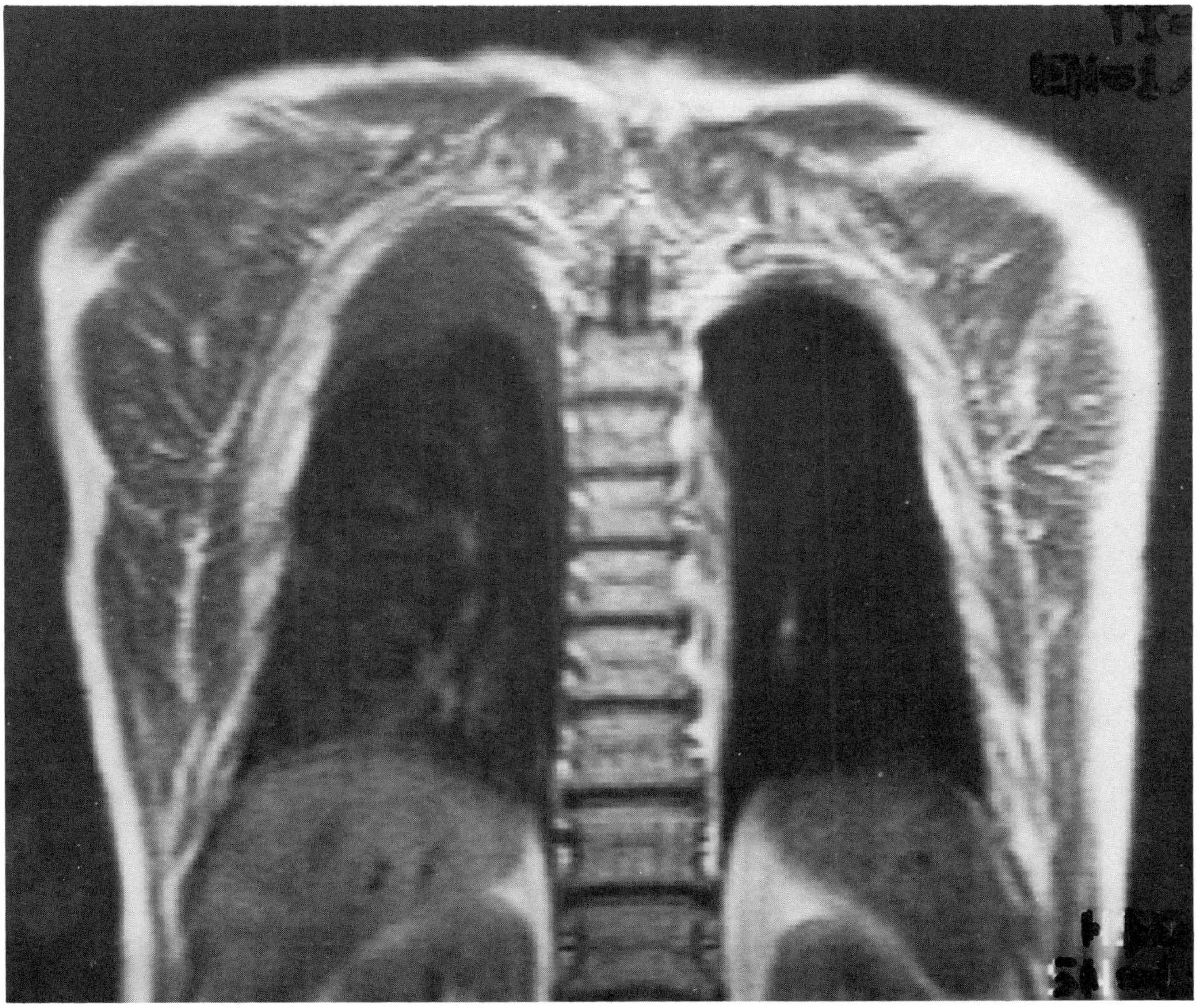

Figure 9.4. Coronal T_1 weighted MR image showing extensive pleural thickening in apex of right lung with low signal intensity.

LOCALIZED OR DIFFUSE PLEURAL THICKENING

Localized pleural thickening at the lung apices is commonly seen and it may be related to aging. Focal pleural thickening is generally secondary to inflammation which has healed and leaves fibrotic pleural changes (Figure 9.4). Bilateral pleural thickening should make one suspect inorganic dust pneumoconiosis such as asbestosis, silicosis and talcosis.

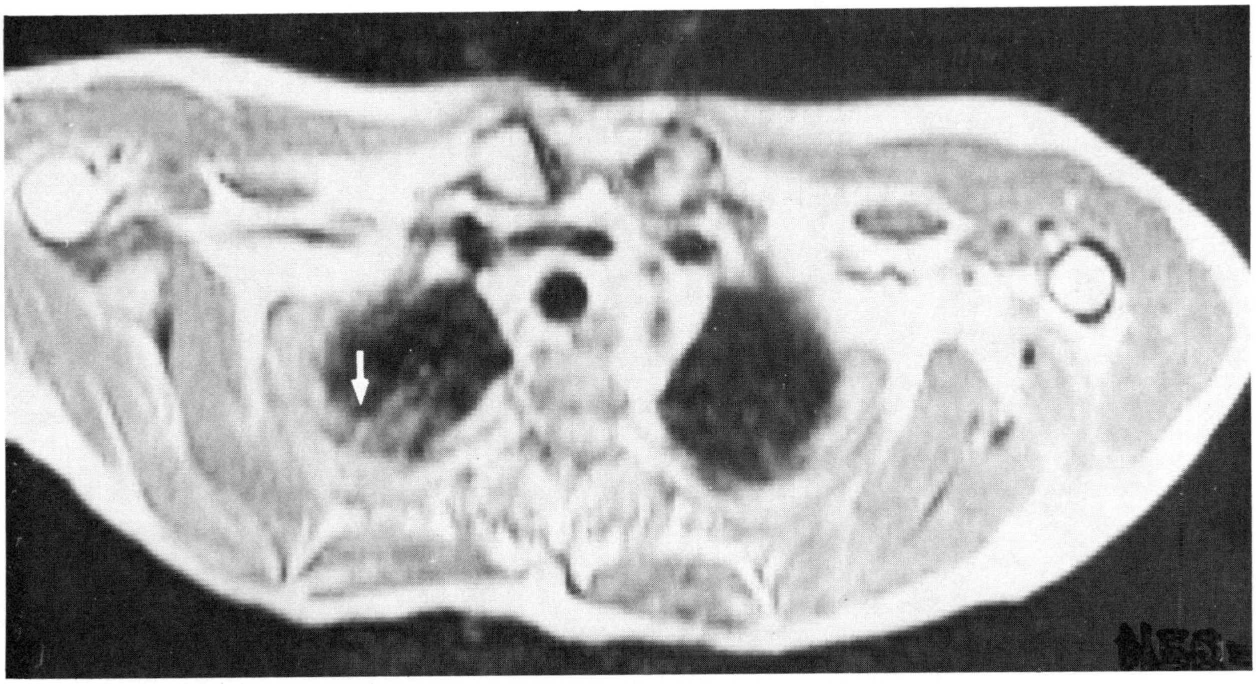

Figure 9.5. Axial slice through upper lungs shows minimal pleural thickening (arrow) together with slight intraparenchymal changes in a patient known with anthraco-silicosis. The lesions were mainly located on the right side.

MRI shows this type of pleural thickening with intermediate signal intensity which does not increase significantly on T_2 pulse sequences. We investigated, by MRI, a patient with known anthraco-silicosis who showed some pleural thickening bilaterally and mainly in the upper halves of both lungs (Figure 9.5). Pleural calcifications, as occurring in asbestosis, are not as easily depicted by MRI as by CT scanning due to their very low signal intensity which can not readily be separated from the low signal intensity lungs.

NEOPLASTIC DISEASES

Whenever a localized pleural change is discovered radiographically, the possibility of the presence of a pleural tumor — either a mesothelioma or a metastatic deposit — has to be excluded. Local mesotheliomas are usually pedunculated and originating from the visceral pleura in most of the cases. Diffuse mesotheliomas are highly invasive malignant tumors, frequently occurring after exposure to asbestos. This neoplasm infiltrates the entire pleural cavity and encases the lung. These tumors may appear as very large and lobulated pleural masses causing extreme compression of the lung,

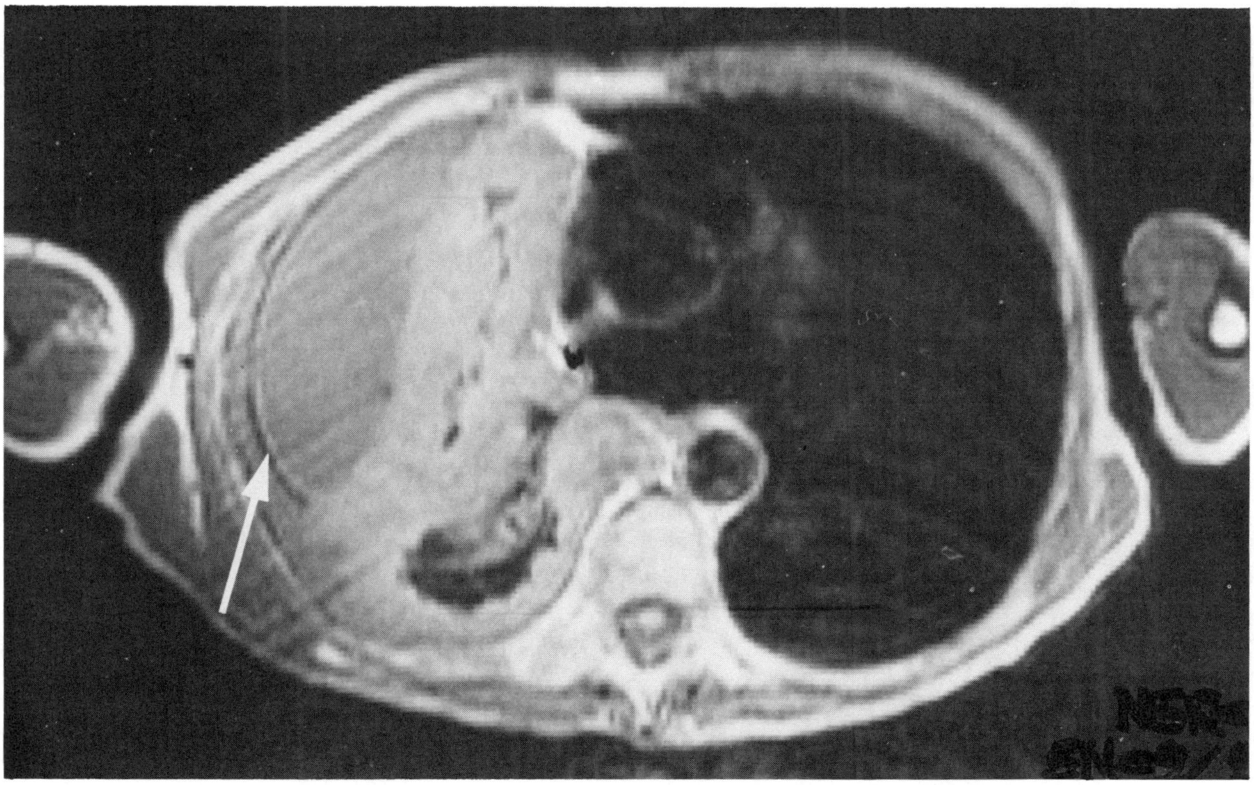

Figure 9.6. T_1 image demonstrates extensive malignant pleural mesothelioma on the right with enclosed fluid collection which is seen with relatively low signal intensity (arrow).

sometimes invading the mediastinum or associated with ipsilateral pleural fluid collections (Figure 9.6). These tumors are seen with intermediate signal intensity on T_1 weighted images and show some increase of their signal intensity on T_2 weighted images while pleural fluid generally shows very intensely increased signal intensity (see Figure 7.13). This fluid may have a high bloody content in many cases, therefore a high signal intensity can be observed on both T_1 and T_2 weighted images.

Pleural metastases originate from a variety of primary lesions, often from bronchial and mammary carcinomas as primary tumors, less frequently malignant lymphomas may produce metastatic infiltration of the pleura and chest wall. As shown in Figures 10.22–10.24 pleural metastases have intermediate signal intensity on T_1 weighted images and denote intense increase in signal intensity on T_2 weighted images.

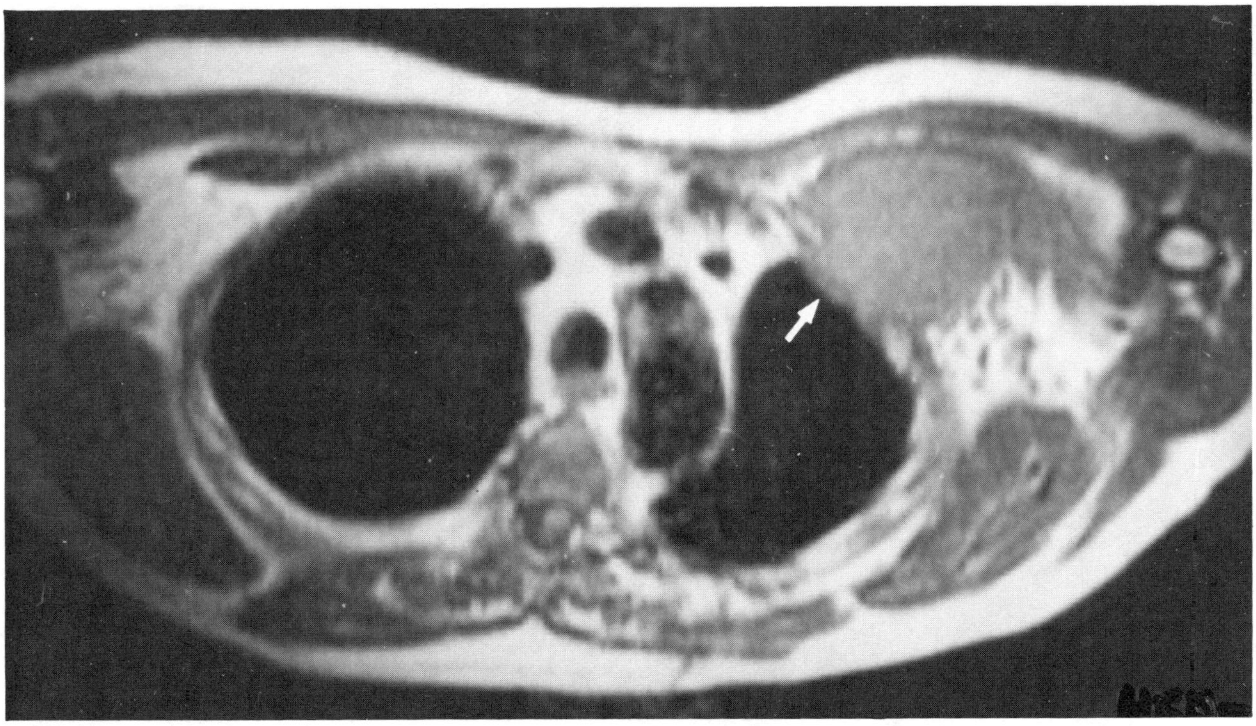

Figure 9.7. Patient with fibrous histiocytoma of the left anterior chest wall shows direct malignant infiltration of pleura (arrow).

In some cases, primary neoplasms of the chest wall may cause malignant infiltration of the adjacent pleura. These neoplasms have intermediate signal intensity on T_1 weighted images and the pleural component has similar signal intensity to the primary mass (Figure 9.7). In the presented case, the mass was caused by a fibrous histiocytoma and invasion of the chest wall was confirmed by surgery. Due to local change in the signal intensity of the intercostal space and of the pleural layers when compared to adjacent structures, malignant invasion of these tissues can easily be recognized by MRI.

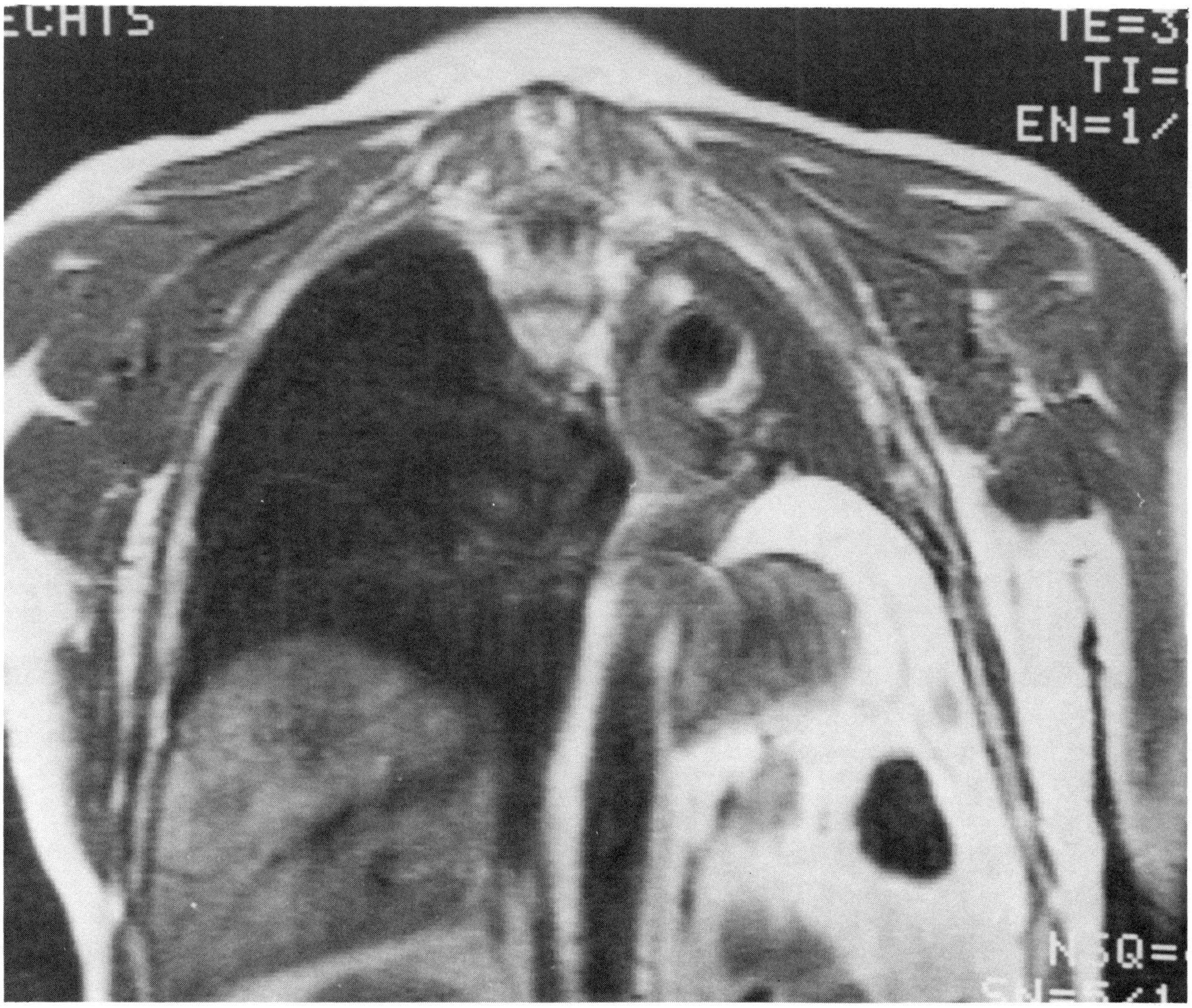

Figure 9.8. Post-pneumonectomy space on the left is filled up by a small amount of fluid. Left diaphragm is elevated. Notice shift of cardio-mediastinal structures and upward displacement of intra-abdominal contents.

Pleural abnormalities are frequently detected on MRI examinations of the thorax and upper abdomen performed for other indications. This statement is even more true for the diaphragm, as primary lesions or neoplasms of the diaphragm are exceedingly rare. Elevation of the diaphragm is the most frequently encountered abnormality which may be due to a number of various causes. Among them, a common reason is the post-pneumonectomy state when elevation of the diaphragm occurs together with cardio-mediastinal shift towards the affected side to fill up the pneumonectomy space. Coronal MRI is particularly suited to visualize accurately cardio-mediastinal structures, the elevated diaphragm and the displaced intra-abdominal contents. These structures can easily be separated from fluid which fills up the post-pneumonectomy cavity (Figure 9.8).

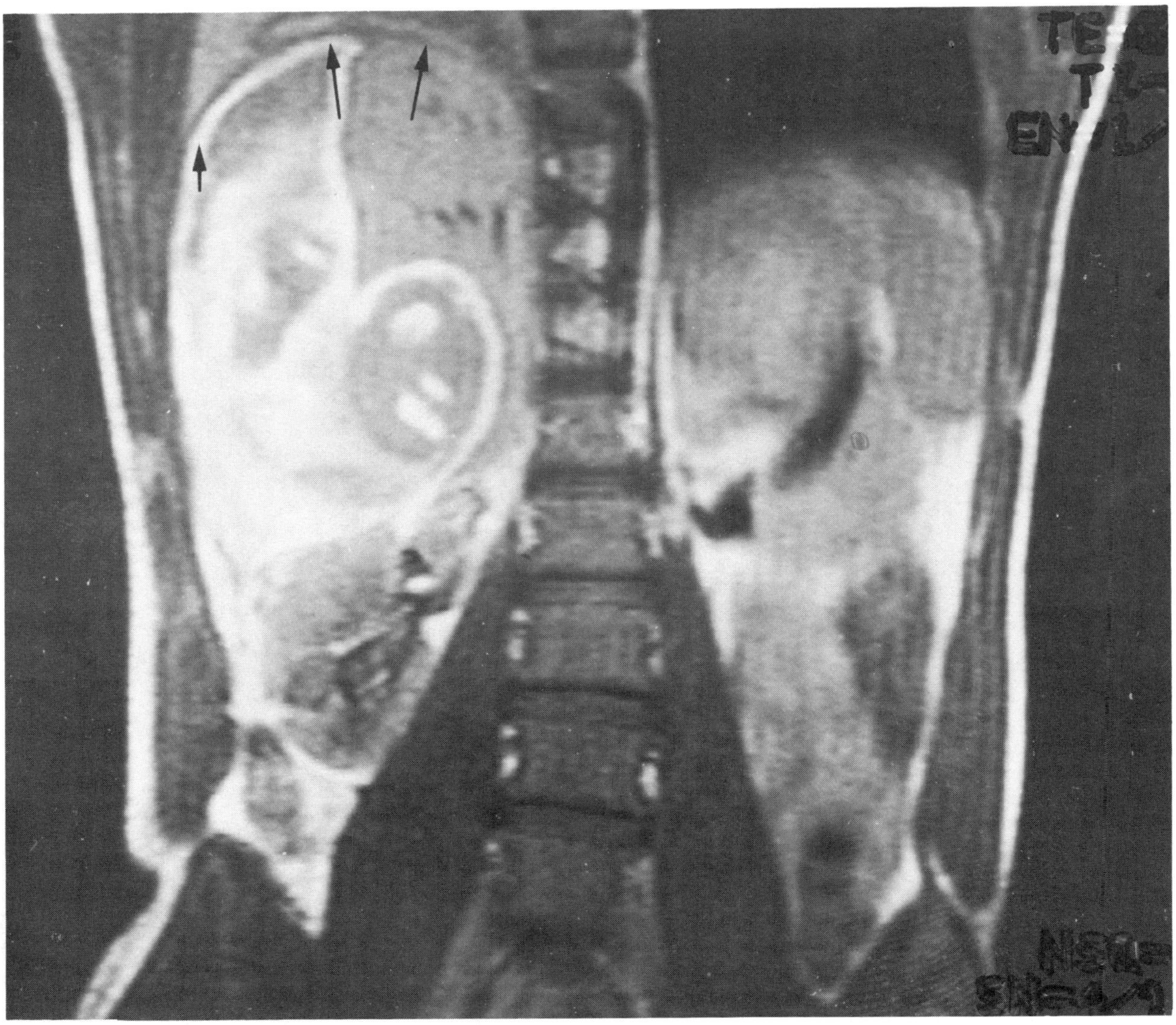

Figure 9.9. Coronal (T_1) image shows extensive subcapsular hematoma of liver. Heterogeneous high signal intensity components of hematoma are easily separated from normal liver parenchyma and right diaphragm (arrows) which is somewhat elevated. Notice supra-diaphragmatic pleural changes.

A different common cause is the presence of sub-diaphragmatic masses or fluid collections. They are frequently represented by liver tumors and subphrenic abscesses. We had a patient showing marked elevation of the right diaphragm caused by a very extensive subcapsular hematoma of the liver. MRI investigation was carried out 10 days after the initial trauma had occurred and the high signal intensity hematoma could easily be differentiated from liver parenchyma on one hand, and from the diaphragm and supra-diaphragmatic changes on the other hand (Figures 9.9, 9.10).

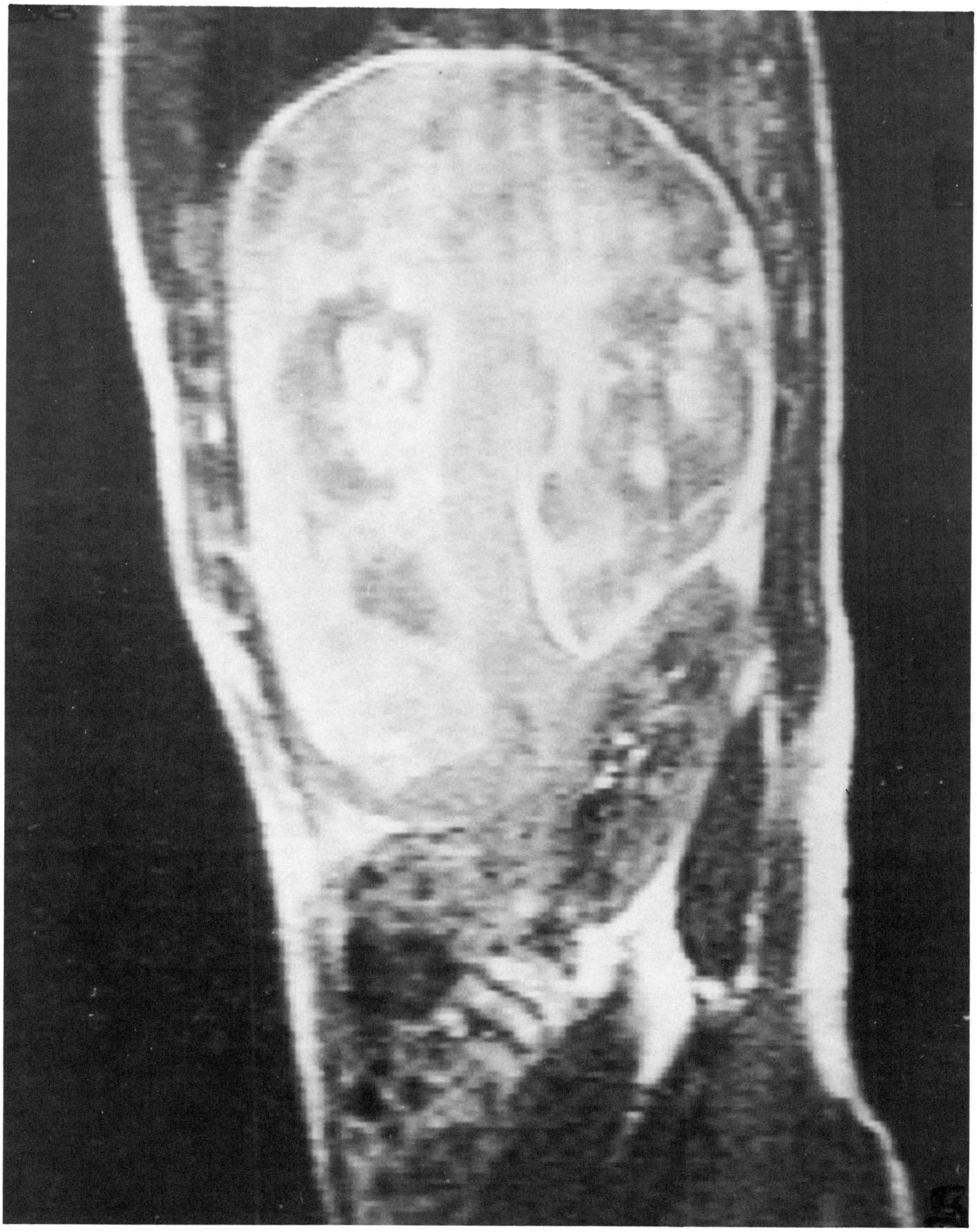

Figure 9.10. Sagittal image illustrates heterogeneous consistency of hematoma, the right diaphragm is obviously elevated. Notice pleural changes posteriorly.

Similarly, we investigated, by MRI, a patient showing extensive changes in the left lower lung. However, due to the presence of pleural fluid and partial atelectasis of the lower lobe, CT scanning was unable to provide sufficient information concerning the underlying pathology. This 20-year-old woman had been operated for an osteosarcoma of the humerus, had undergone irradiation treatment concomitant with chemotherapy. Metastatic disease to the lower chest wall was suspected. For incremental information about this mass and in a view to be able to separate it from the associated pulmonary and pleural changes on the left side, MRI was requested.

Sagittal images using a short TR (300 msec) show a very extensive soft tissue mass of relatively low signal intensity at the postero-basal aspect of the left lung (Figure 9.11), but its location and composition could not be assessed in a more precise manner. T_1 weighted coronal images show obvious atelectasis of the lower lobe, elevation of the diaphragm by an underlying mass of relatively heterogeneous consistency (Figure 9.12). This mass denounced intense increasement of its signal intensity on T_2 weighted images (Figure 9.13). Furthermore, axial images through the upper half of the thorax demonstrated quite massive left-sided thickening of heterogeneous consistency due to pleural effusion and malignant tissue formation (Figure 9.14). This woman had massive subphrenic metastatic spread causing elevation of the diaphragm. Because of tissue changes in the adjacent supra-diaphragmatic region, both components were not easily differentiated from each other and from the diaphragm. For this purpose, coronal and sagittal T_1 and T_2 weighted images are particularly helpful as they permit more accurate determination of the different structures which may be separated from each other in an easier way. For the same reason, we believe that herniations and traumatic ruptures of the diaphragm can more easily be recognized by MRI than by conventional transverse CT scanning.

As it seems by now, MRI has some value in the evaluation of pleural, thoracic wall and diaphragmatic abnormalities, major benefit arising from the existent possibilities of multiplanar imaging. Also, the inherent high contrast resolution of MRI may serve as an adjuvent in the often difficult diagnosis of complex pathological findings in these areas.

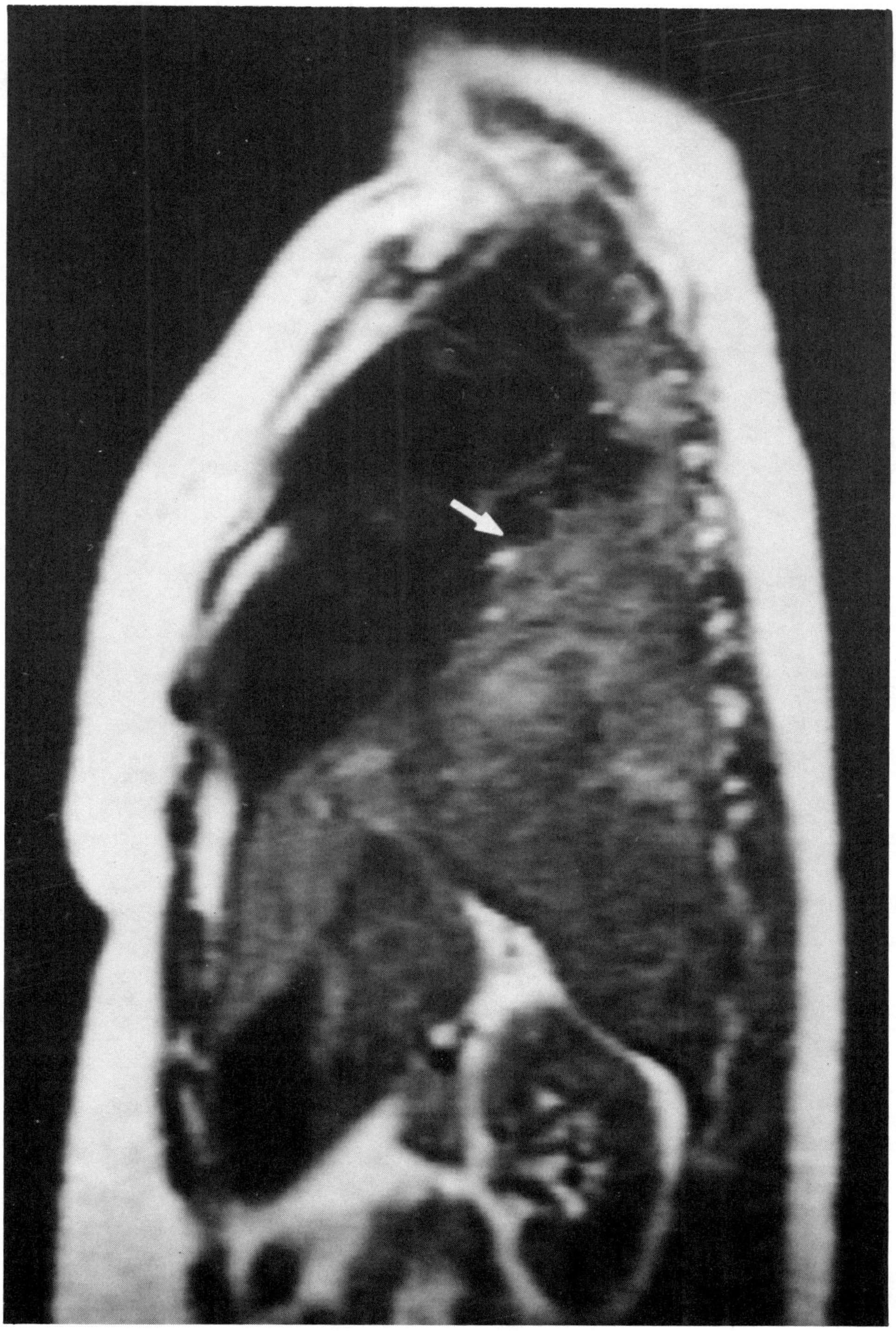

Figure 9.11. Patient showing extensive soft tissue mass at postero-basal aspect of the left lung on sagittal MR slice (arrow).

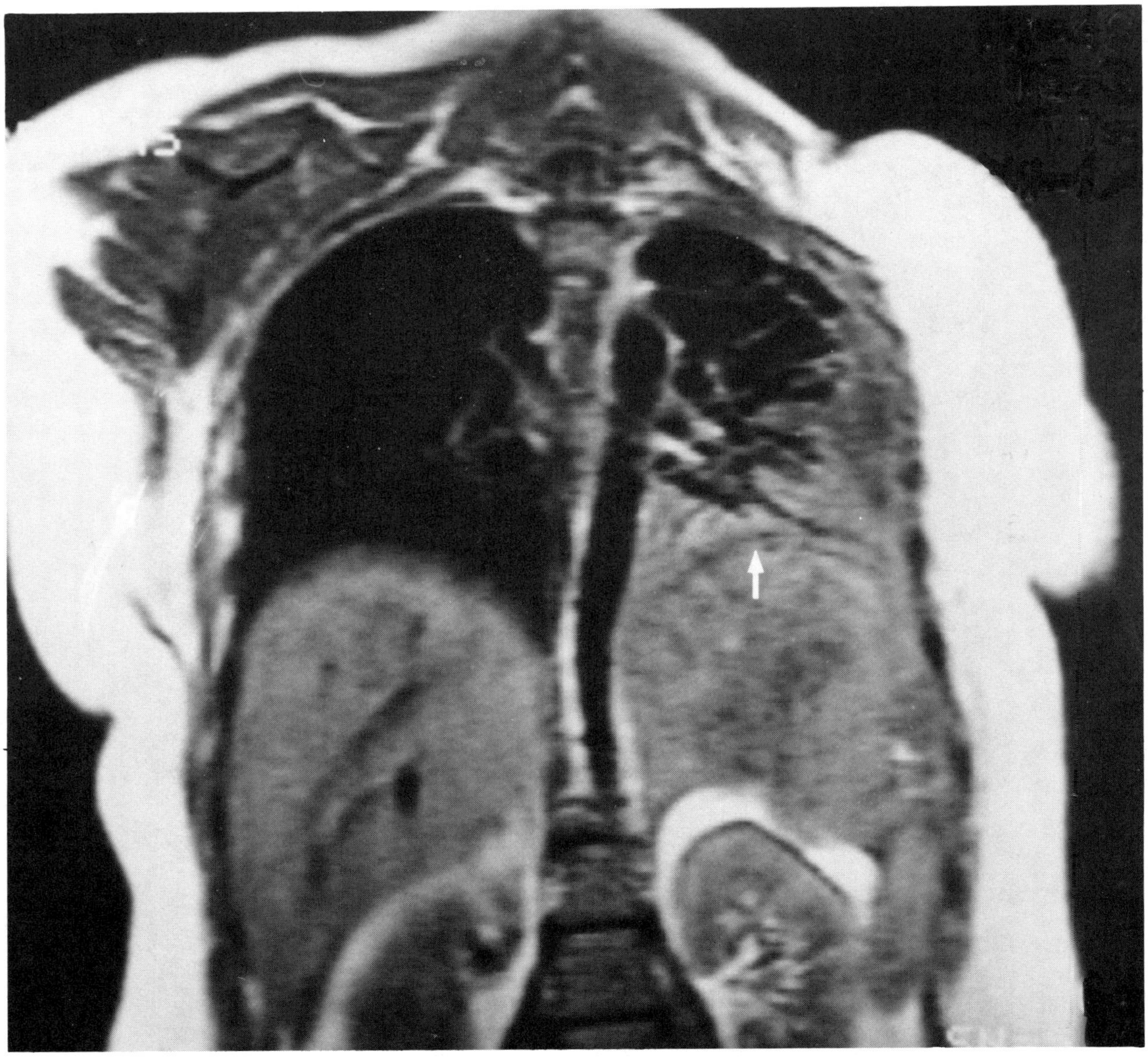

Figure 9.12. Coronal T_1 image shows lower lobe atelectasis and large heterogeneous mass elevating the diaphragm (arrow).

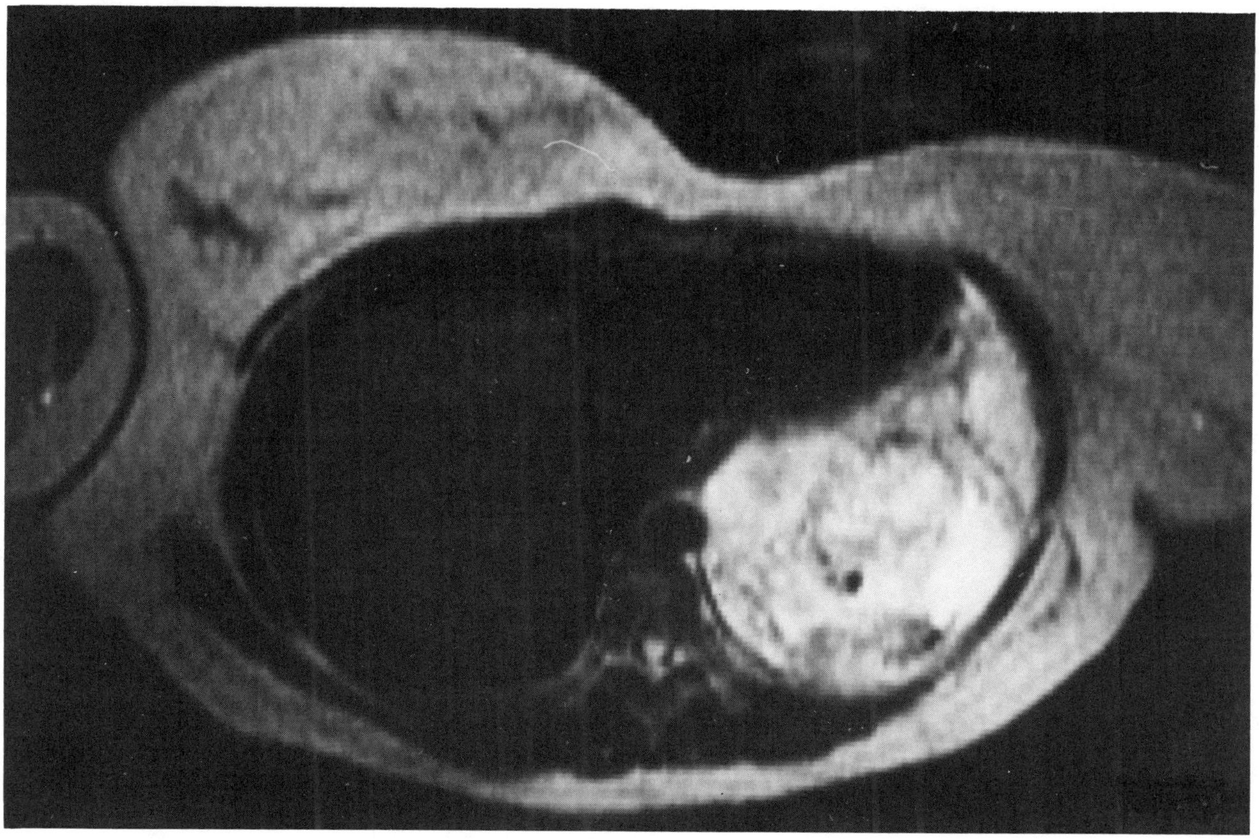

Figure 9.13. Axial T_2 image shows markedly increased signal intensity of mass and its consistency is much more heterogeneous than on Figure 9.12.

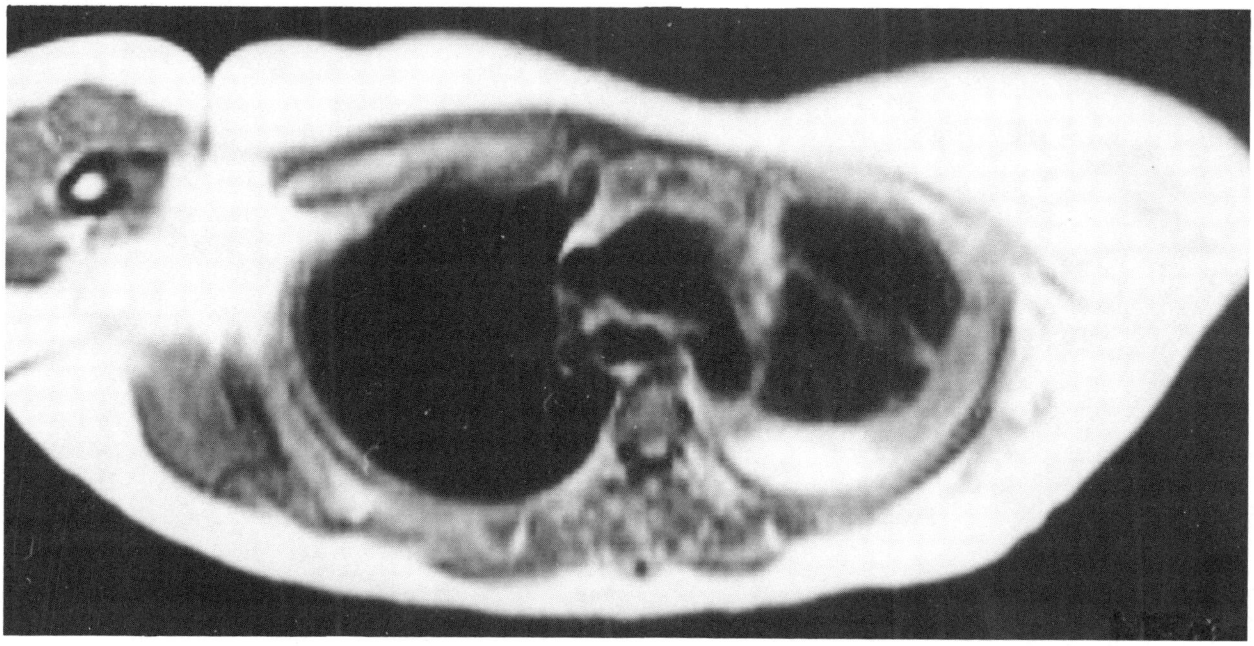

Figure 9.14. Left-sided pleural thickening due to pleural effusion and malignant tissue infiltration.

REFERENCES

1. Revel D, Terrier F, Hricak H, Higgins CB: Determination of the nature of pleural effusions with MR imaging. RSNA Scientific Program, Washington, DC, Radiologic Society of North America, 1984.

2. Brown JJ, van Sonnenberg E, Gerber KH, Strich G, Wittich GR, Slutsky RA: Magnetic resonance relaxation times of percutaneously obtained normal and abnormal body fluids. *Radiology, 154:*727-731, 1985.

10

Selected Cases

CASE 1

A 55-year-old man was known with longstanding shoulder pain on the left side. Conventional x-rays of the cervical spine and of the left shoulder provided no evident explanation for this pain.

Since MRI is a diagnostic tool capable of providing very accurate imaging of the musculo-skeletal system, MRI investigation of the thoracic wall was requested. The posterior thoracic wall on the left side was very accurately examined by MRI, and image zooming was performed in this area to optimalize the anatomical representation. Spin echo images using a short TR (500 msec) and cardiac gating showed no abnormalities of the musculo-skeletal system on the left, but an obvious anterior mediastinal mass with relatively low signal intensity was also demonstrated at the superior edge of the image (Figure 10.1). This mass was located just in front of the main mediastinal vessels. Sagittal MR imaging showed the mass with intermediate signal intensity, thus confirming the previous findings on transverse slices. The lesion had homogeneous consistency, regular outlines and there was no evident compression of the mediastinal vessels (Figure 10.2). On T_2 weighted images using a TR 3000 msec and four delayed echoes (32, 64, 96, 128 msec) the signal intensity of this mass did not show obvious increasement (Figure 10.3) while it became relatively more inhomogeneous.

At this stage, an MRI diagnosis of an anterior mediastinal mass of unknown etiology was made. This mass did not compress the surrounding structures. Conventional films of the chest showed the presence of a metallic foreign body in the region of the right pulmonary hilum (Figure 10.4).

The patient was a hunting sportsman enthusiast and other metallic foreign bodies were disseminated throughout his body. One shot was located behind the left scapula and was eventually responsible for the patient's pain. We believe that the anterior mediastinal mass of intermediate signal intensity is due to fibrotic changes along the pathway followed by a shot through the patient's chest occurring during a hunting accident. It has to be

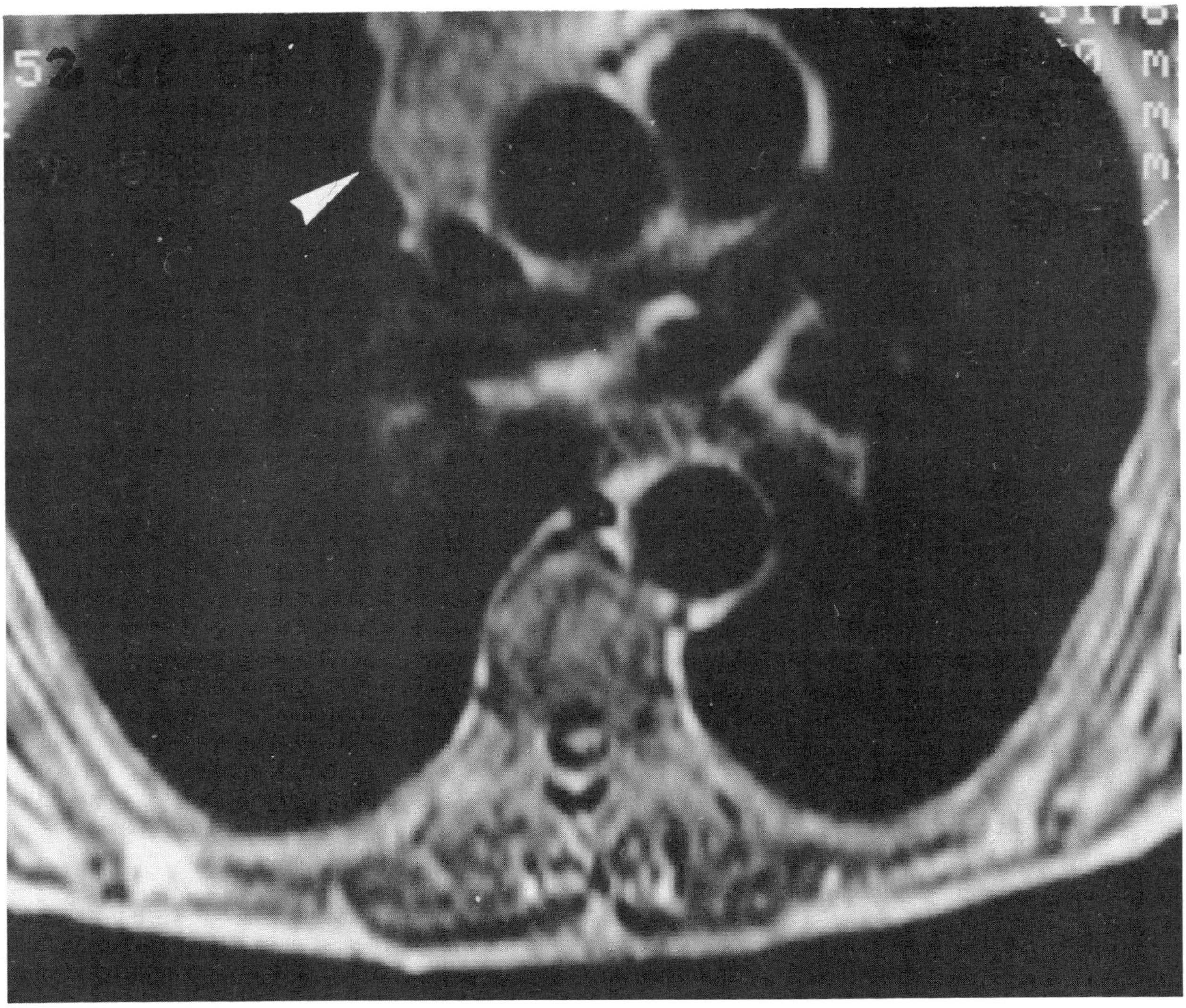

Figure 10.1

noted that this foreign body was not delineated by MRI as it consists of lead, a non-magnetic material. It has inherent low signal intensity and cannot be separated from surrounding structures by MRI. In this particular case, MRI was able to delineate a lesion at a distant site from the area of original interest and its benign nature could be confirmed.

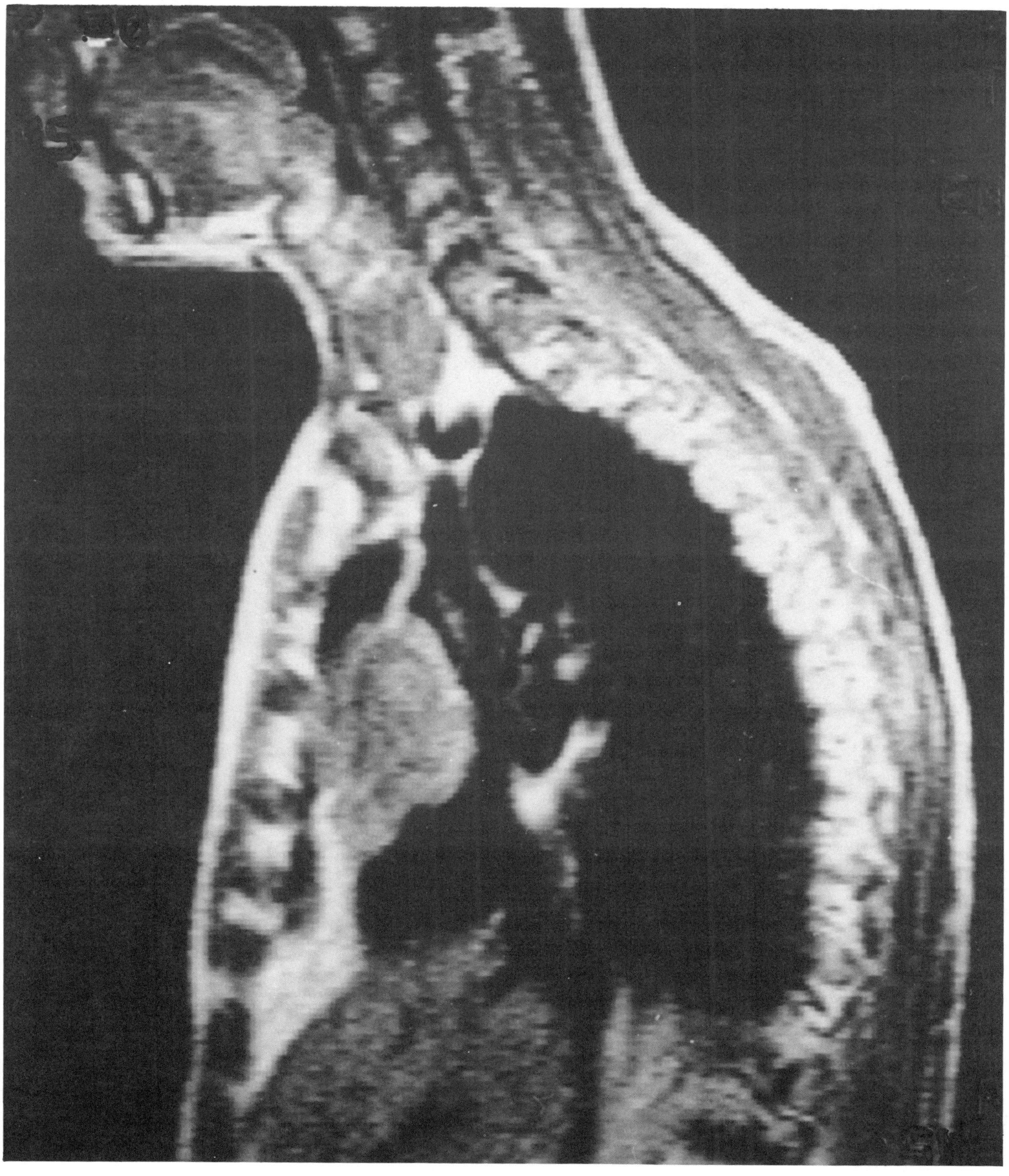

Figure 10.2

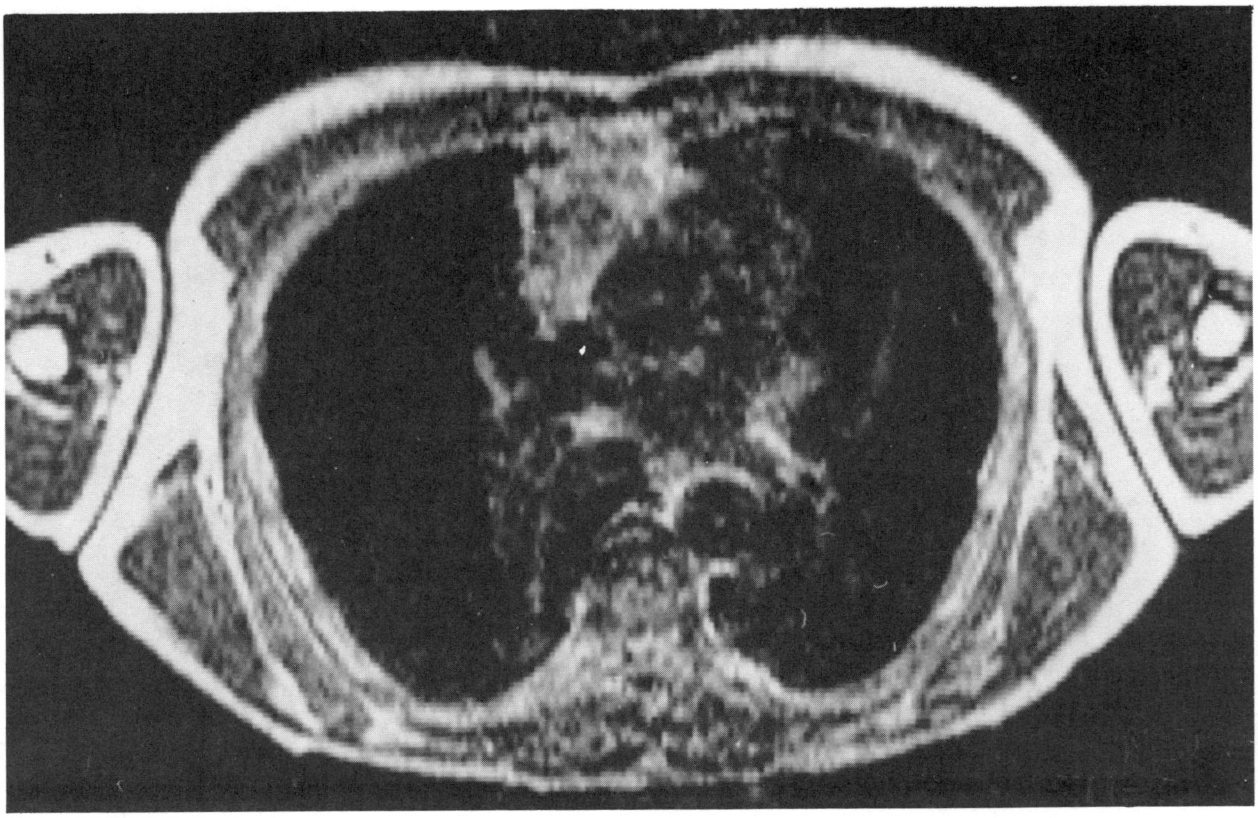

Figure 10.3

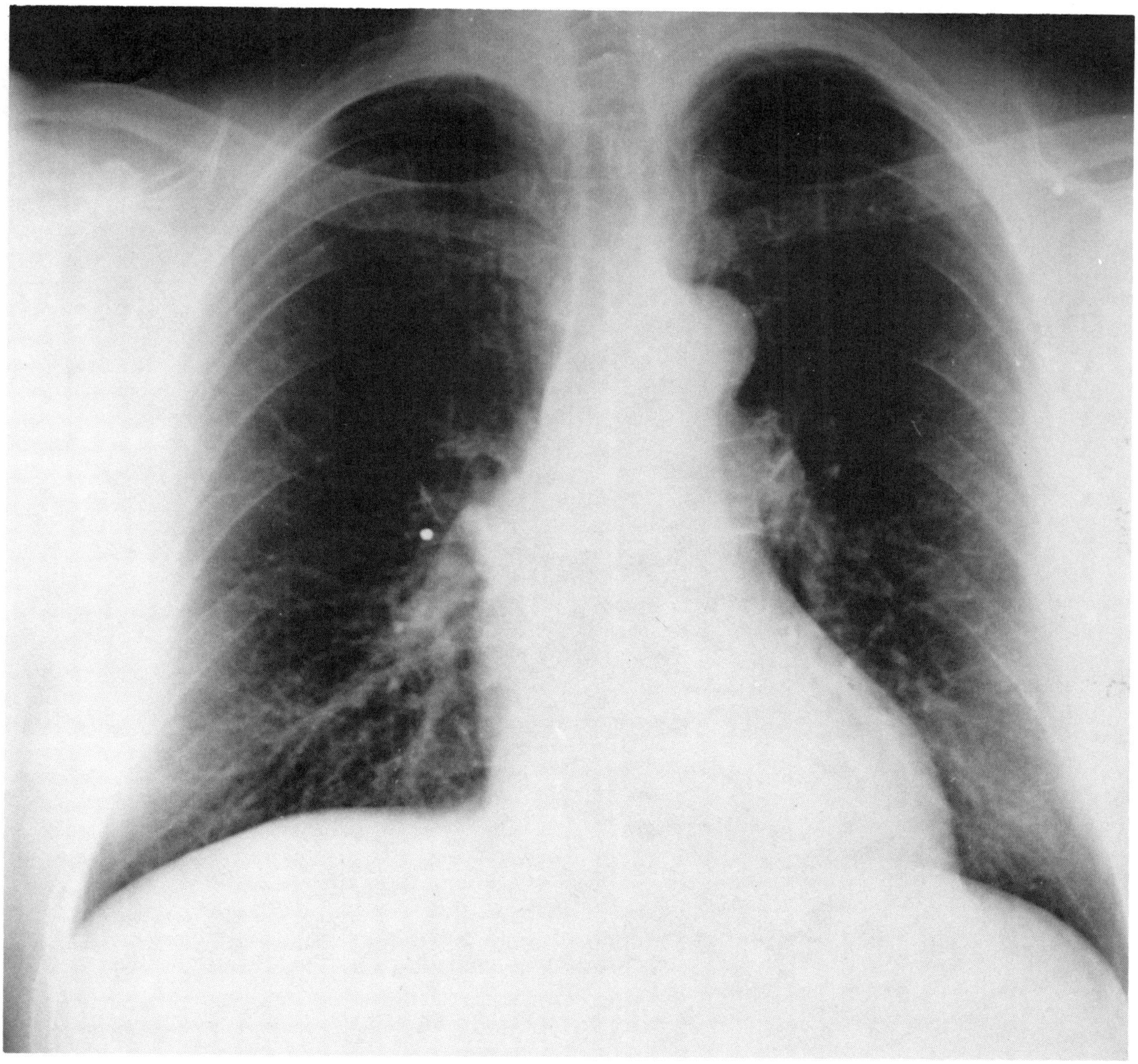

Figure 10.4

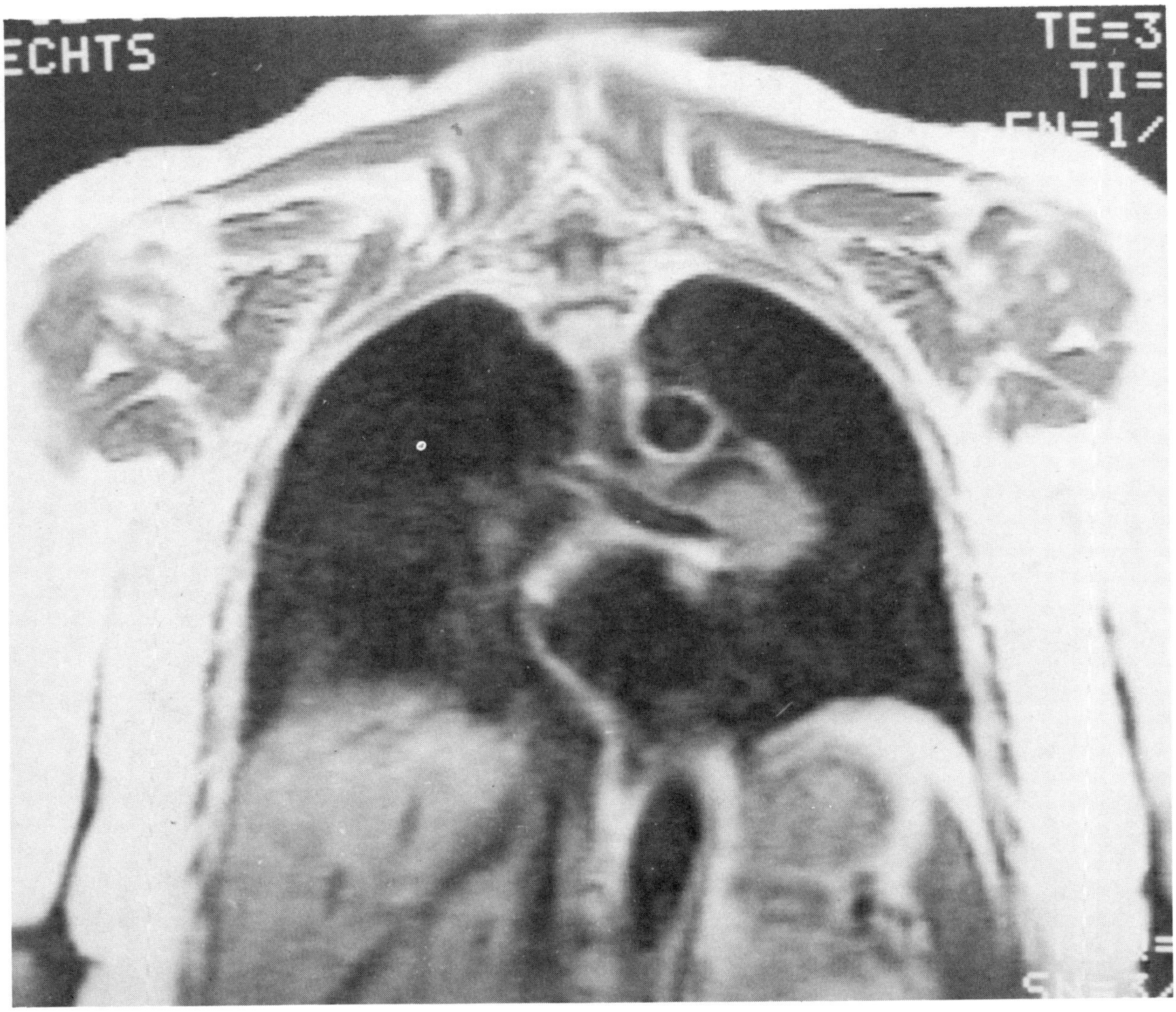

Figure 10.5

CASE 2

A 64-year-old man was found to have a hilar tumor with post-stenotic atelectasis of the left upper lobe. For incremental information, the patient was referred to our clinic for MR imaging of the chest, in the hope that additional data concerning preoperative staging of the lesion could be obtained. A three-planar MRI examination of the thorax using short TRs was performed since the main interest was on the mediastinum. As stated in chapter 5, mediastinal masses and/or lymphadenopathy are most accurately visualized in T_1 weighted images, since they are imaged with intermediate signal intensity by these pulse sequences. Consequently, they can easily be separated from the broncho-vascular tree on one hand, and from mediastinal fat on the other hand.

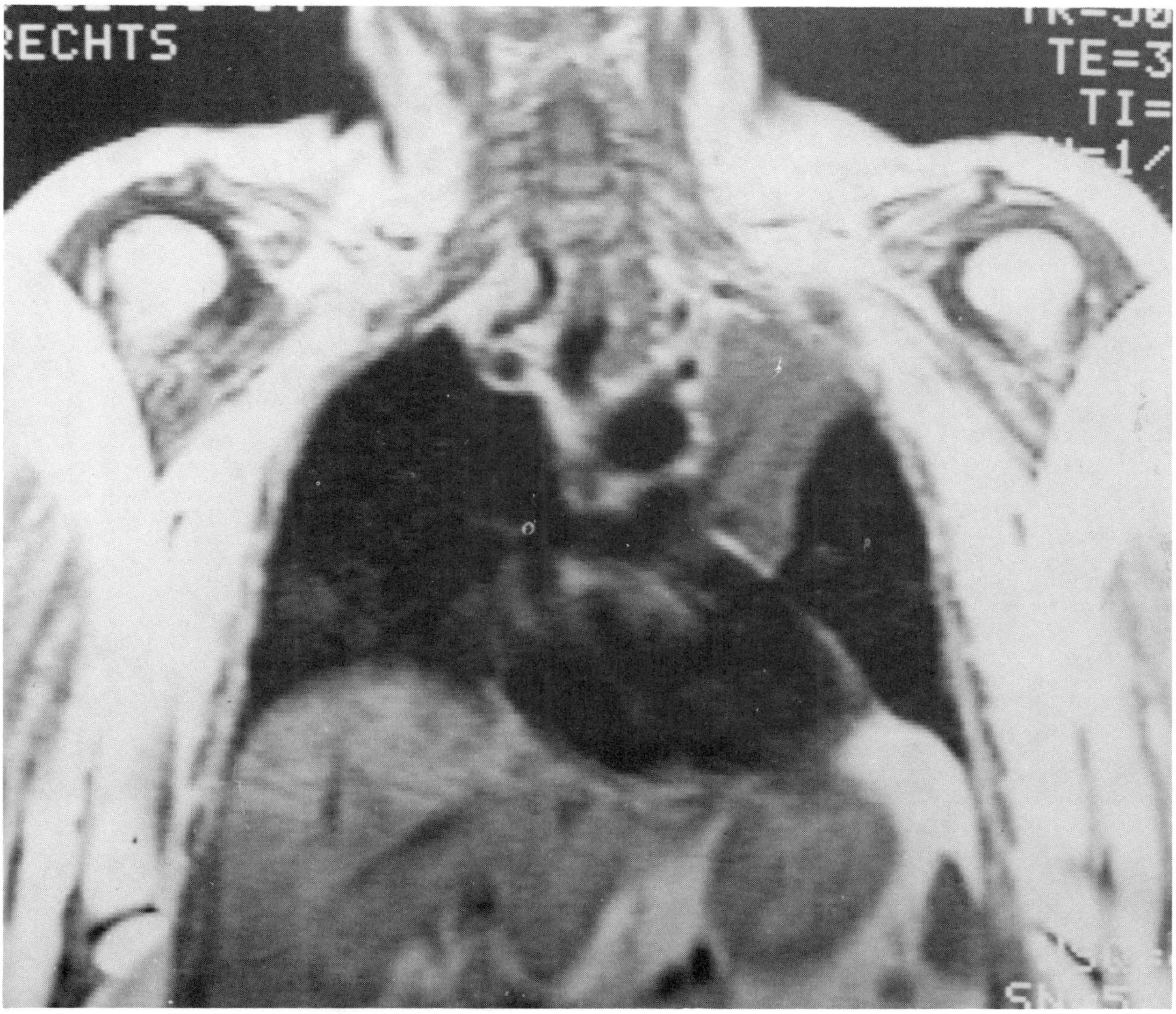

Figure 10.6

Coronal MR images demonstrated very clearly the hilar tumor which appeared to invade the mediastinum (Figure 10.5). Atelectasis of the left upper lobe was also outlined, the signal intensity of collapsed lung being very similar to the signal intensity of tumor (Figure 10.6). Axial slices confirmed mediastinal invasion by the tumor, they also demonstrated compression of the broncho-vascular structures within the left hilum, mainly of the left pulmonary artery (Figure 10.7). Axial images passing through the upper mediastinum showed obvious paratracheal lymphadenopathy (arrow) (Figure 10.8). This case illustrates that MRI may play an important role in the preoperative staging of bronchogenic carcinoma in the future.

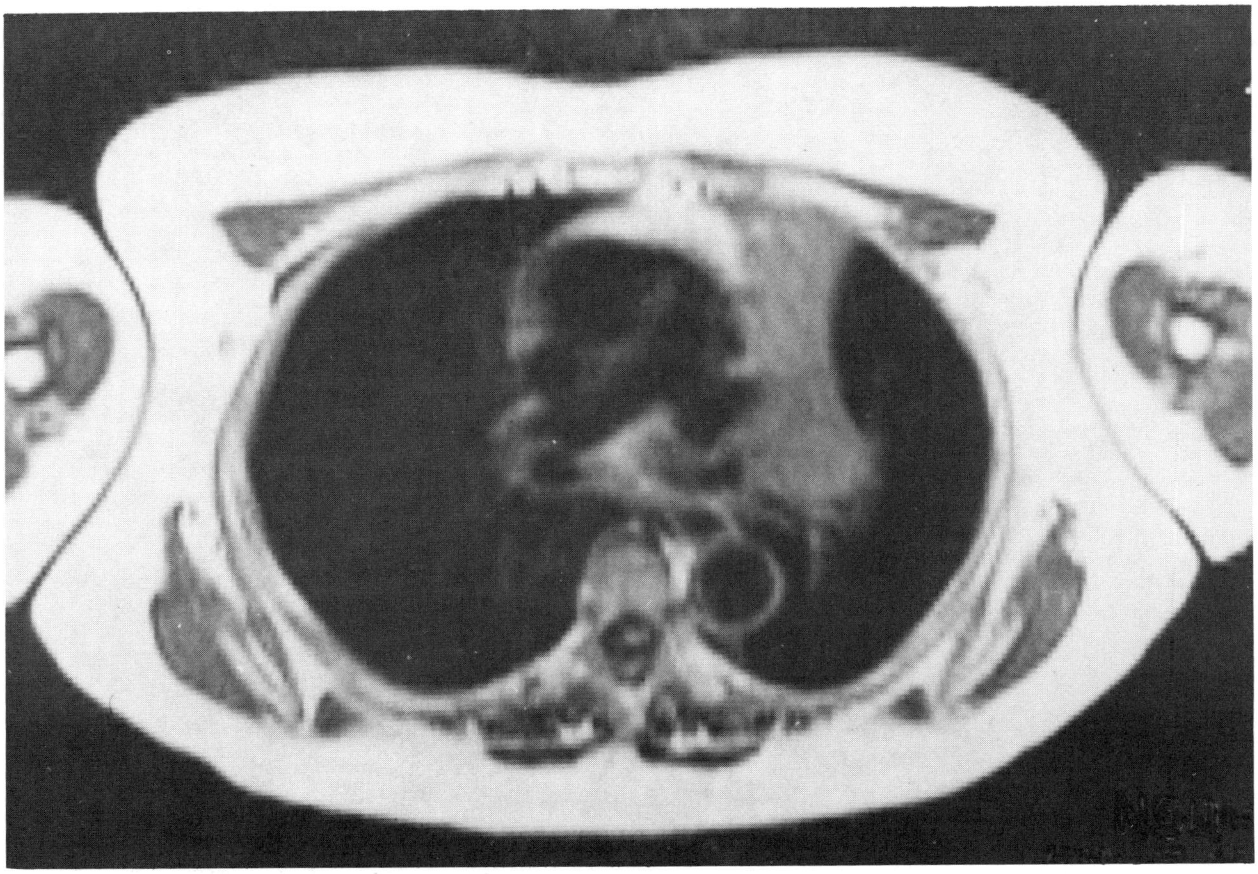

Figure 10.7

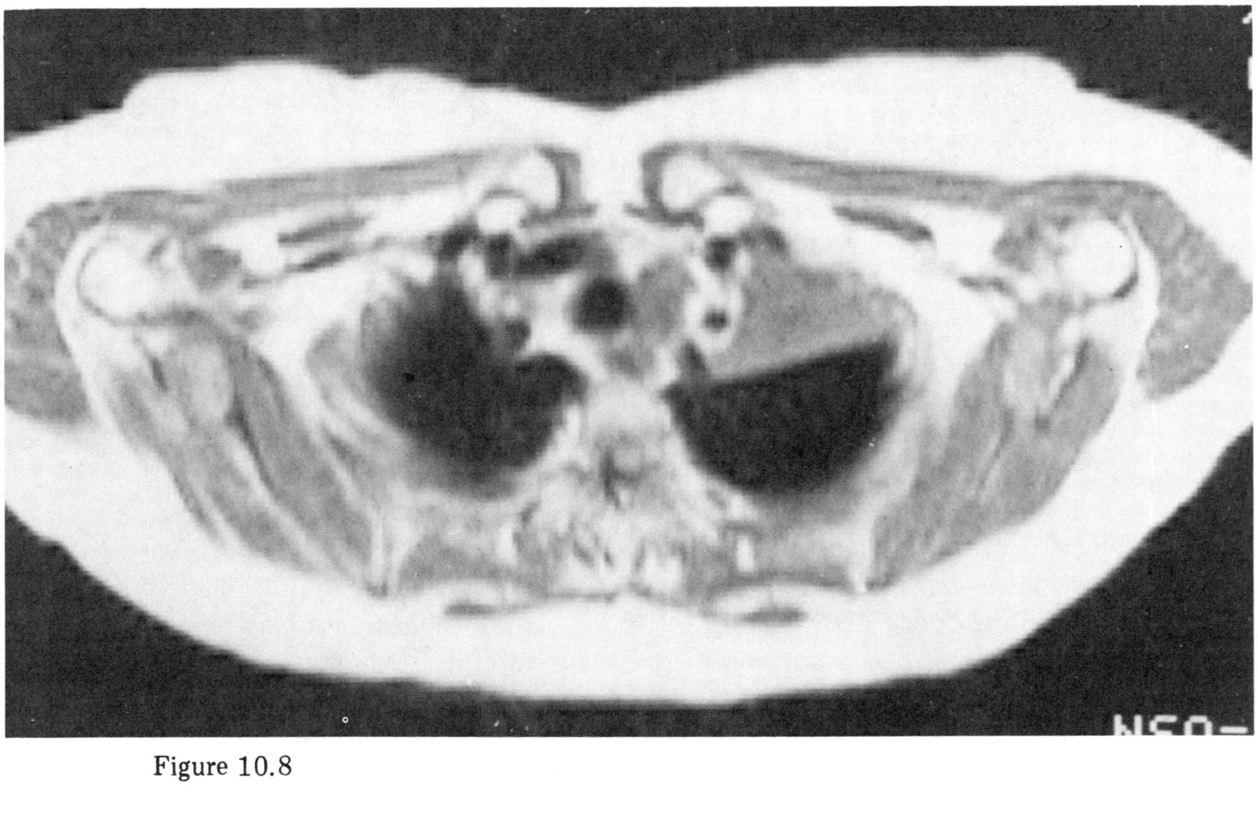

Figure 10.8

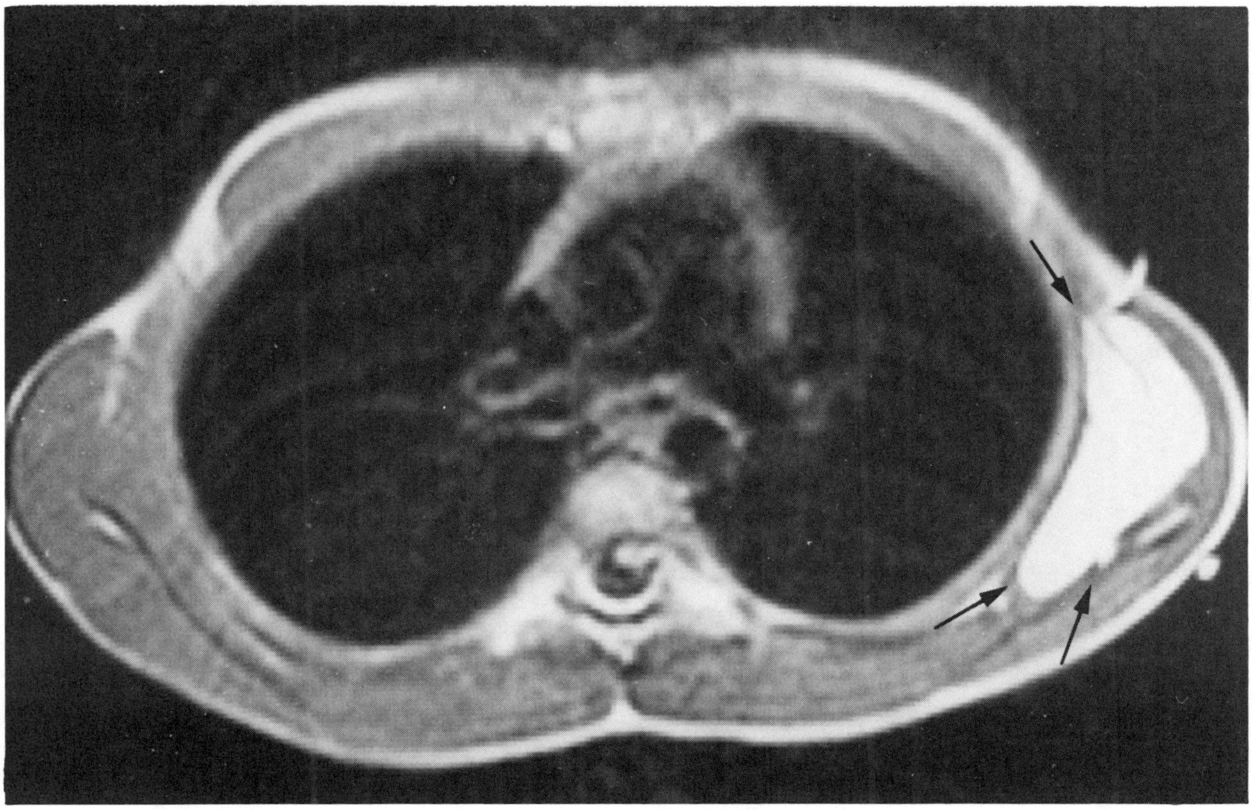

Figure 10.9

CASE 3

A 12-year-old boy presented with a painless soft tissue swelling located at the postero-lateral aspect of the left thoracic wall. Preoperative evaluation of this thoracic mass was requested and MRI appeared to be an adequate non-invasive diagnostic tool to evaluate the lesion presented by this young patient. It was believed that MRI could provide additional information about etiology and precise location of this mass.

MR imaging was performed in the axial and sagittal planes. Axial images using a short TR (630 msec) and a 192 x 256 matrix clearly demonstrated a relatively large and sharply delineated soft tissue mass located between the muscular layers of the postero-lateral portion of the left chest wall. This mass showed very high signal intensity, had homogeneous consistency and did not invade surrounding tissues (Figure 10.9). T_2 weighted images (TR 3000 msec, TE 32 and 90 msec) showed no significant increase of the

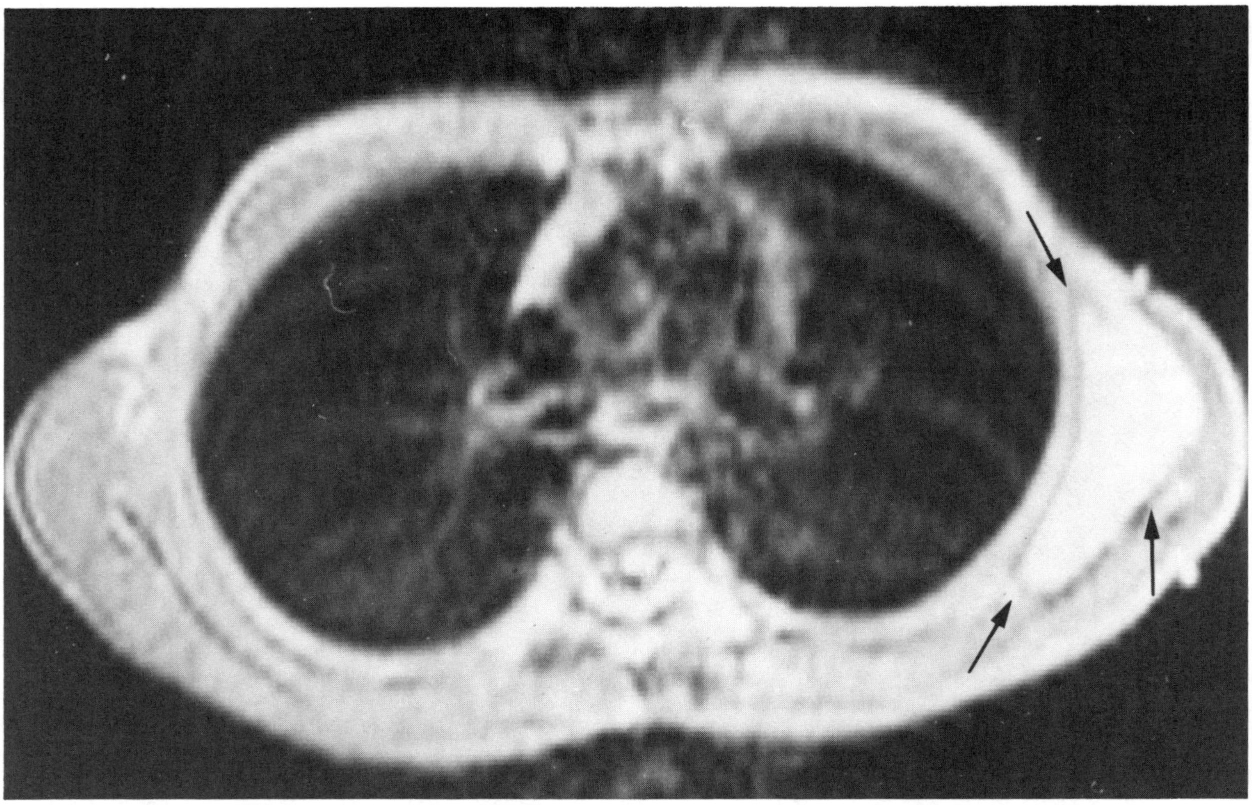

Figure 10.10

signal intensity of this mass which remained homogeneous in appearance (Figure 10.10). Sagittal images showed the exact location of this mass as it was located under the subscapular and infraspinatus muscles (Figure 10.11). The mass showing high signal intensity on both T_1 and T_2 weighted images (short T_1 and T_2 relaxation times), a differential diagnosis between a lipoma and a post-traumatic hematoma had to be considered. The mass also had very regular outlines and no trauma could be traced in the patient's anamnesis so that a presumptive diagnosis of an intramural lipoma was made. This diagnosis was confirmed by subsequent surgery.

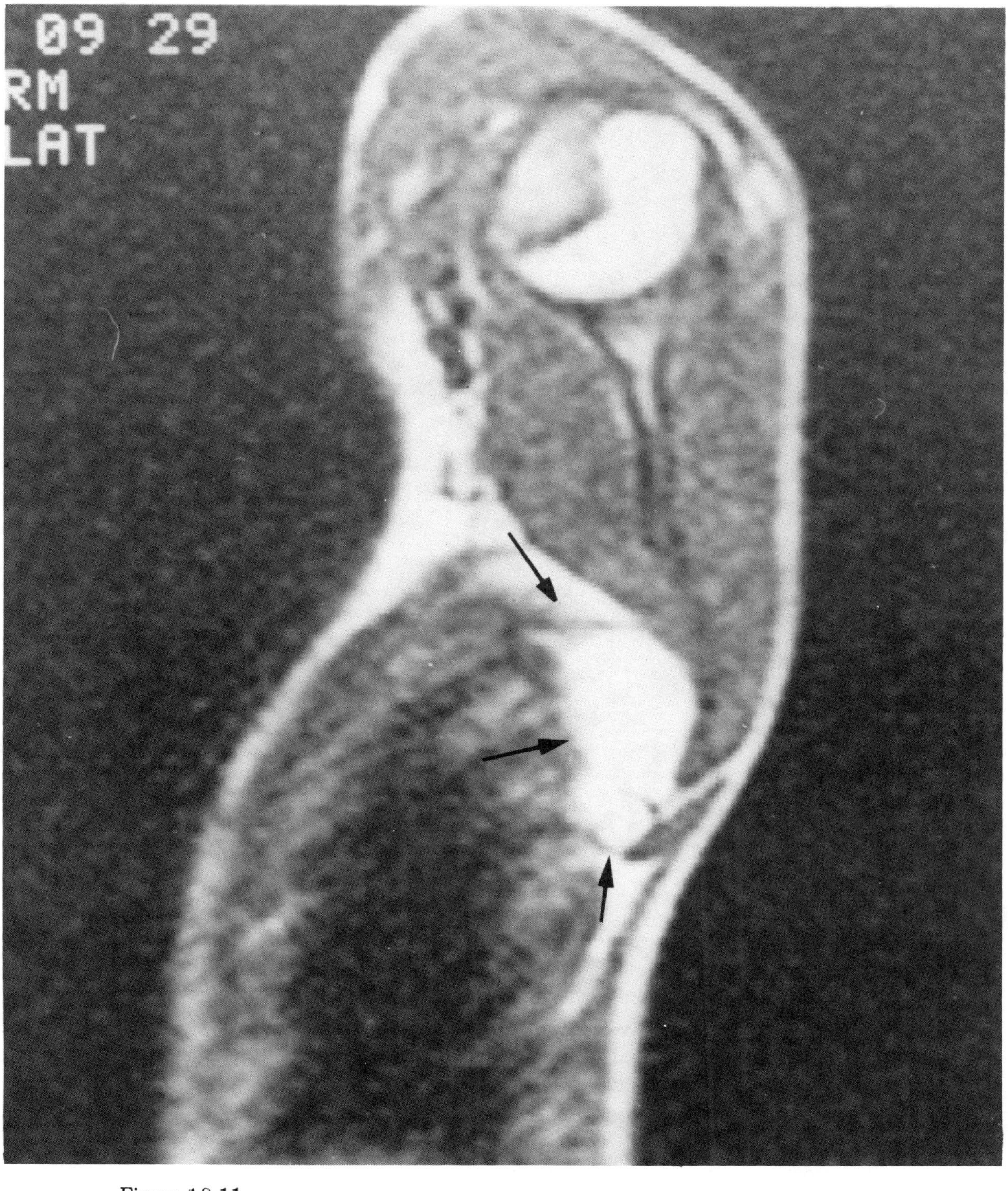

Figure 10.11

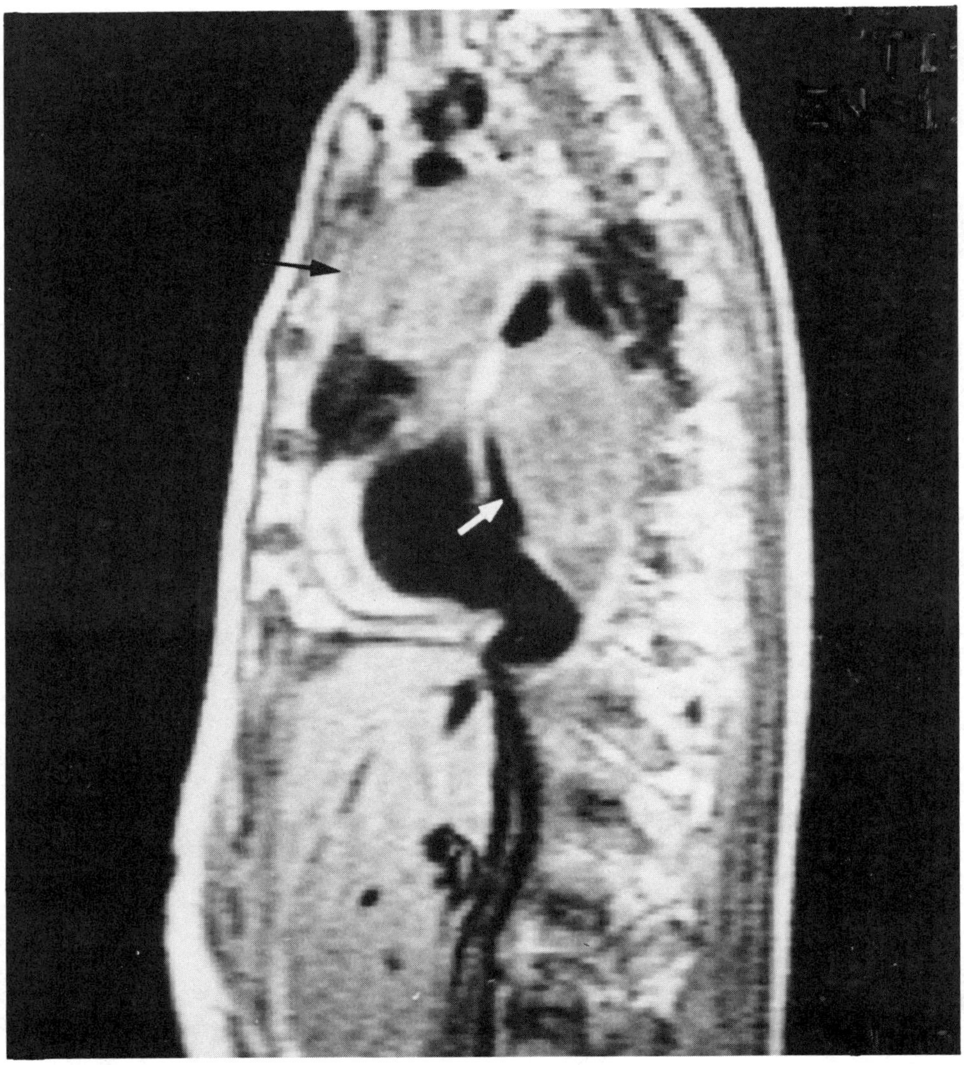

Figure 10.12

CASE 4

A 24-year-old woman had been operated on for a sarcoma of the right anterior chest wall which was surgically resected. Two years later she was admitted again since a tumor recurrence was suspected. Conventional radiography and computed tomography of the chest were requested. Standard films demonstrated an opaque lower hemithorax on the right side and the cardiac silhouette appeared to be somewhat enlarged. The patient had also undergone irradiation treatment and a clinical diagnosis of pericarditis with right pleural effusion was made. CT of the chest showed, moreover, a right paraspinal soft tissue mass which was obviously not related to the spine. In a view to obtain further information about this mass, mainly concerning tissue characterization, MRI of the chest was performed.

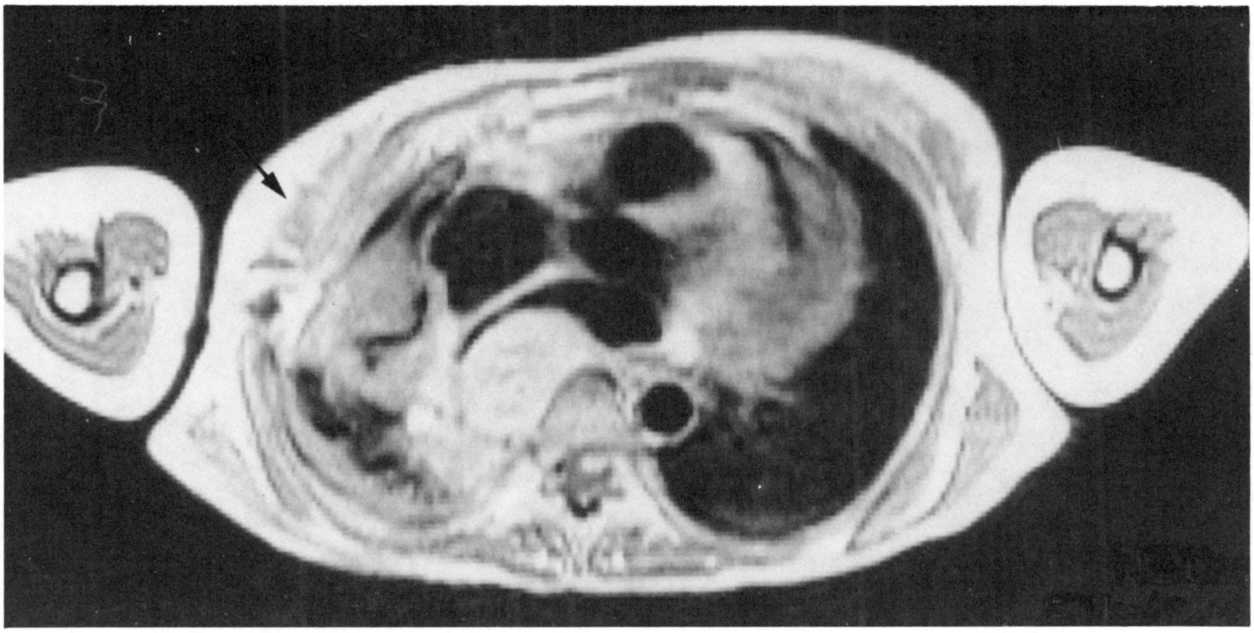

Figure 10.13

Sagittal images using cardiac gating demonstrated an obvious mass of intermediate signal intensity just in front of the right costovertebral gutter (Figure 10.12). Furthermore, another soft tissue mass of intermediate signal intensity was seen within the upper mediastinum. This lesion had regular boundaries, had a slightly inhomogeneous consistency and was located just behind the sternum (Figure 10.12). T_1 weighted axial slices with cardiac gating outlined the right paravertebral mass which compressed and displaced the main bronchus. Postoperative changes were found (arrow) on the anterior chest wall on the right side (Figure 10.13). A quite large tumor mass of intermediate signal intensity was outlined within the upper mediastinum (Figure 10.14). T_2 weighted images (TR 3000 msec, TE 32, 64, 96 and 128 msec) without cardiac gating showed a markedly increased signal intensity of all these masses (Figure 10.15). Malignant tissue showing high signal intensity was also found in the right parahilar region. The appearance on T_1 and T_2 weighted images seemed to be typical for malignant disease and a diagnosis of intrathoracic metastatic spread was made. Sternotomy was performed and a biopsy confirmed the MRI diagnosis of metastatic seeding. The patient died two months later.

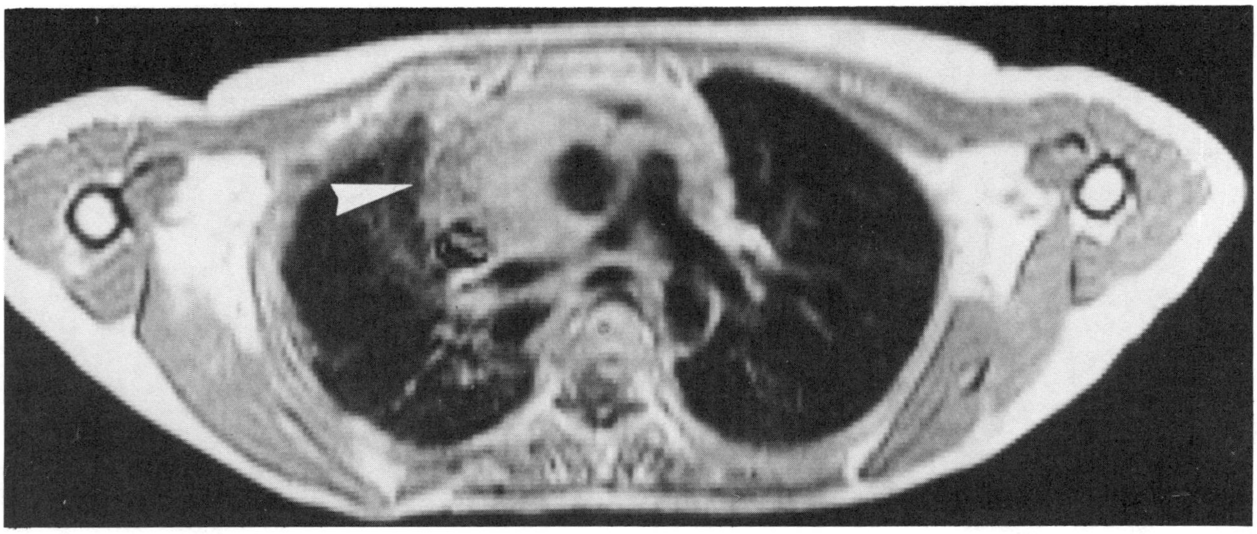

Figure 10.14

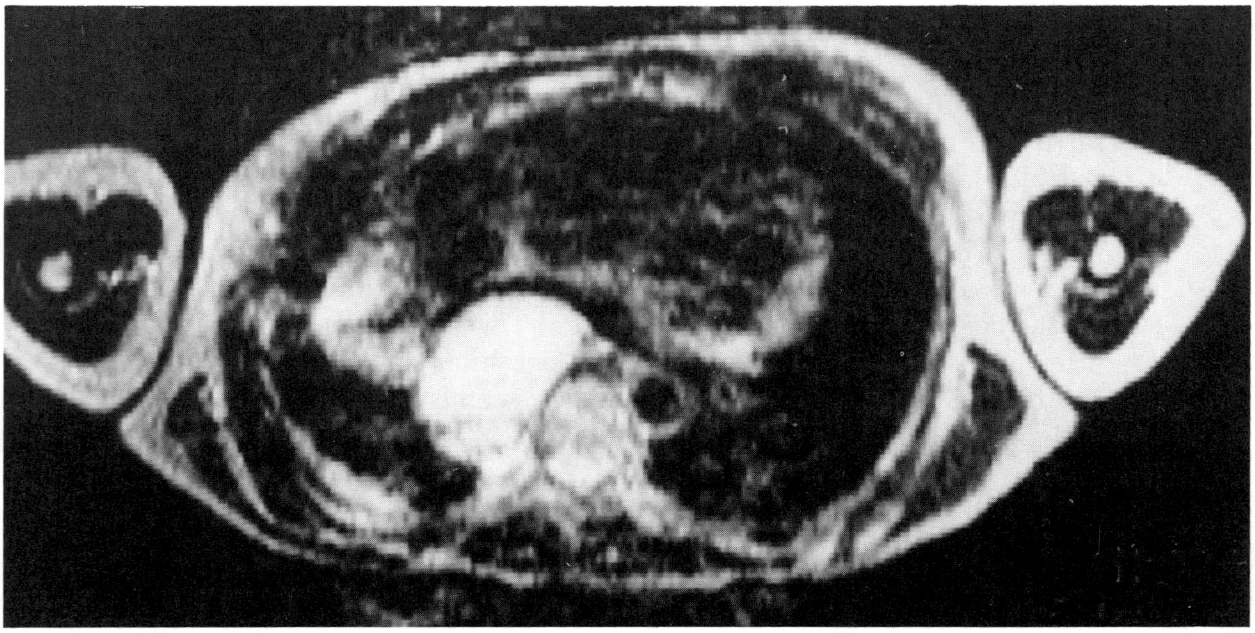

Figure 10.15

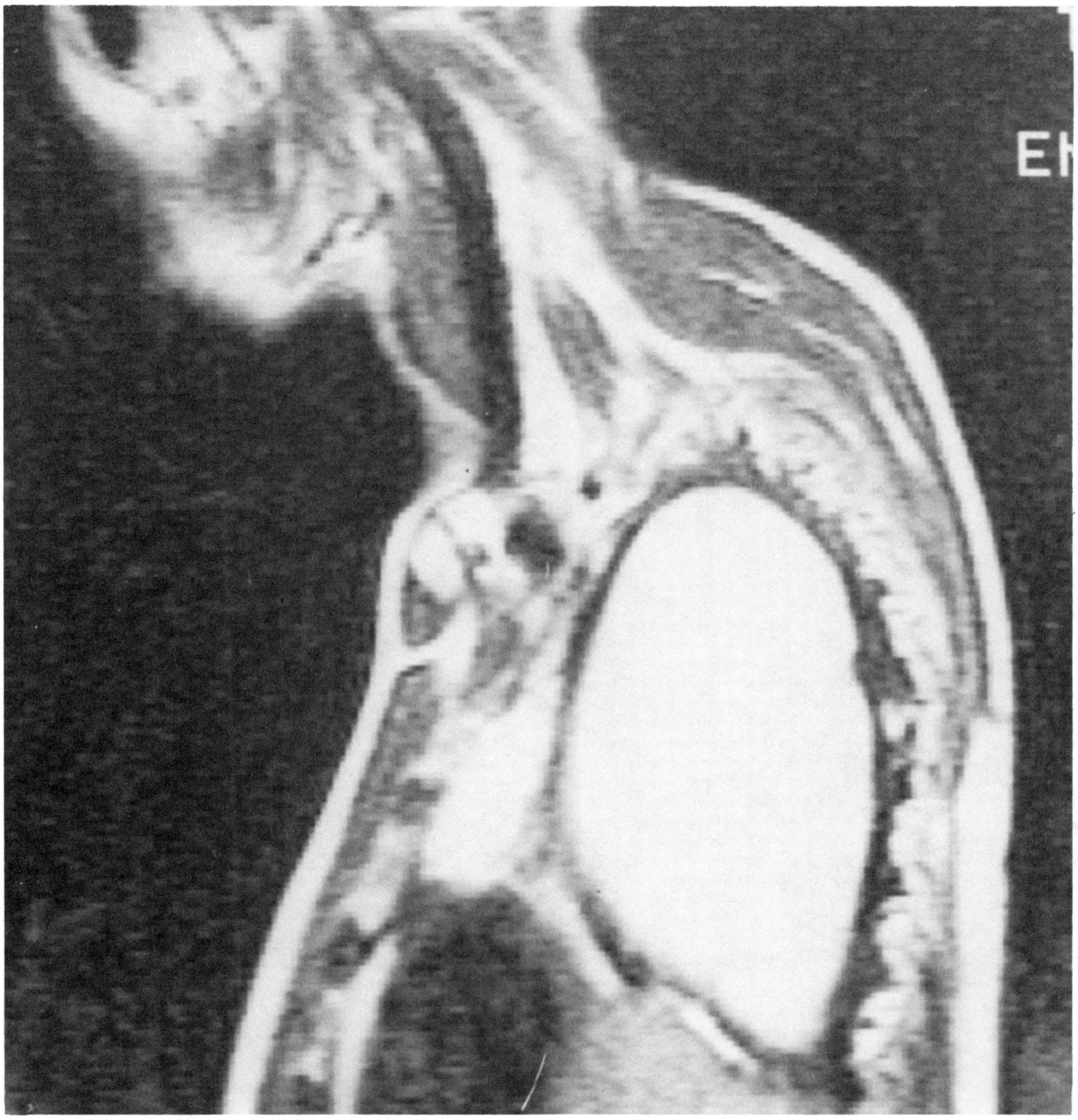

Figure 10.16

CASE 5

A 52-year-old man had undergone pneumonectomy for a bronchogenic carcinoma on the right side. Follow-up conventional radiographs of the patient showed an opaque hemithorax on the right side, but no signs of a recurrent tumor or metastatic spread were found. In our initial experience with MRI of the chest we hoped to obtain additional information about the post-pneumonectomy space and about the mediastinum with a view to detect tumor recurrency at an early stage.

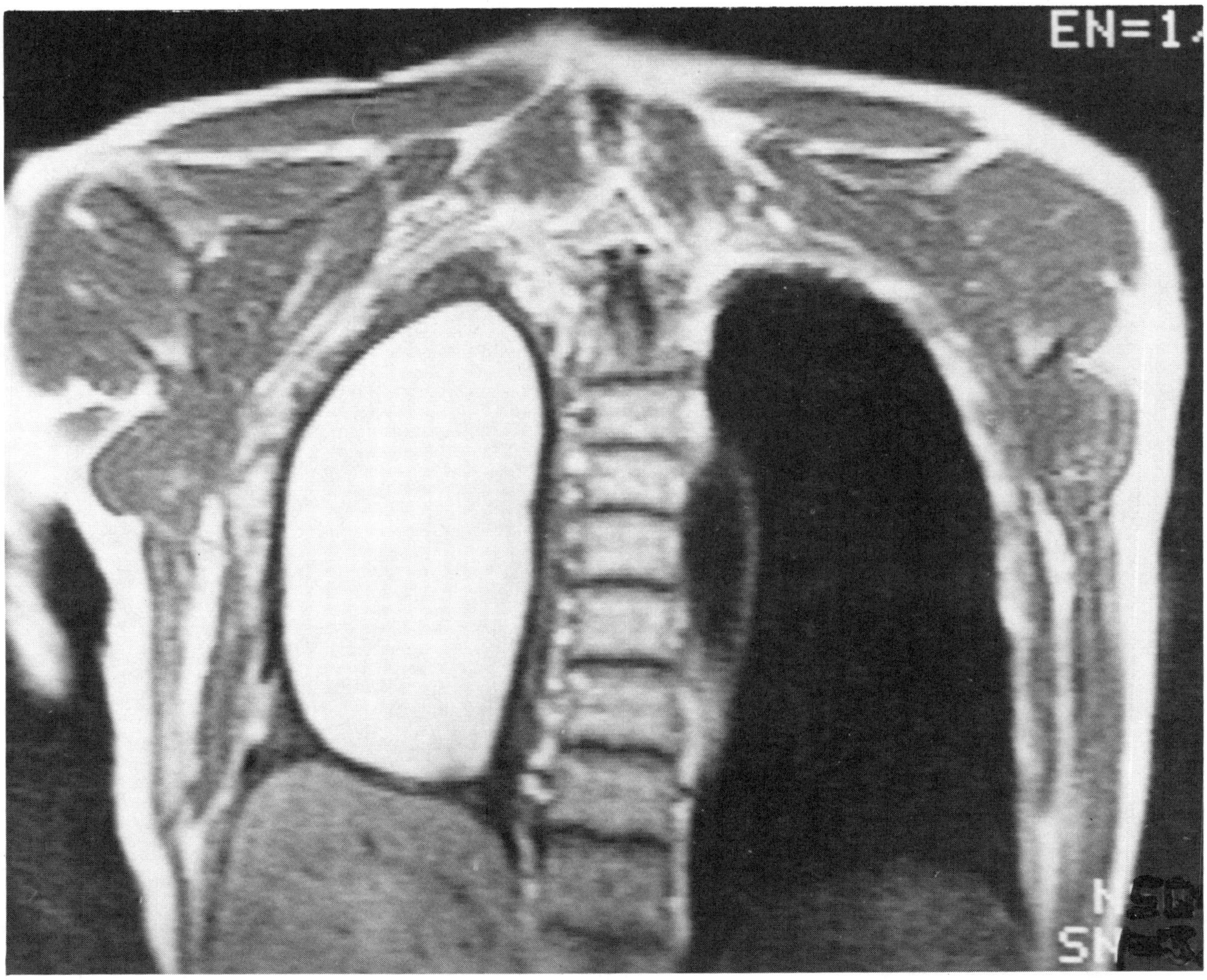

Figure 10.17

Sagittal SE images (TR 300 msec) showed a large structure of very high signal intensity with a smooth low density rim within the pneumonectomy space on the right side (Figure 10.16). Coronal images (TR 500 msec) showed that the structure completely occupied the right post-pneumonectomy space (Figure 10.17). T_2 weighted axial slices (TR 3000 msec, TE 64 msec) showed almost no change of the signal intensity of this mass which had very smooth boundaries (Figure 10.18). The mediastinum was in normal location and no metastatic spread could be detected.

Since both T_1 and T_2 weighted images showed this structure on the right side with high signal intensity, the possibility of an old hemothorax or of an empyema was raised. But the mass had very homogeneous consistency and its borders were too sharply delimited, and for these reasons the possibility that the structure could be due to a paraffin-endoprosthesis was advocated. The

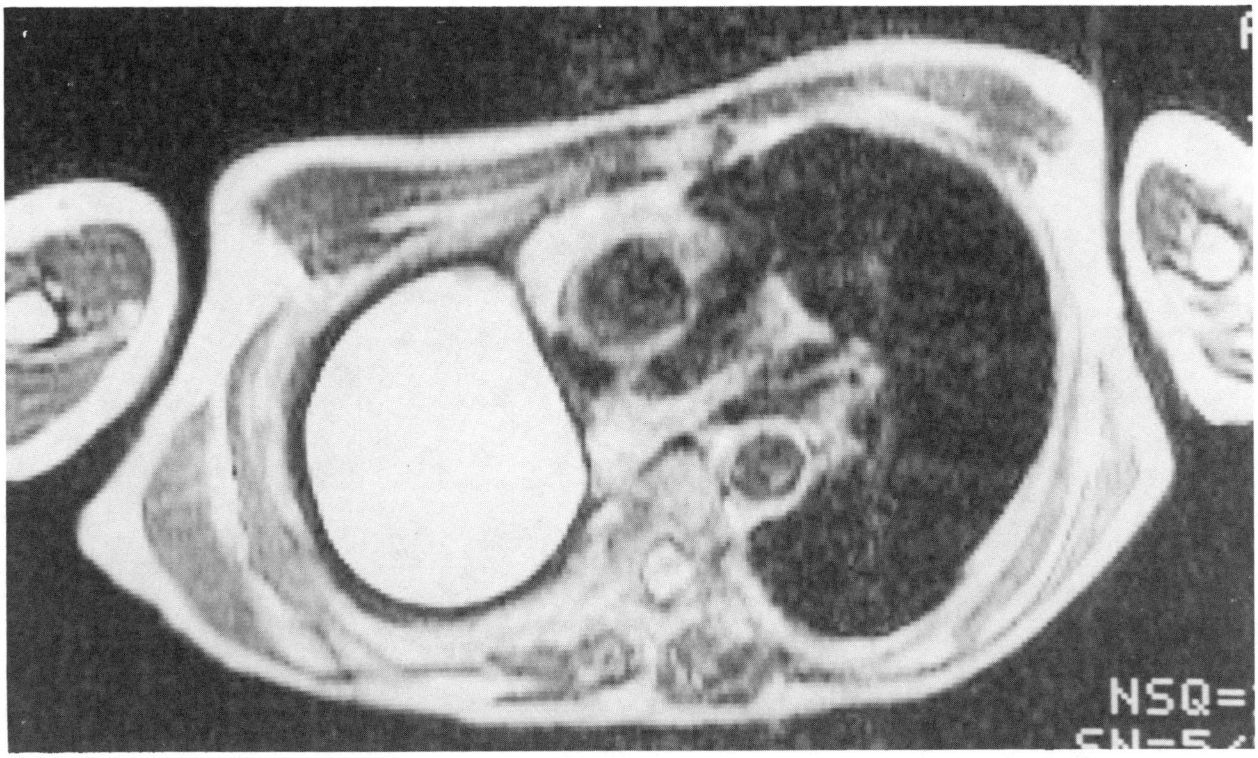

Figure 10.18

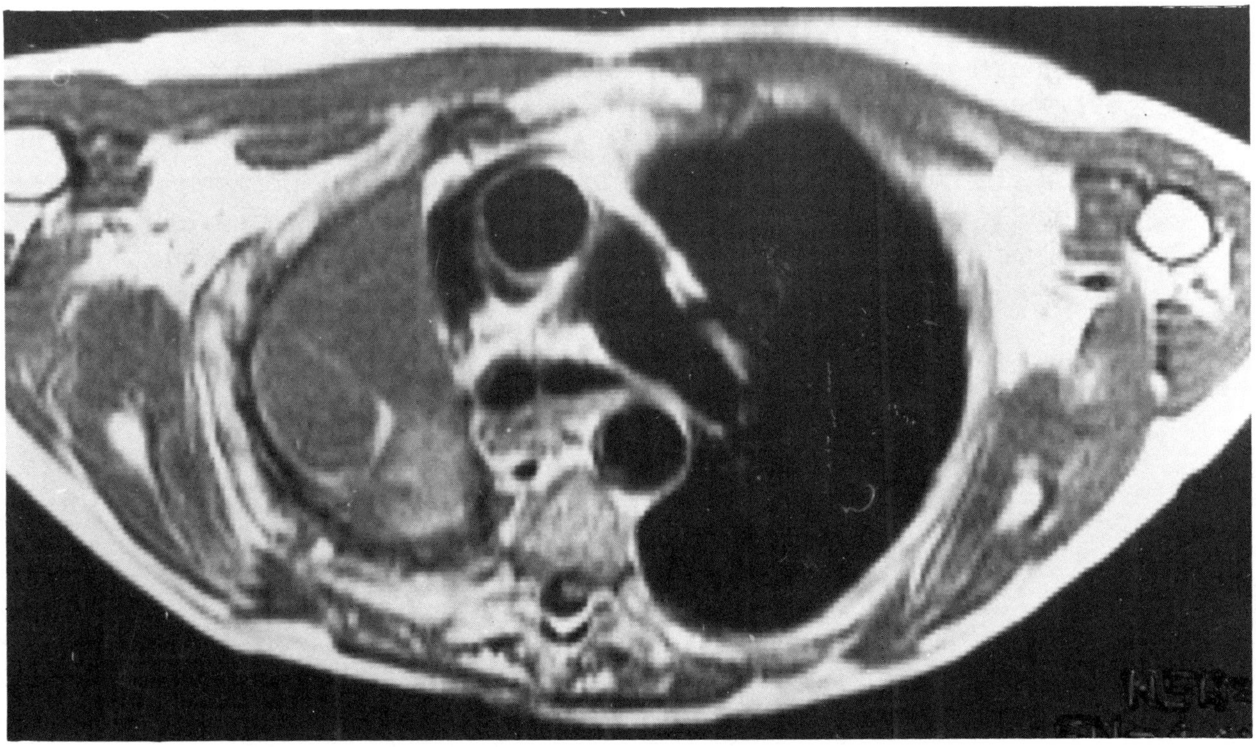

Figure 10.19

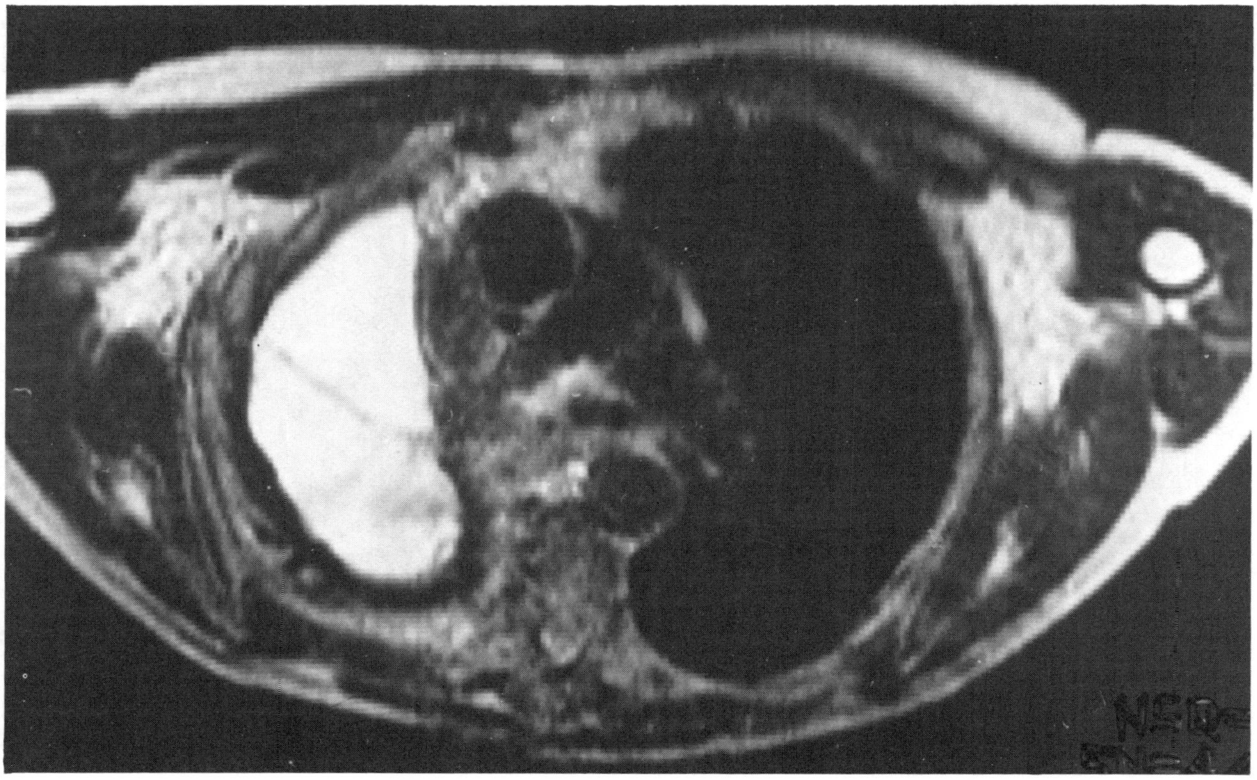

Figure 10.20

patient had been operated on at another clinical center and no further information could be obtained about the surgical procedure.

For comparison, we show a patient in which the post-pneumonectomy space is filled by fluid which is seen with relatively low signal intensity on T_1 weighted images (Figure 10.19), and marked increasement of its signal intensity on T_2 weighted images is observed (Figure 10.20). Furthermore, it is less homogeneous in appearance and it is not so regularly delimited. In the present case, differentiation between a paraffin-endoprosthesis and fluid of atypical consistency could not definitely be made by MRI, but tumor recurrency and metastatic disease were excluded.

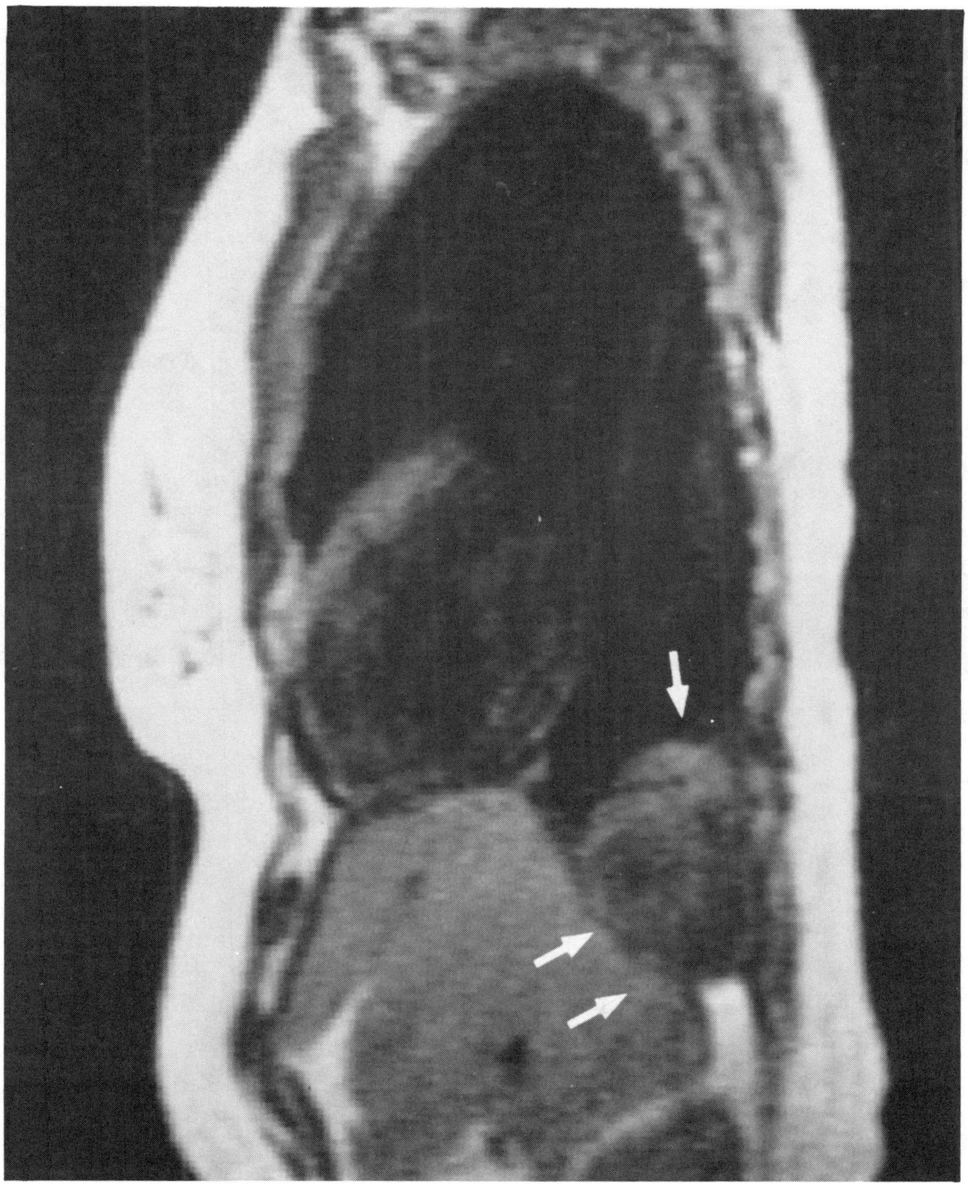

Figure 10.21

CASE 6

A 40-year-old woman presented with a metastatic lesion in the left lower lobe. Amputation of her left leg had been performed two years prior to the examination. Resection of a previous metastasis from the left lower lung had already been done a year later. In the actual treatment of the recurrent lesion on the left side, chemo- and radiotherapy were considered. For pretreatment planning, MRI of the chest was requested with a view to obtain incremental information about location and extension of the disease.

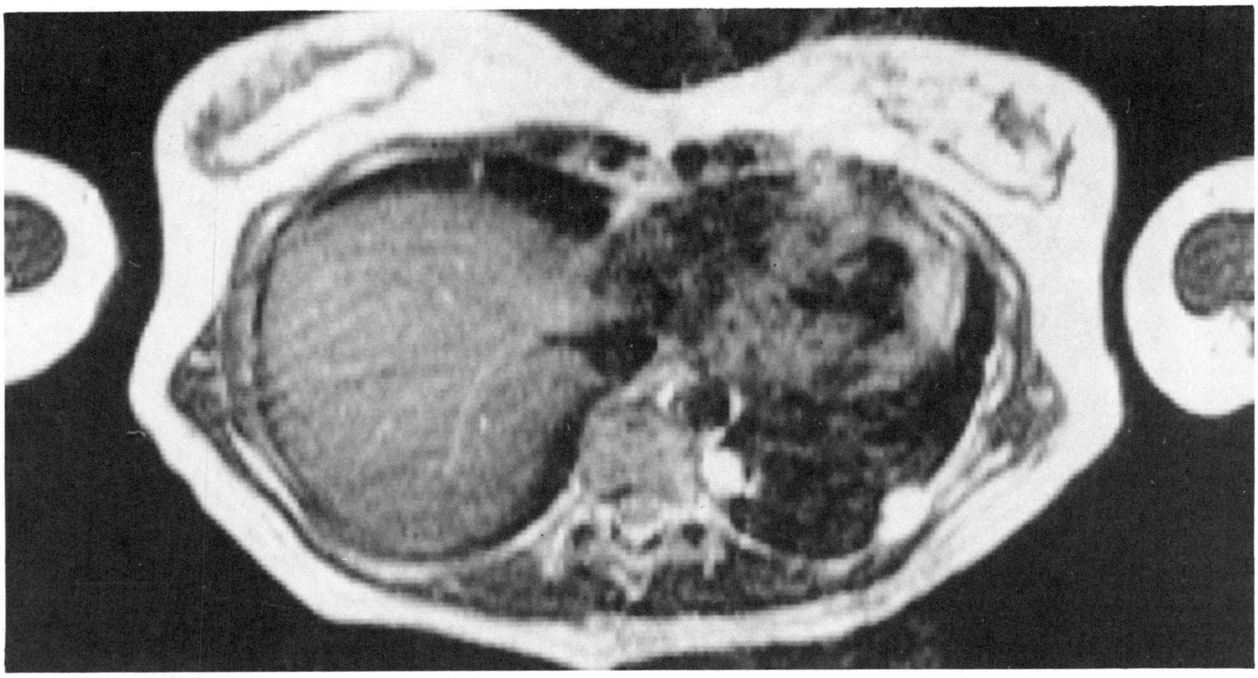

Figure 10.22

T_1 images in the sagittal plane demonstrated a mass of relatively low signal intensity located within the postero-basal segment of the left lower lobe (Figure 10.21). This mass was compressing the posterior portion of the left diaphragm and the spleen was displaced somewhat anteriorly. T_1 weighted images in the axial plane showed a relatively heterogeneous pleural mass on the left side (Figure 10.22). T_2 weighted images (TR 3000, TE 64 msec) showed a markedly increased signal intensity of this mass (Figure 10.23), but smaller metastatic deposits were also detected in the left paravertebral gutter (Figure 10.24) and another deposit was lying just above the diaphragm and against the posterior border of the heart (Figure 10.23 arrow). This information was important for treatment planning. This case illustrates the value of T_2 weighted images in the detection of malignant pleural nodules, which show intermediate signal intensity on T_1 weighted images. In this way, they can hardly be separated on T_1 weighted images from surrounding structures having similar signal intensity. On T_2 images, malignant nodules show marked increasement in signal intensity, while other tissues show only very slight increase of their signal intensity. Easy separation of malignant nodules from surrounding anatomical structures is thus easily possible.

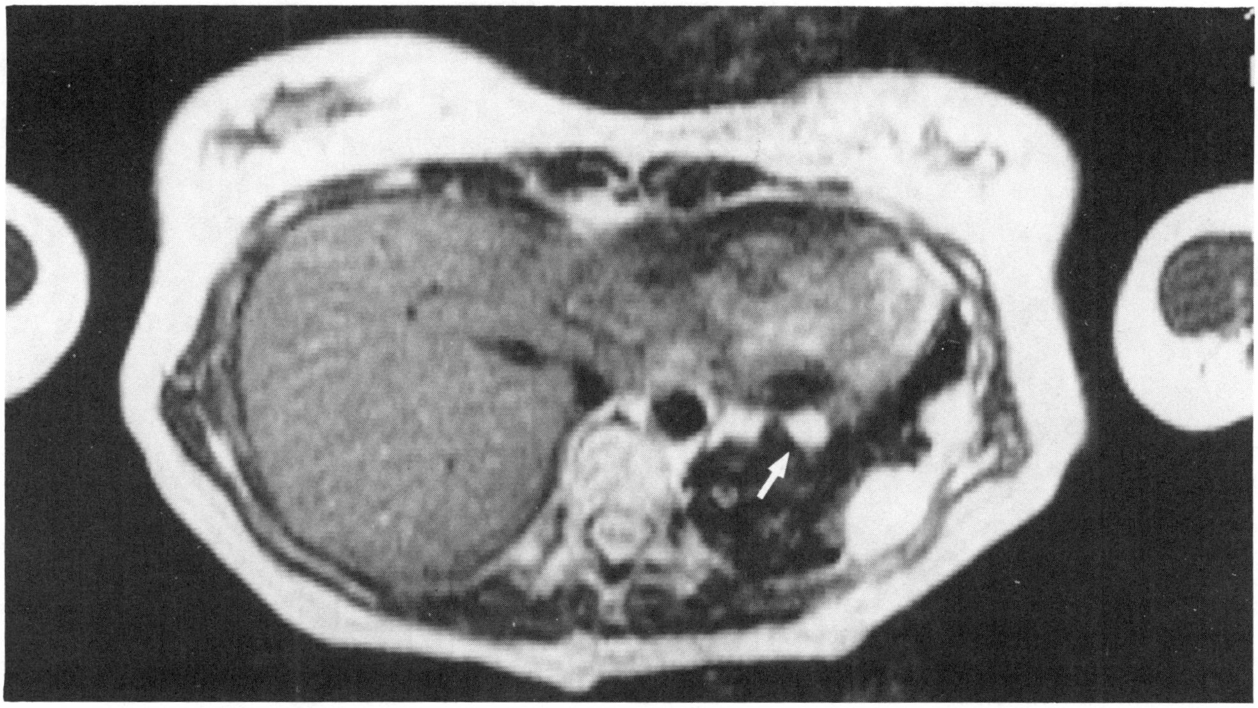

Figure 10.23

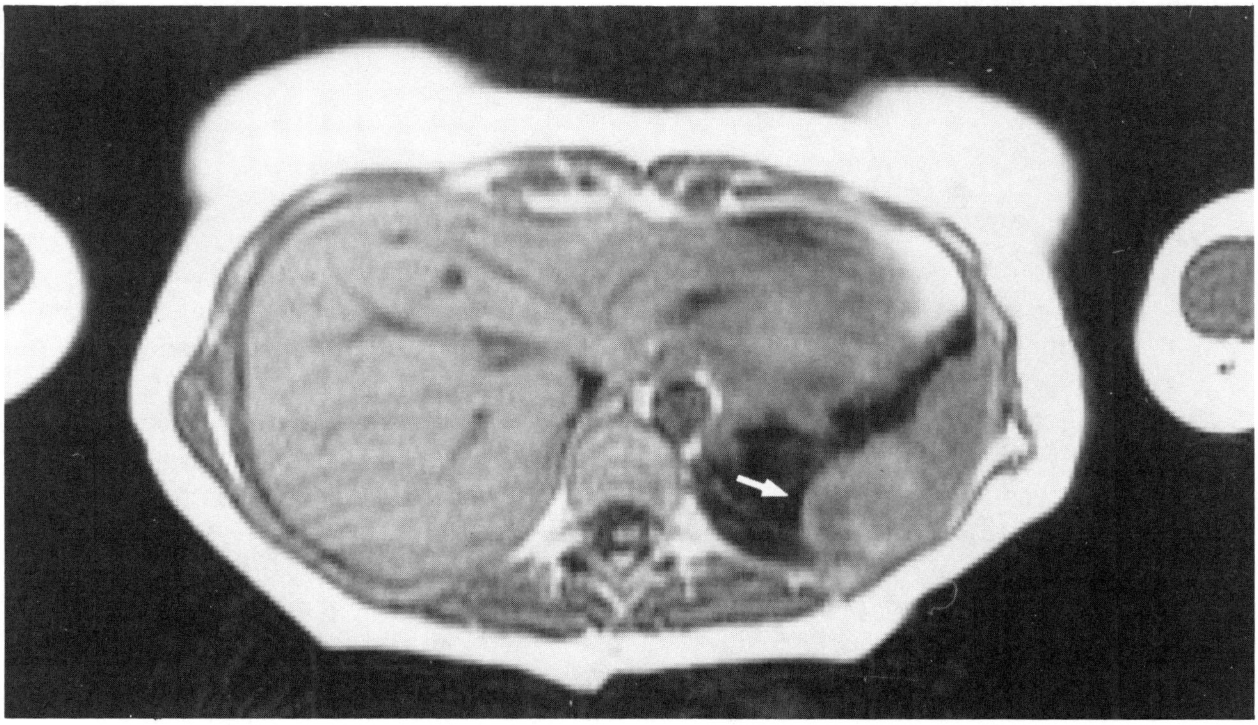

Figure 10.24

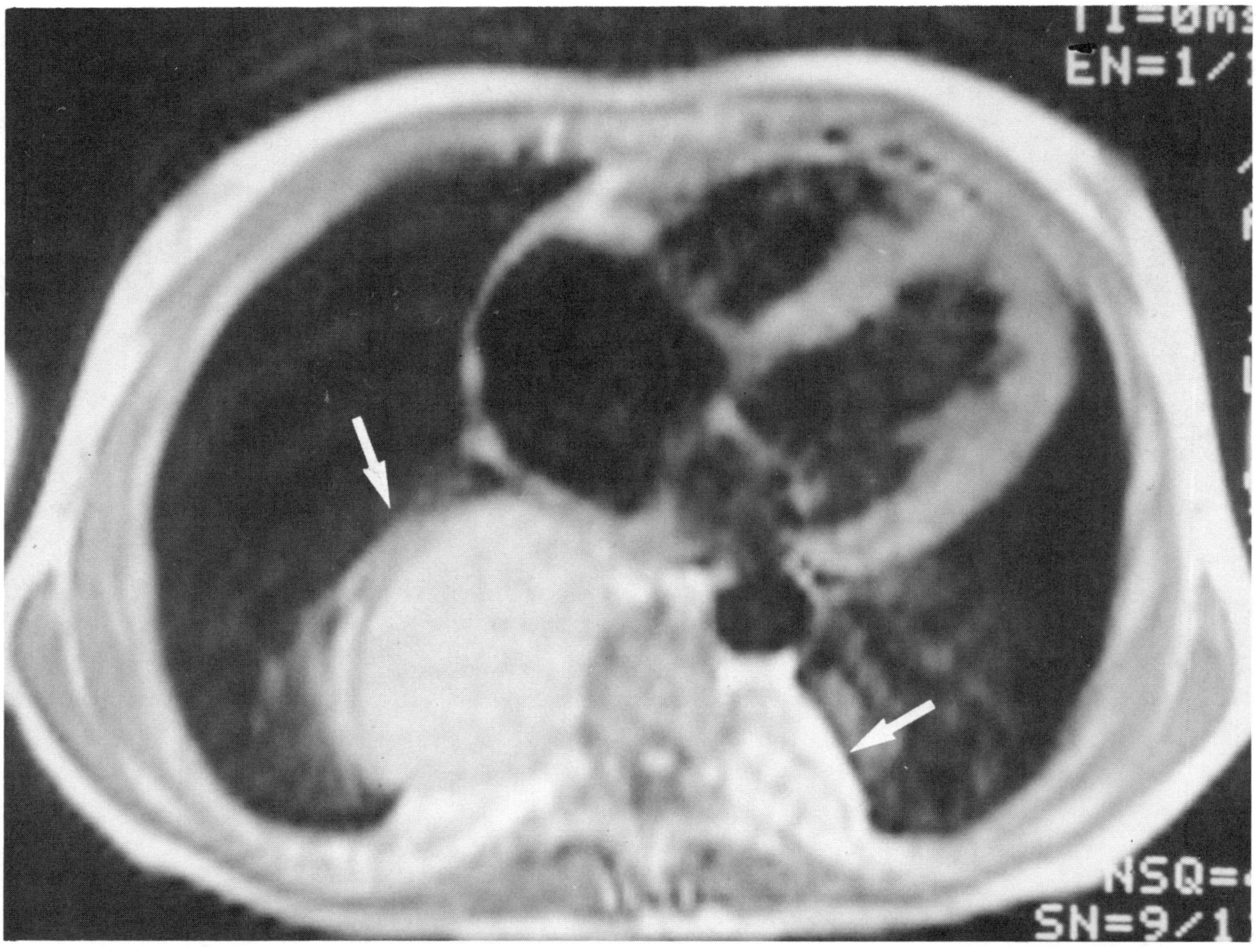

Figure 10.25

CASE 7

A 37-year-old man was known for many years with HBE thalassemia. He also had diabetes mellitus and was infertile due to primary and secondary hypogonadism. He had undergone splenectomy earlier and had received frequent blood transfusions. CT of the abdomen showed a relatively dense liver parenchyma consistent with hemochromatosis. Conventional films of the chest showed a posterior mediastinal mass. For further evaluation of this mediastinal lesion, MRI examination was done. T_1 weighted images in the transverse plane using cardiac gating (TR 500 msec) show a relatively sharply marginated mass in the paravertebral space on both sides, mainly on the right (Figure 10.25, arrows). The paravertebral mass lesions were shown with intermediate signal intensity and were considered to be characteristic for extramedullary hematopoiesis.

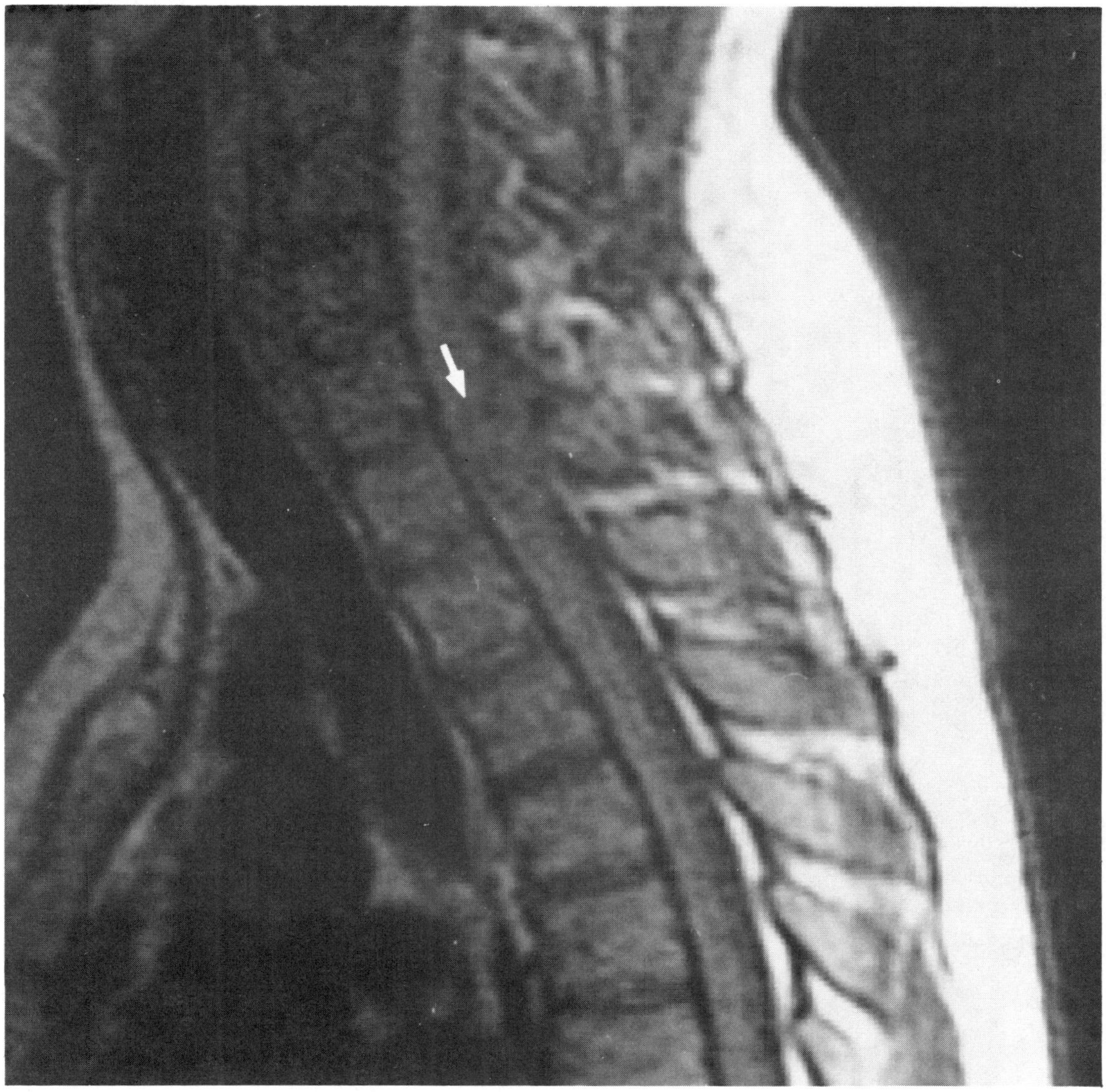

Figure 10.26

CASE 8

A 26-year-old man complained about progressively increasing back pain located at the upper thoracic level, numbness and later paresthesias of the right arm and shoulder. Conventional films and plain CT scans of the lower cervical region had shown no abnormalities.

MRI of the cervical and upper dorsal region was requested. Sagittal images using a short TR (550 msec) faintly demonstrated a low signal intensity lesion in the vertebral canal at the level Th 1-2 (Figure 10.26 arrow). Sagittal slices passing through the right paravertebral area clearly outlined a soft tissue mass located

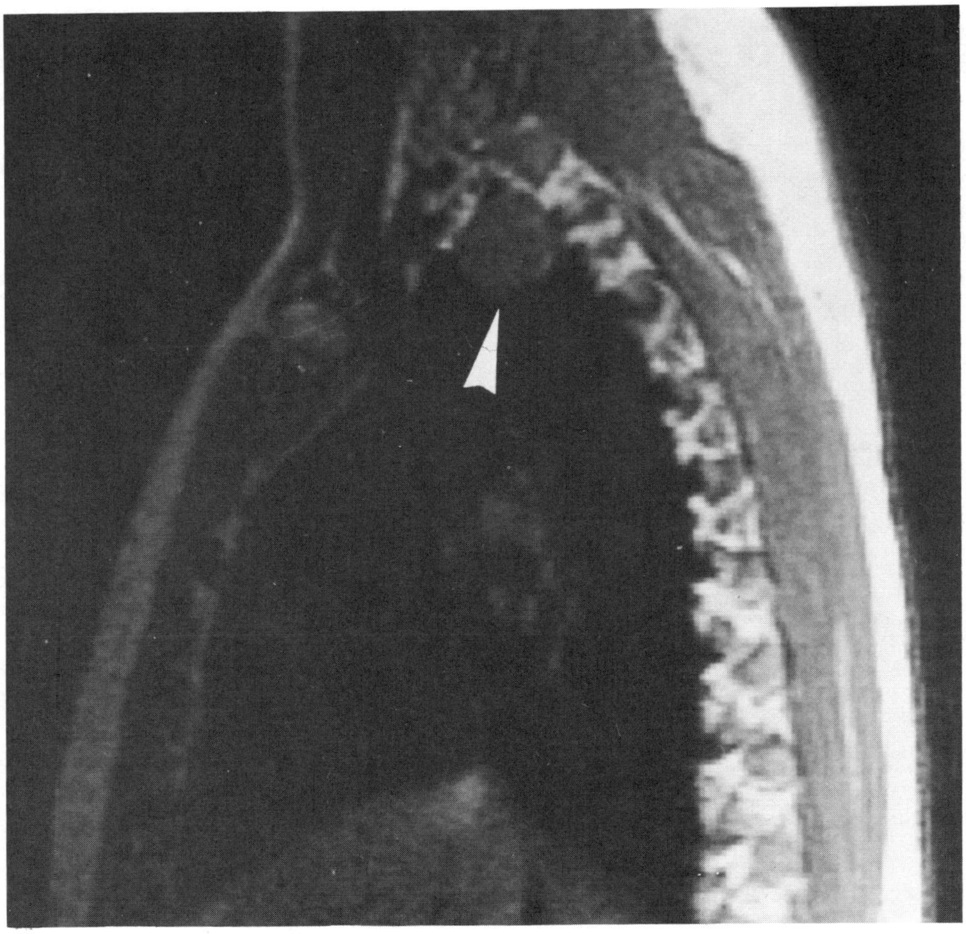

Figure 10.27

at the dome of the right hemithorax (Figure 10.27 arrowhead) which had intermediate signal intensity. On T_2 weighted images this mass showed some increase in signal intensity and its consistency became less homogeneous. At this stage a presumptive diagnosis of an intraspinal tumor extending into the apex of the right hemithorax was made and it was decided to perform intravenous injection of Gadolinium-DTPA. At first, sagittal images using the same pulse sequence parameters as in Figure 10.26 were done which showed a well defined mass lesion inside the canal at the level Th 1-2 with obvious enhancement in comparison to its appearance on previous images (Figure 10.28). After this series, axial images were generated (TR 350 msec) which showed marked increasement of the signal intensity of the content of the spinal canal together with enhancement of a relatively large mass located within the paravertebral region (Figure 10.29). Coronal images also demonstrated the mass with marked enhancement after injection of Gd-DTPA and the connection between the intraspinal and intrathoracic components was obviously shown (Figure 10.30).

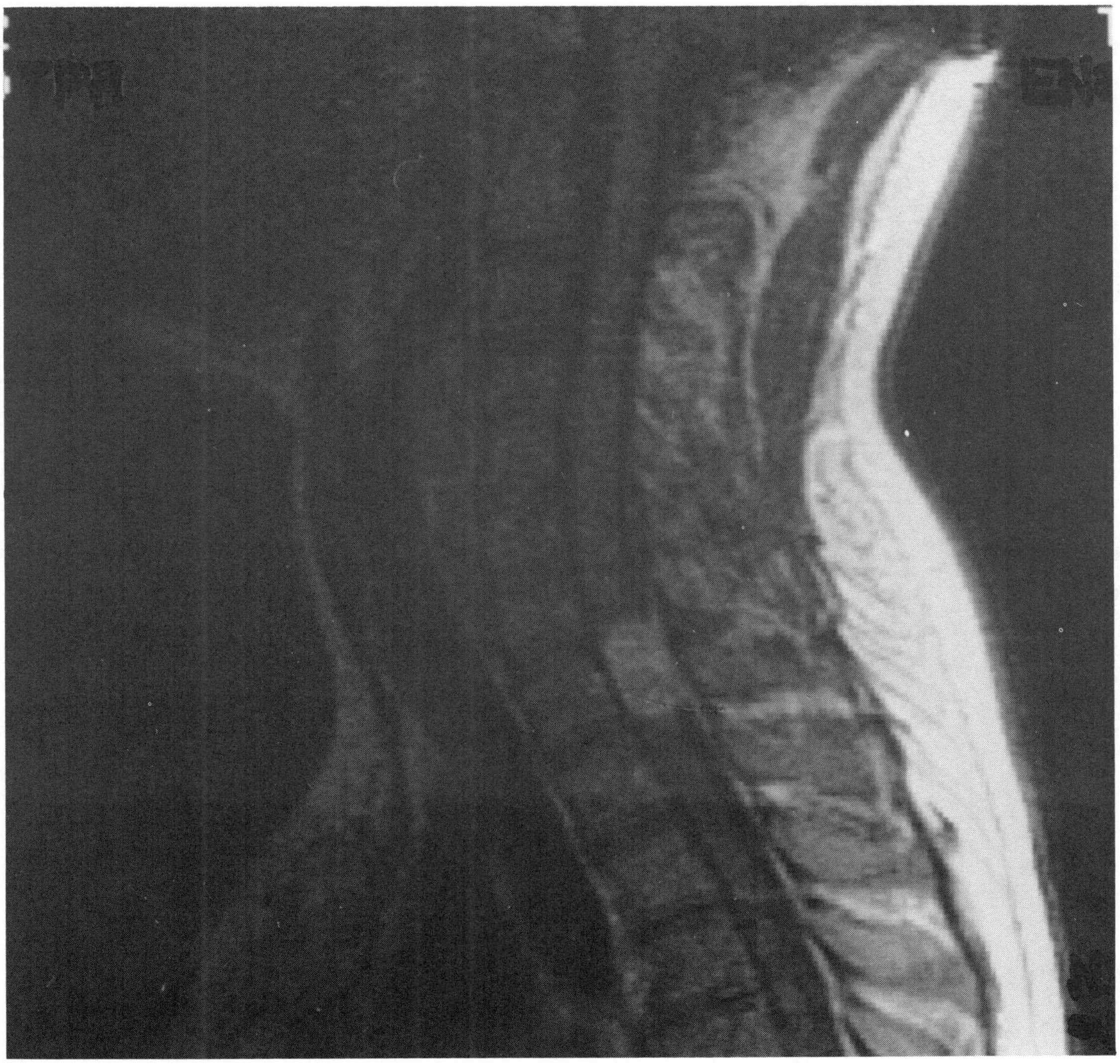

Figure 10.28

This case exemplifies the usefulness of surface coils in the study of thoracic or mediastinal masses which are in relationship with the spine or intraspinal contents. By using paramagnetic contrast agents, scanning times can be significantly reduced as shorter pulse sequences may be selected and enhancement of tumor tissue facilitates separation of the lesion from surrounding structures.

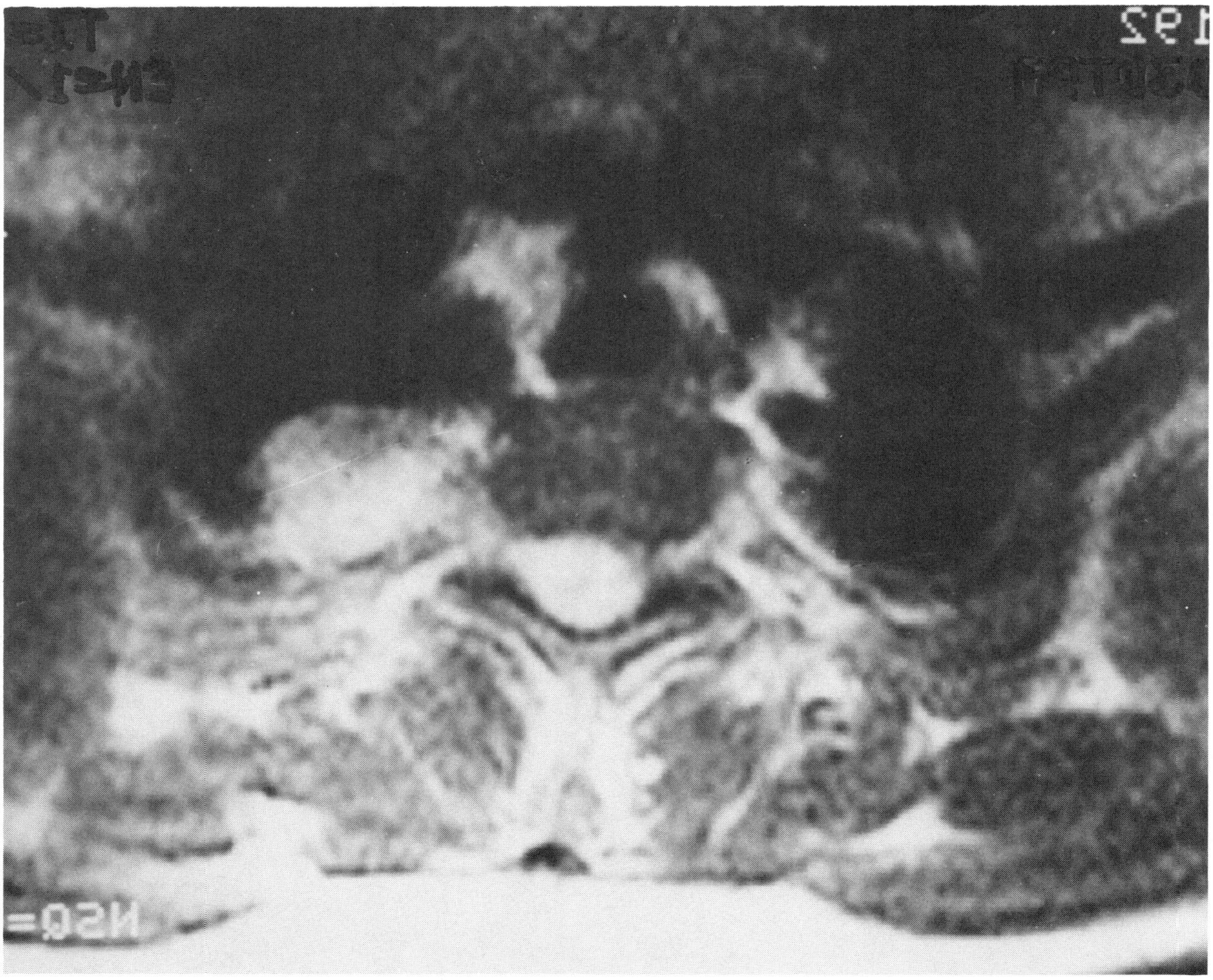

Figure 10.29

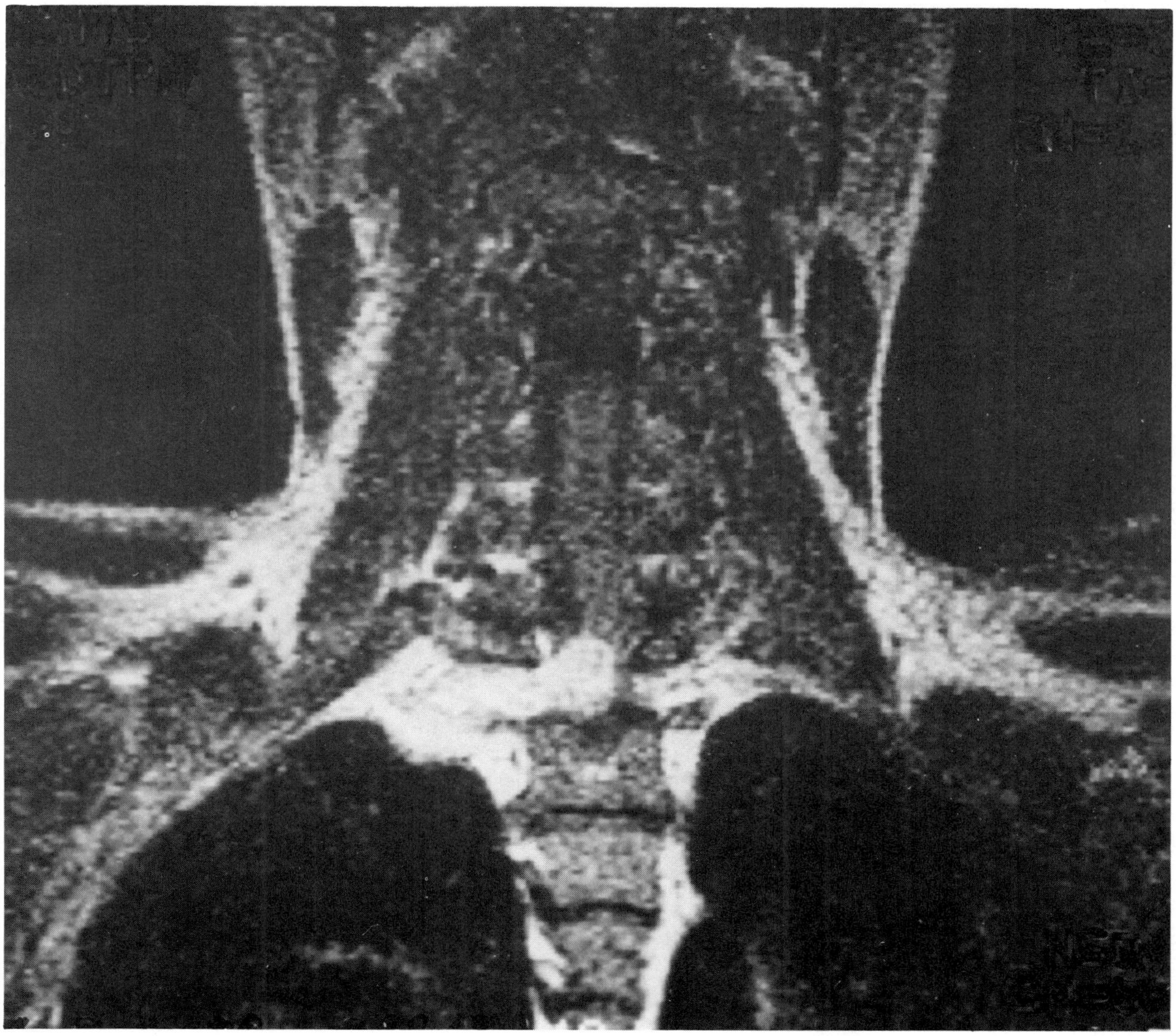

Figure 10.30

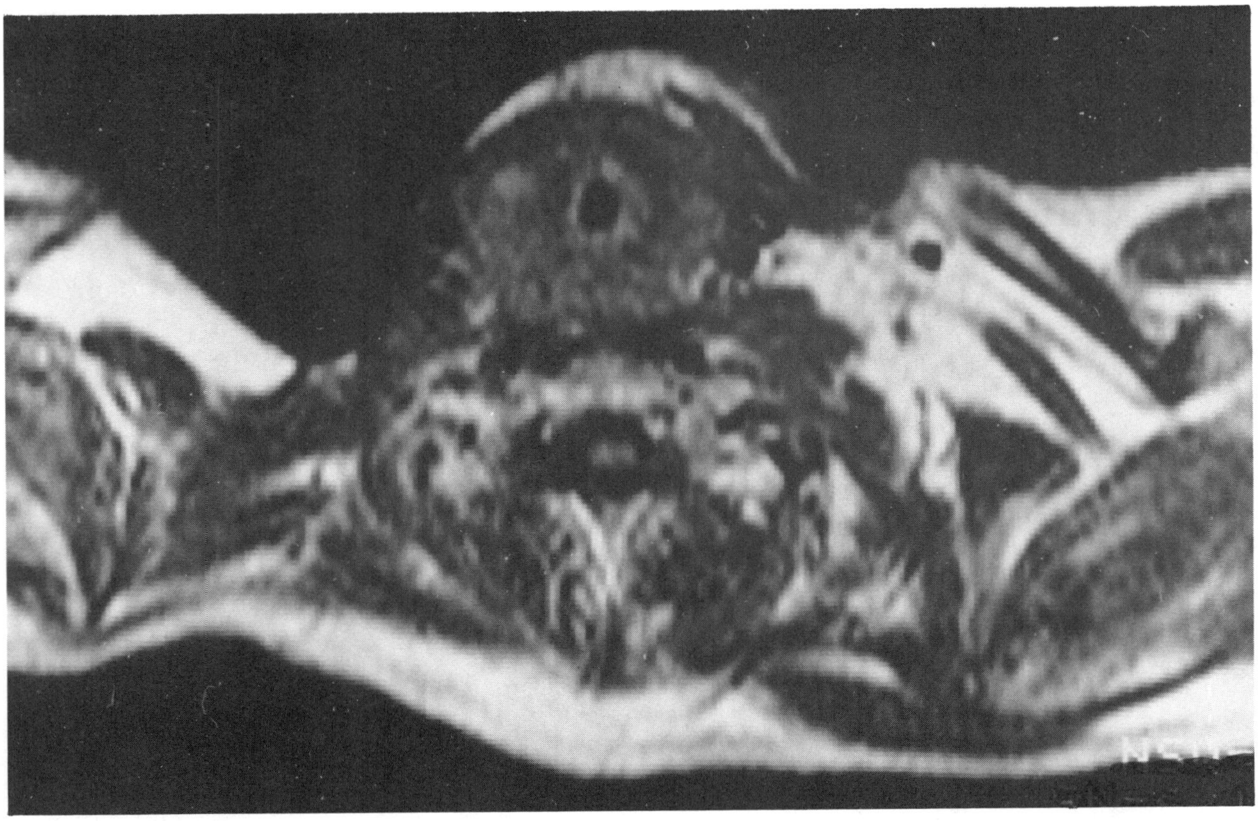

Figure 10.31

CASE 9

A 49-year-old man was admitted in emergency because of stridor apparently due to a swelling found within the region of the right thyroid gland. Tracheostomy was done and CT examination of this region did not provide useful information due to motion artifacts. This patient had undergone neck dissection for a carcinoma of the base of the tongue 9 years prior to the examination and subsequently he underwent irradiation treatment. Biopsy of the right thyroid gland revealed a relatively well differentiated carcinoma. In view to obtain additional information about eventual intrathoracic extension of this tumor MRI of the thorax and lower neck were requested. Axial T_1 weighted images revealed the presence of a mass lesion of relatively high signal intensity located within the right thyroid lobe (Figure 10.31). Sagittal images showed tracheostomy and a quite large soft tissue mass of intermediate signal intensity above and posteriorly to the trachea. This mass was supposed to represent post-irradiation fibrosis

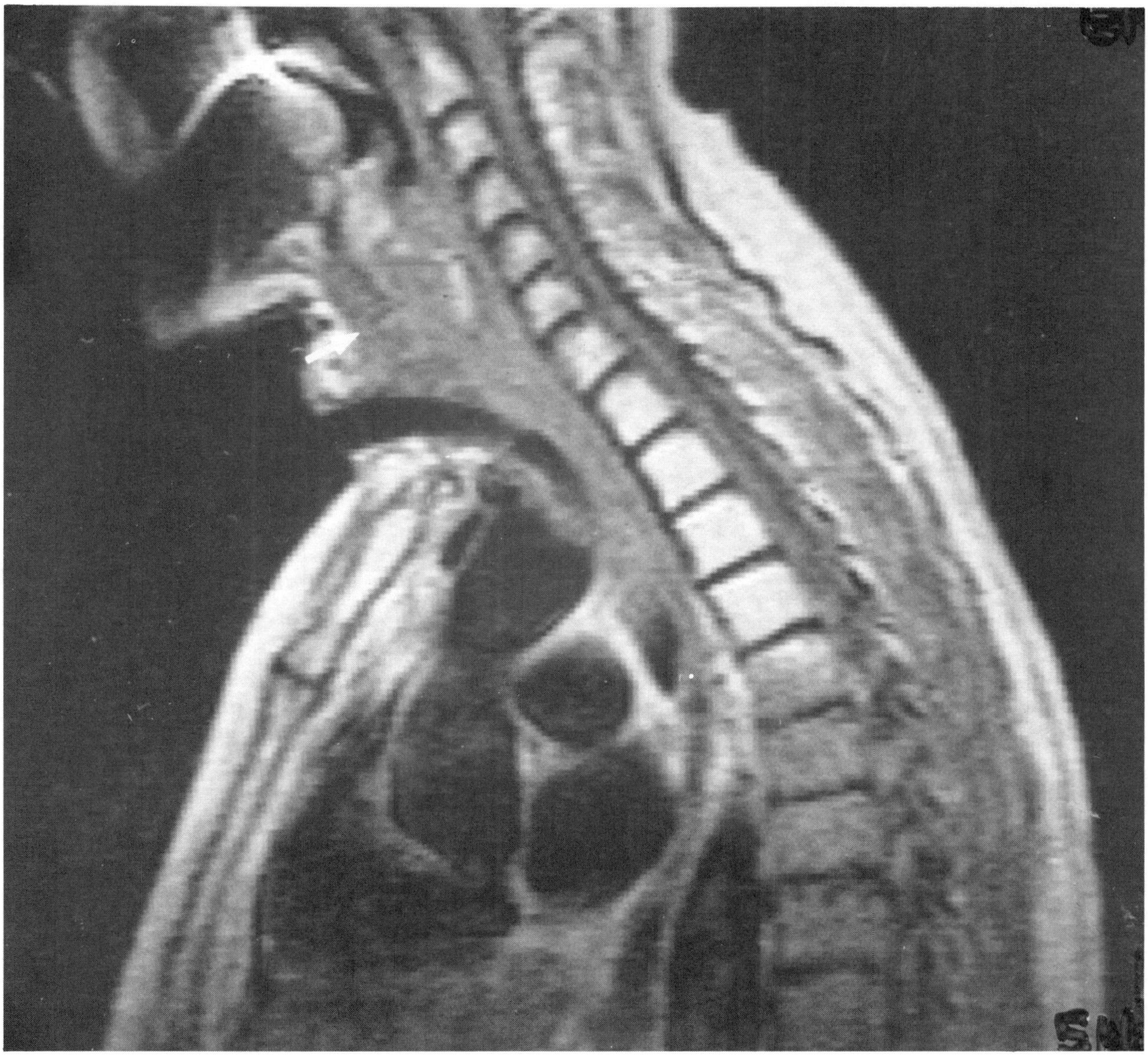

Figure 10.32

(Figure 10.32). Furthermore, a mass lesion was seen at the base of the tongue (arrow). The presence of this mass was also demonstrated by transverse slices (arrows) (Figure 10.33). Intrathoracic extension of the thyroid tumor was not found and there was no metastatic spread into the mediastinum. In fact, the patient had a tumor recurrency at the base of the tongue which could not be differentiated from irradiation fibrosis by MRI scanning. This case taught us that in patients with severe respiratory distress, MRI is able to delineate thoracic and also extrathoracic areas which may eventually be incriminated in the generation of the symptoms presented. This capability of MRI is due to imaging facilities along the long axis of the body offering more information per slice generated than the conventional transverse slices.

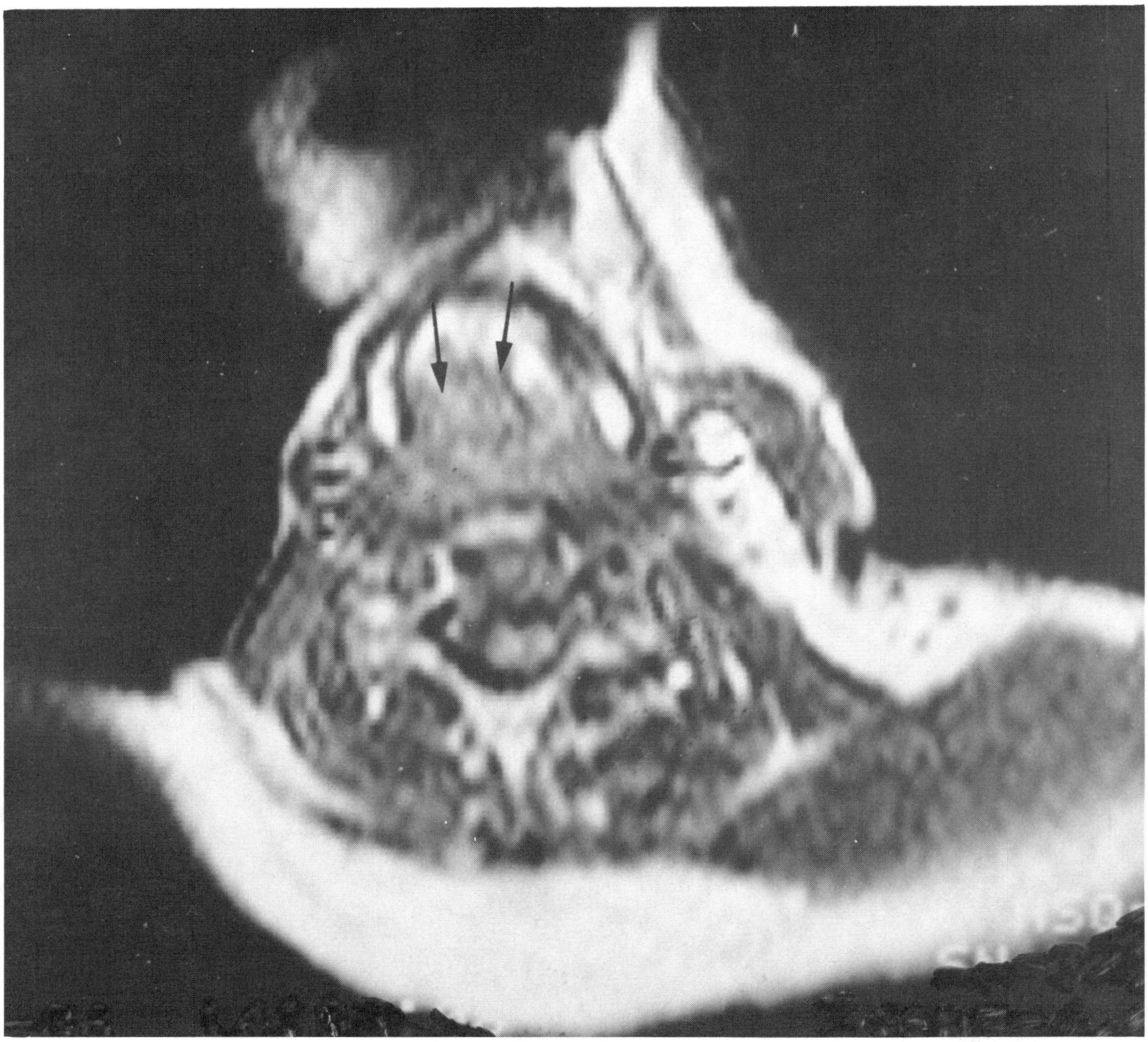

Figure 10.33

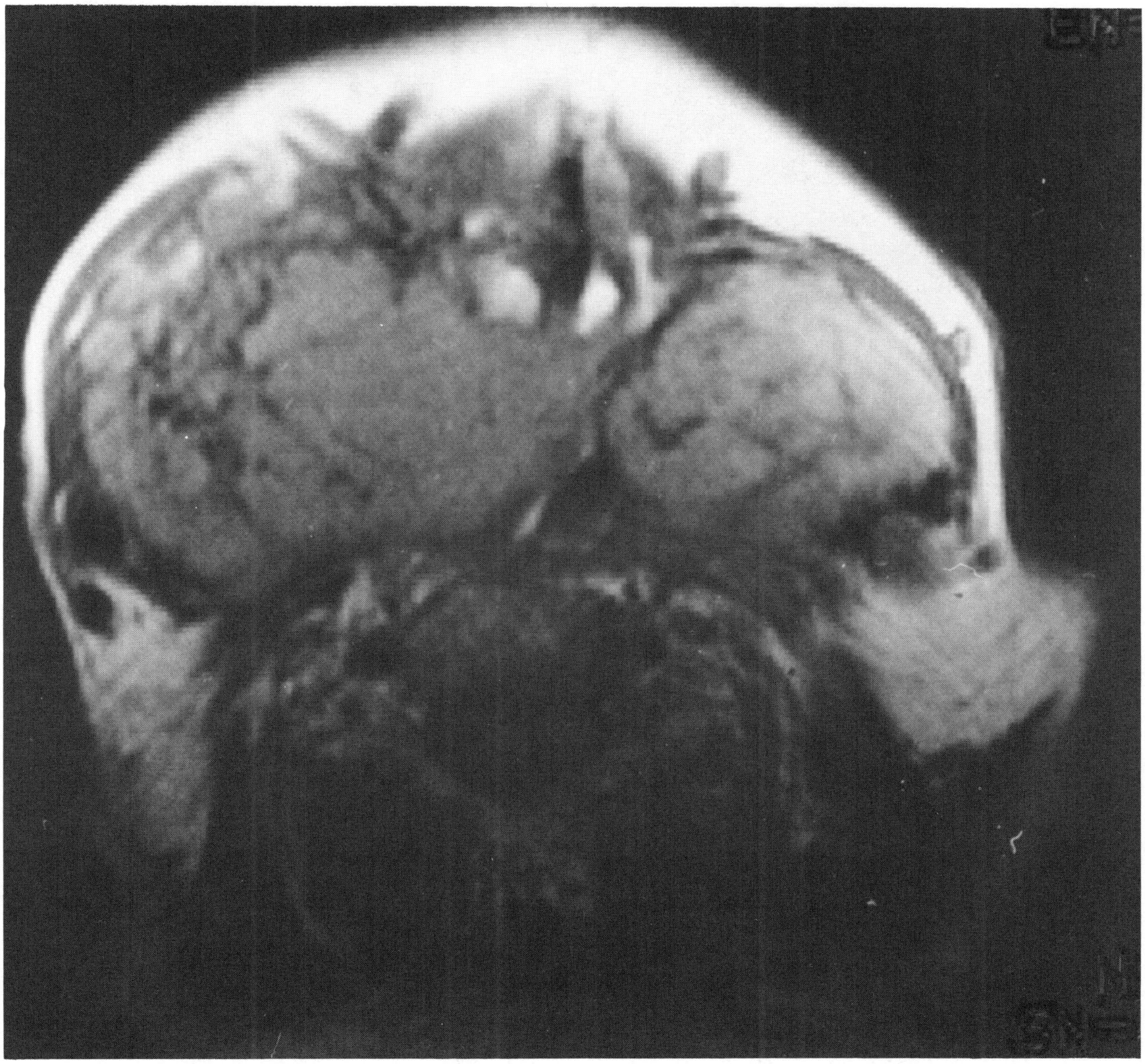

Figure 10.34

CASE 10

An 88-year-old woman had a massive multinodular goiter bilaterally. MRI was requested to determine if intramediastinal extension of this mass existed.

Transverse T_1 weighted images showed a very large bilateral multinodular goiter displacing the vascular structures of the neck laterally (Figure 10.34). This mass had intermediate signal intensity and contained multiple septations. Severe compromise of the upper airways was present. Sagittal images outlined its extension in the cranio-caudal direction, but only slight intramediastinal

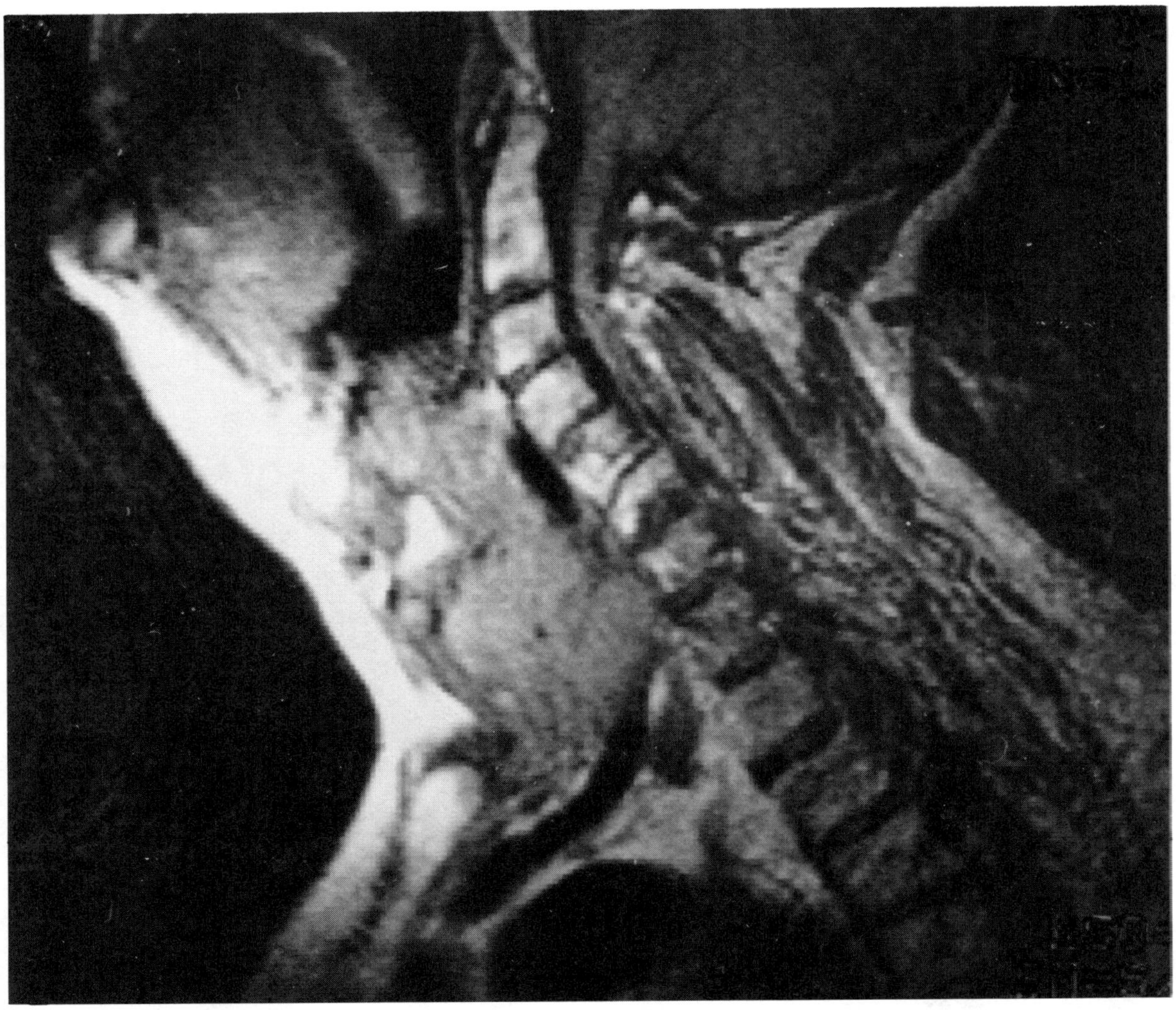

Figure 10.35

ingrowth was noted (Figure 10.35). Transverse MR images confirmed the intramediastinal extension of the goiter on the left side (Figure 10.36). With a TR of 1500 msec and a TE of 90 msec the goiter showed marked inhomogeneity due to significant increasement of its signal intensity and a calcified nodule on the right side was seen (Figure 10.37).

This case exemplifies the statement that MRI examinations are also possible in old patients and under respiratory distress. Although it was not possible to generate heavily T_2 weighted MR images, the diagnostic results were still quite satisfactory as the extension and composition of the mass lesion were well delineated and its relationship to vessels and upper airways was clearly demonstrated. Benign masses of the neck and upper mediastinum show increased signal intensity with both a longer TR and TE in comparison with subcutaneous fat. This increase in relative signal intensity is accompanied by less contrast between the mass and fat.

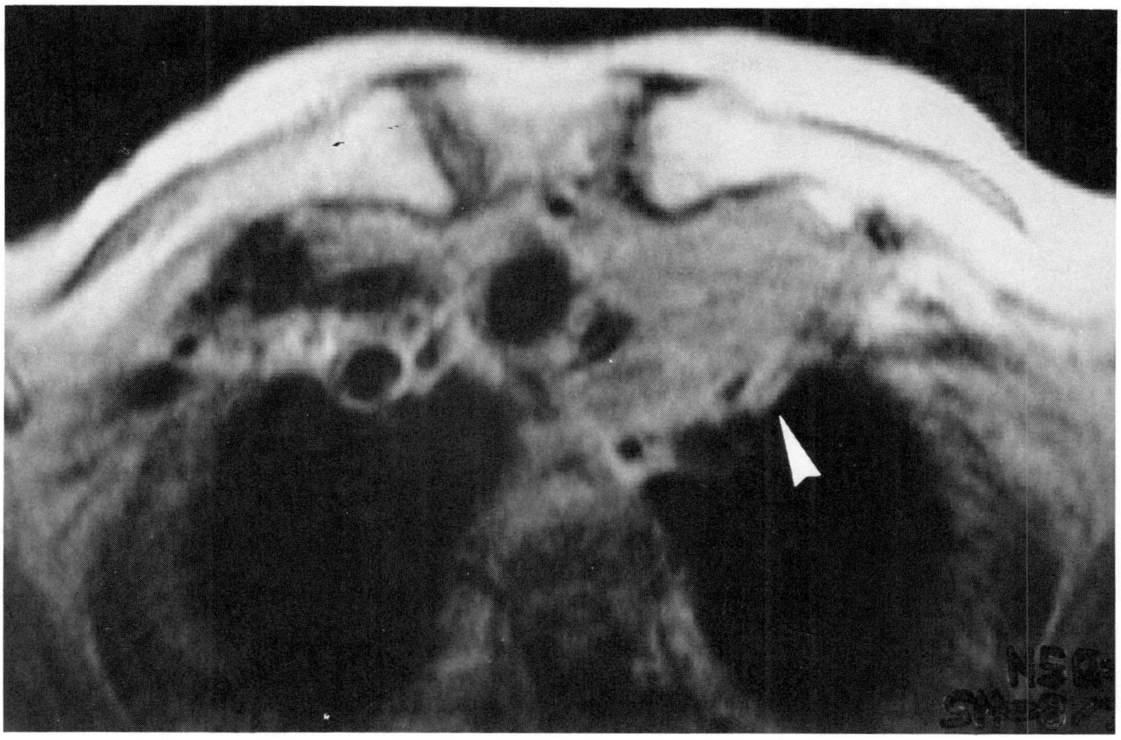

Figure 10.36

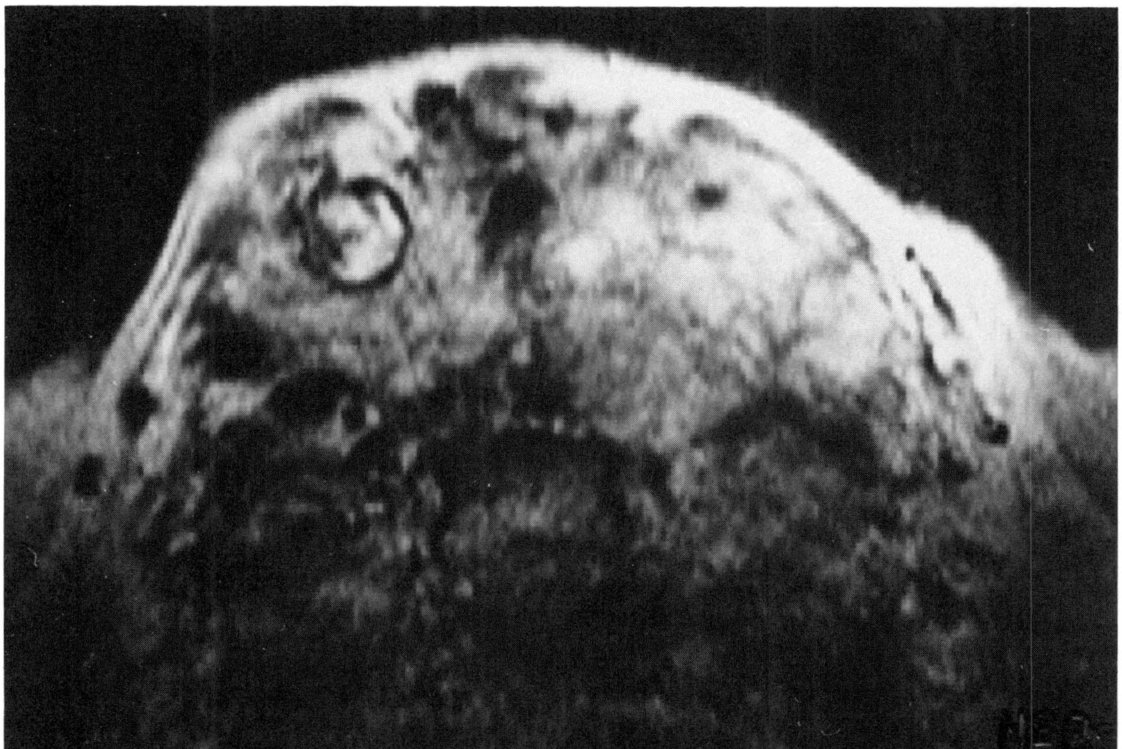

Figure 10.37

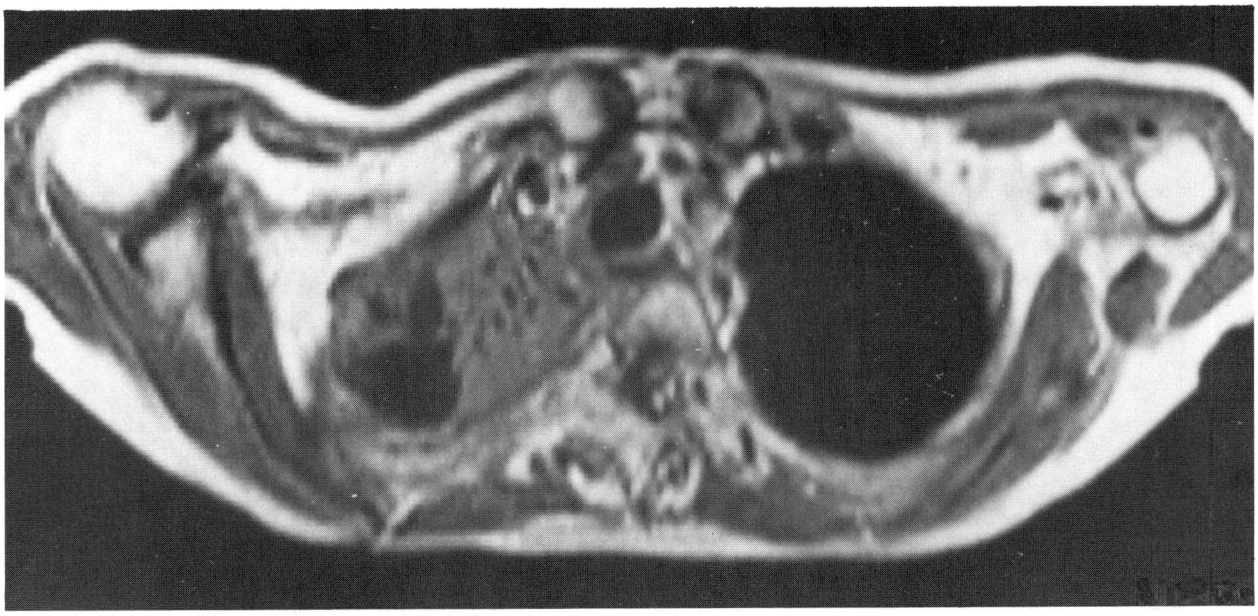

Figure 10.38

CASE 11

A 68-year-old man had undergone lobectomy for a bronchogenic carcinoma of the right upper lobe. During follow-up, he underwent irradiation treatment. One year later, MRI of the thorax was done with a view to be able to find out if recurrent tumor existed among fibrotic changes due to irradiation.

T_1 weighted MR images in the transverse plane demonstrate extensive soft tissue changes of intermediate signal intensity within the apex of the right hemithorax (Figure 10.38). Coronal images confirmed these findings. Furthermore, extension of the fibrotic changes into the mediastinum was also shown (Figure 10.39). T_2 weighted images (TR 3000 msec, TE 96 msec) demonstrate only minimally increased signal intensity of this mass which appeared to be composed by fibrotic changes only, no evidence for tumor recurrency was detected (Figure 10.40). In our experience with MRI in the post-pneumonectomy chest, it was sometimes extremely difficult to separate tumorous tissue from reactive fibrosis due to irradiation treatment. We think that for this particular purpose, the intravenous injection of Gd-DTPA may be of interest in the future in order to enable detection of tumor recurrency at a relatively early stage.

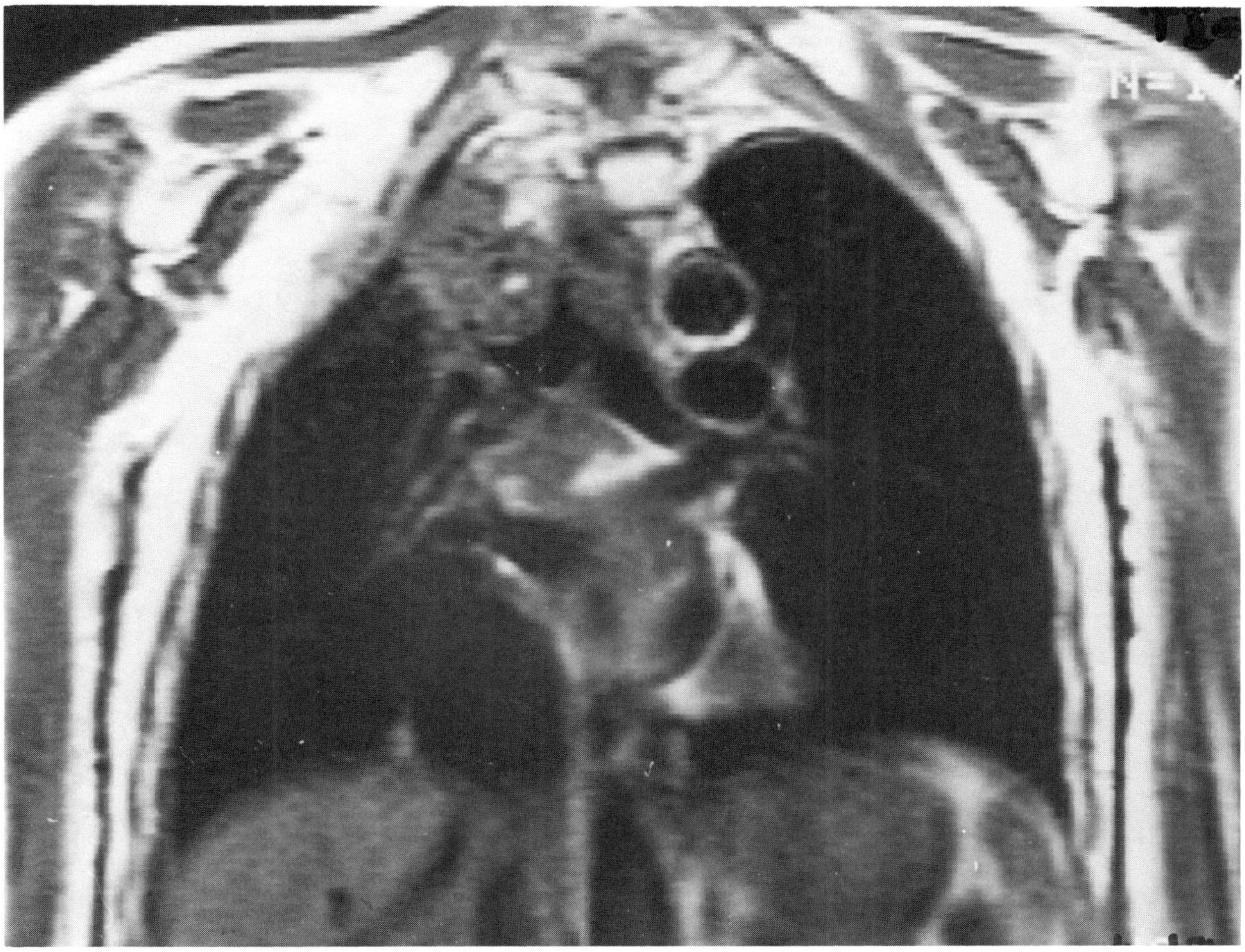

Figure 10.39

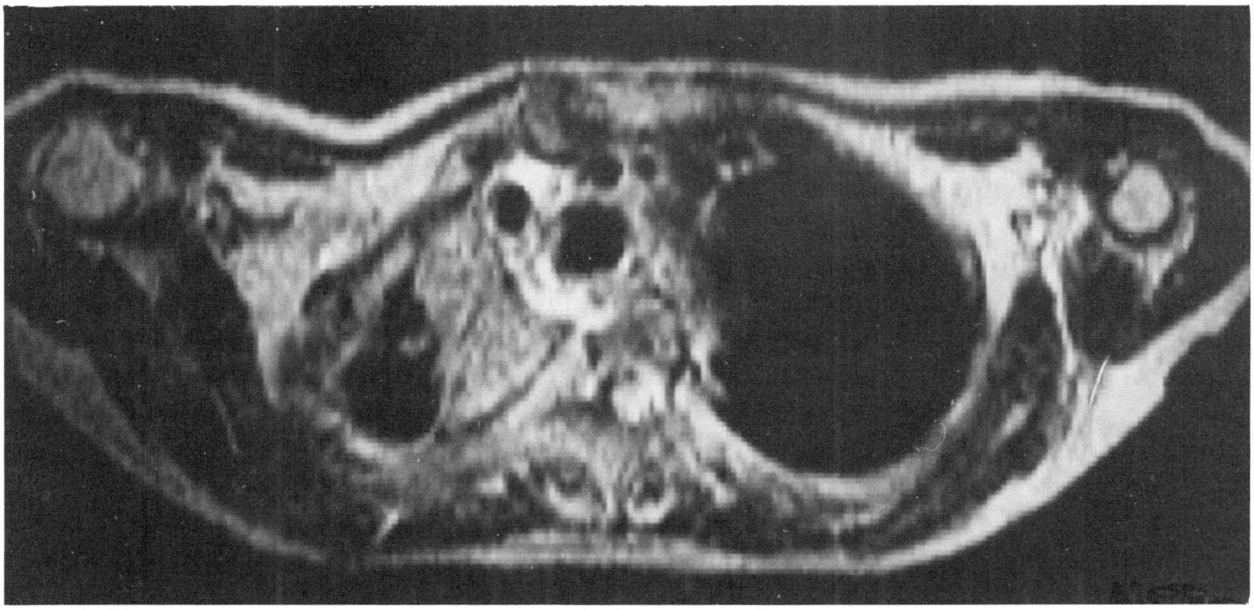

Figure 10.40

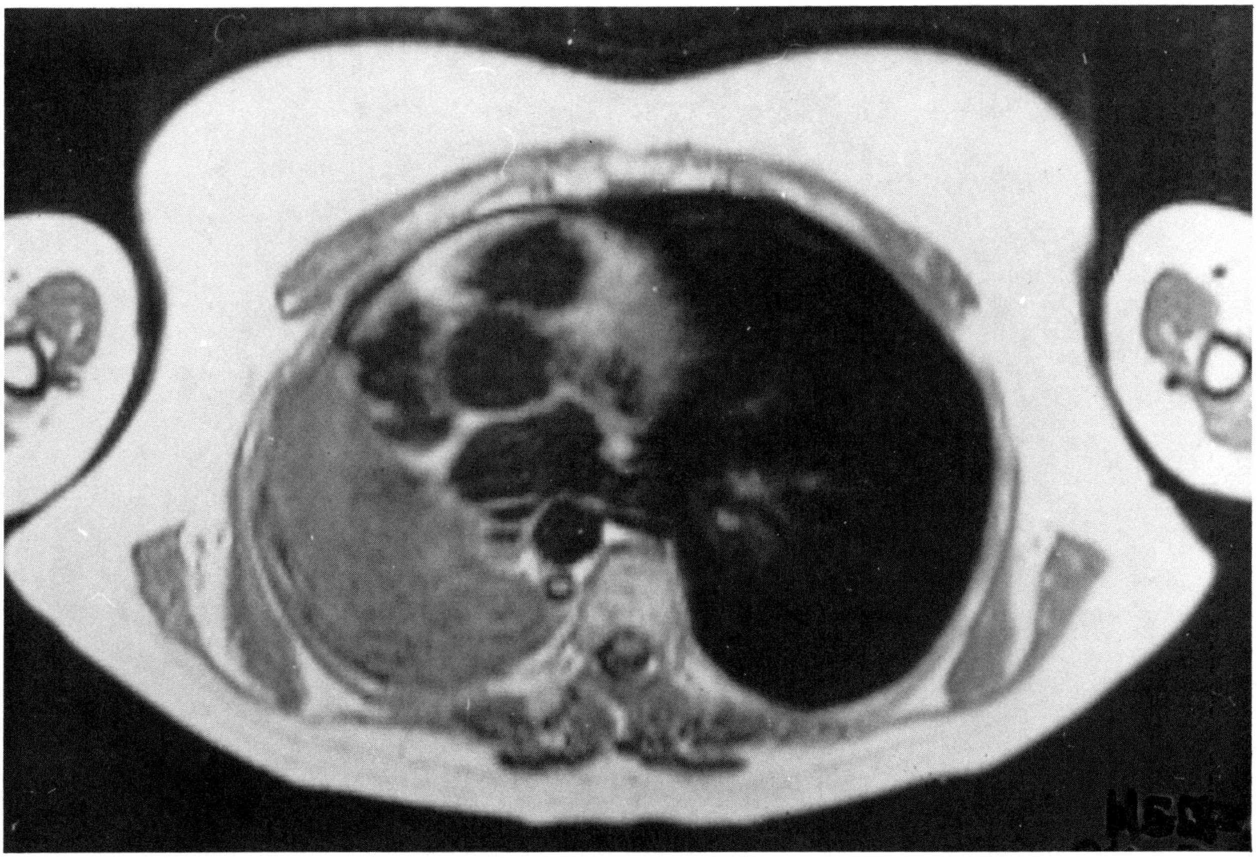

Figure 10.41

CASE 12

A 24-year-old woman underwent pneumonectomy for a primary melanoma of the right lung. T_1 weighted images show that the post-pneumonectomy space on the right is filled up by a relatively low signal intensity structure (Figure 10.41). T_2 weighted images (TR 3000 msec, TE 64 msec) show markedly increased signal intensity within the post-pneumonectomy space which was filled up by fluid (Figure 10.42). Furthermore, a relatively large mass within the anterior portion of the left hemithorax was seen. This round lesion had smooth contours and it showed intermediate signal intensity. On T_1 weighted images this lesion had already been seen with a similar signal intensity (Figure 10.43) and its signal intensity increased only minimally on T_2 weighted images (Figure 10.42). The lesion represented metastatic spread to the left lung.

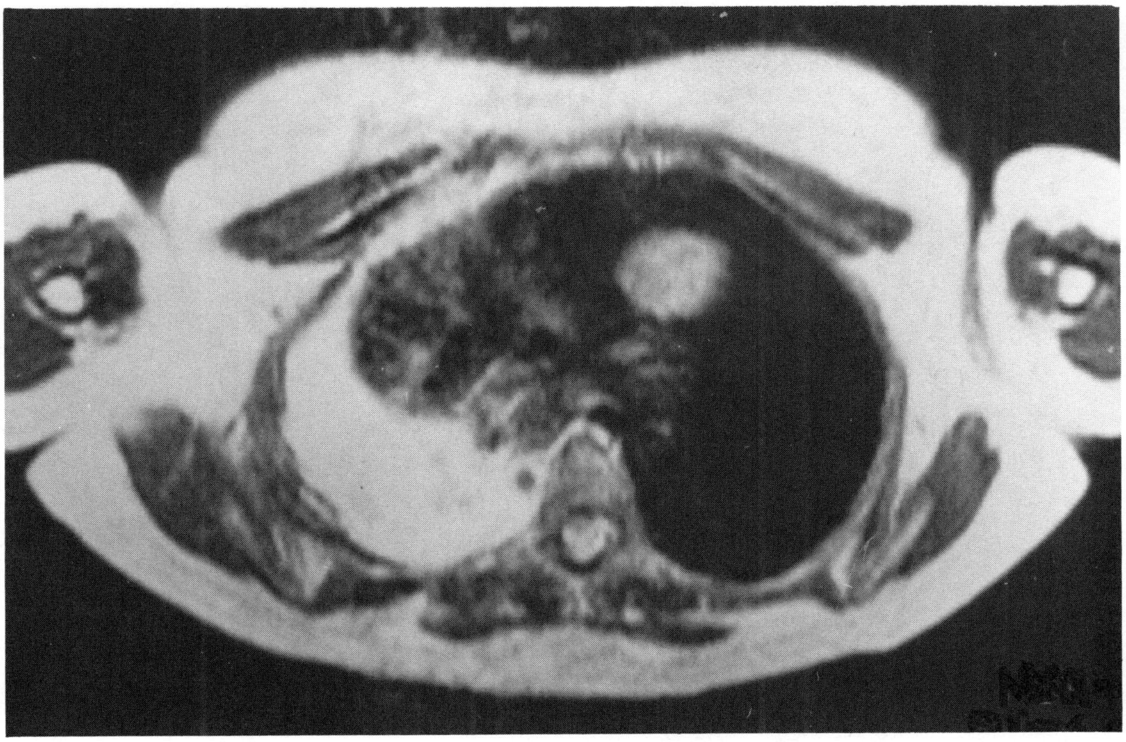

Figure 10.42

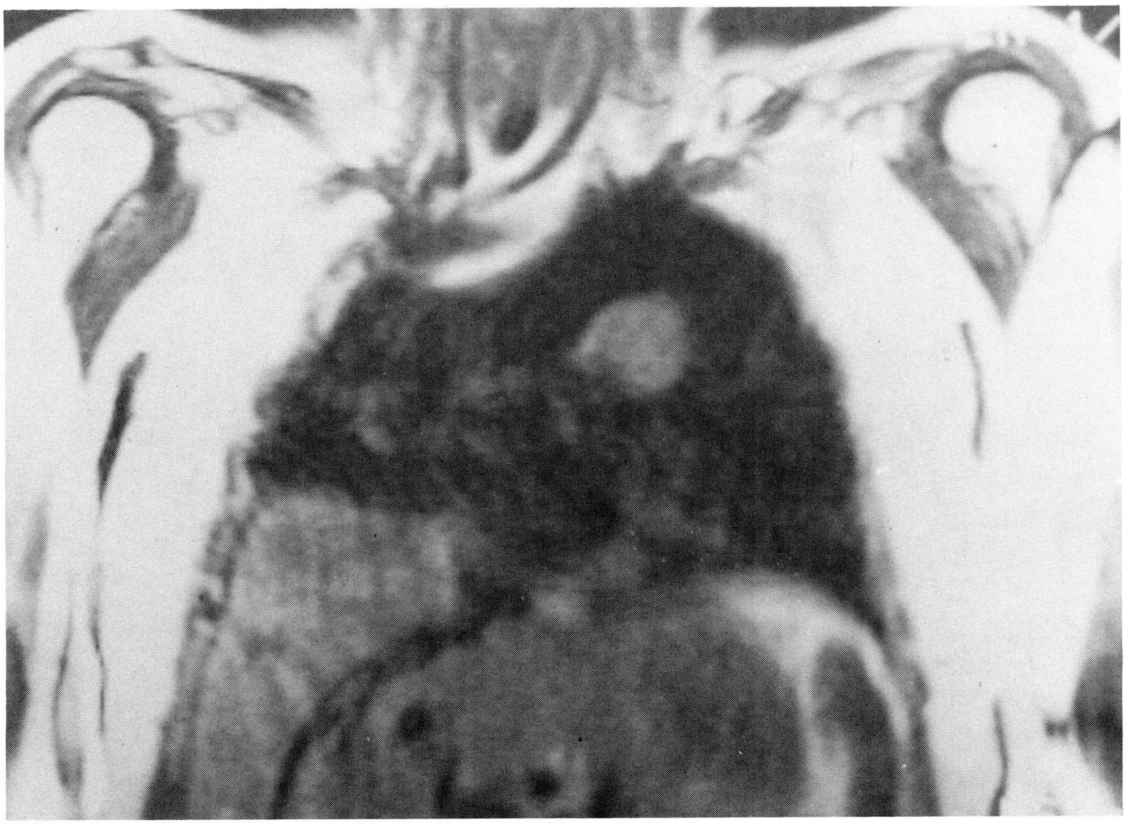

Figure 10.43

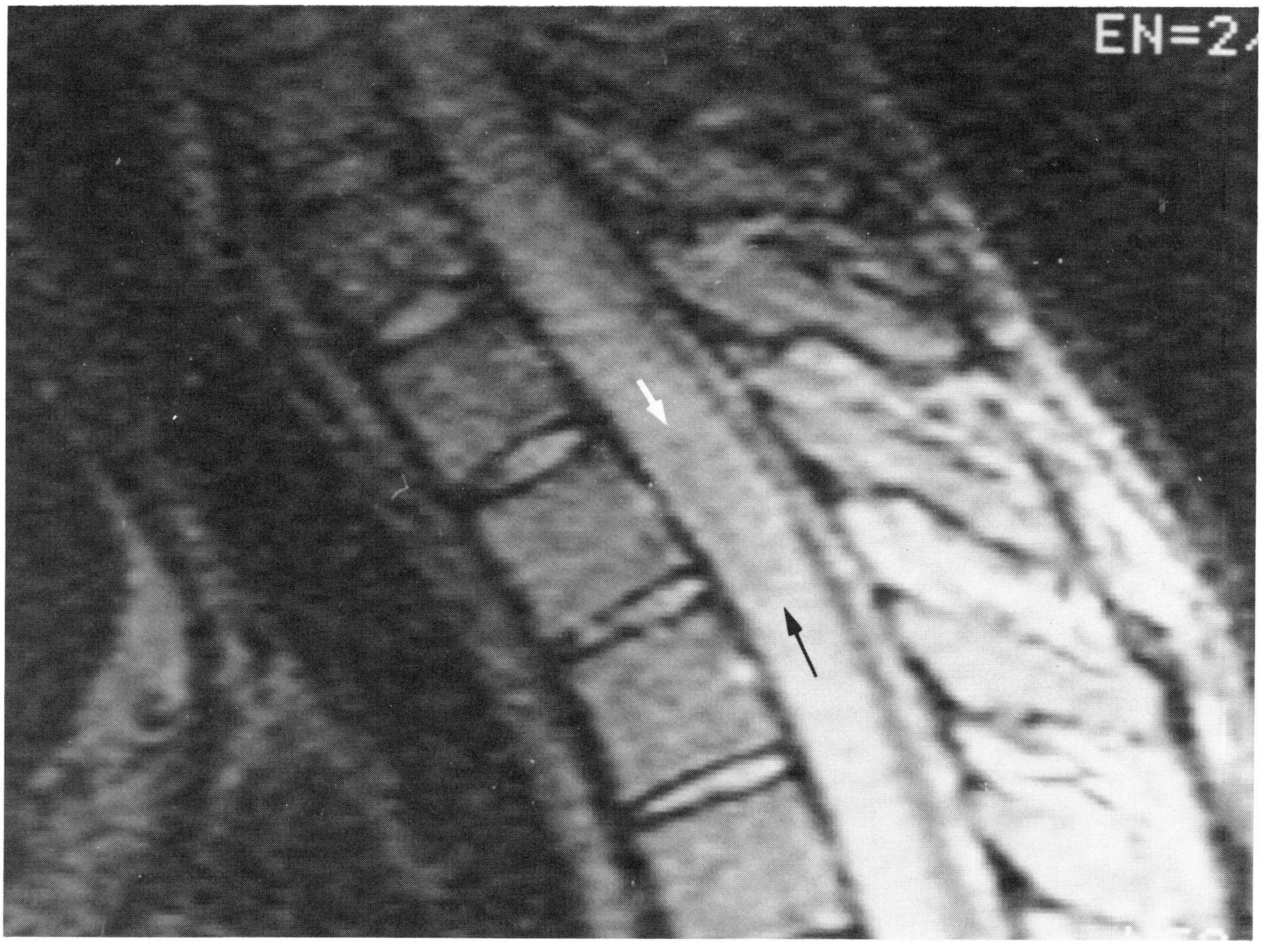

Figure 10.44

CASE 13

A 20-year-old man experienced rapid onset of gait disturbances and he developed tetraplegia within a short time interval. Cervical myelography and secondary CT myelography showed no abnormalities. Consequently, MRI of the cervical spine was requested.

At the level of the cervical cord no abnormalities were seen, but at the level D2 - D3 an intradural lesion could faintly be delineated on a sagittal image obtained with a TR 1500 msec and a TE 70 msec (arrows) (Figure 10.44). This MRI finding required further elucidation and intravenous injection of GD-DTPA was performed. Sagittal images of the cervico-thoracic junction demonstrated an intensely enhancing rim which surrounded a central area showing intermediate signal intensity (Figure 10.45).

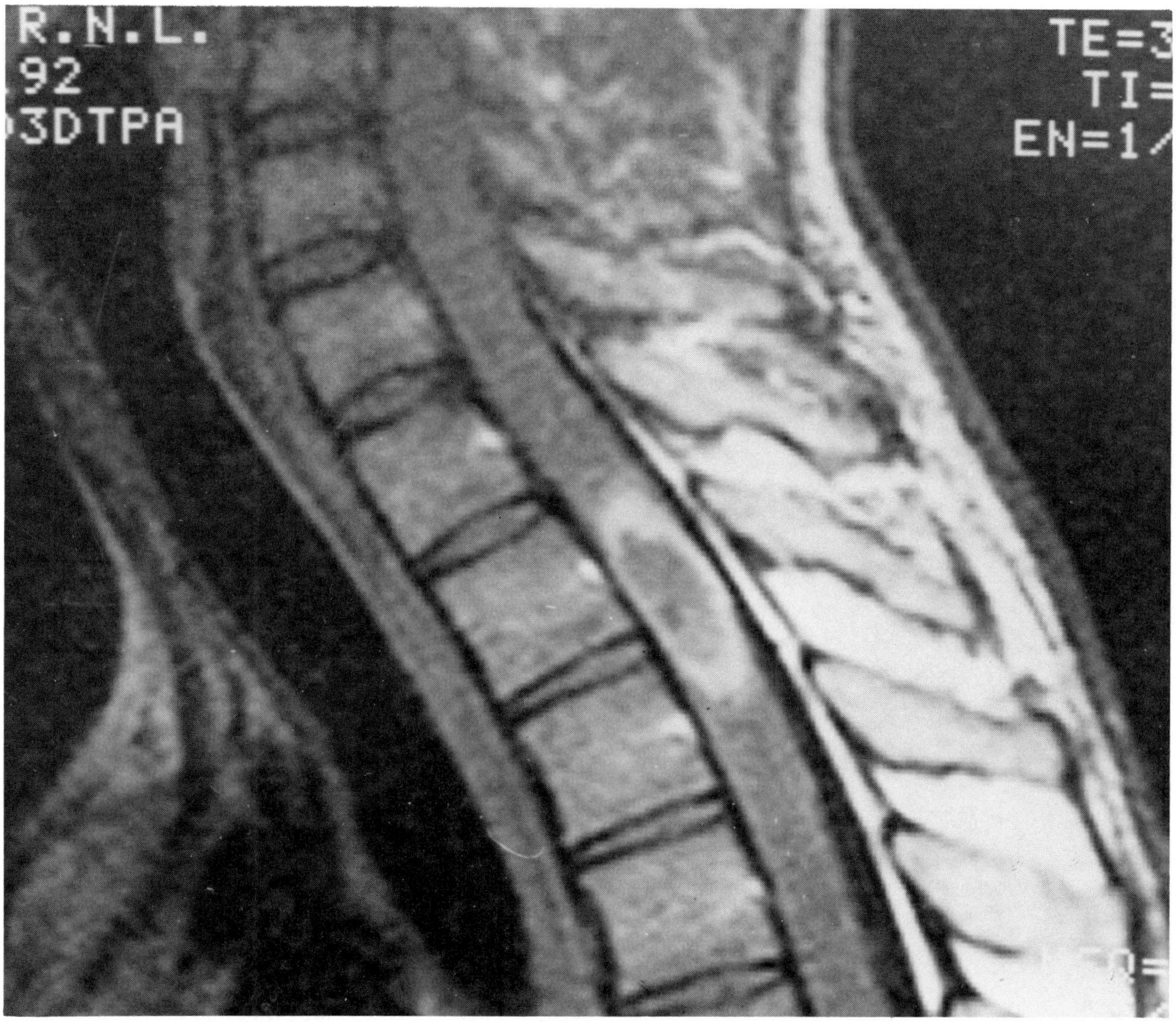

Figure 10.45

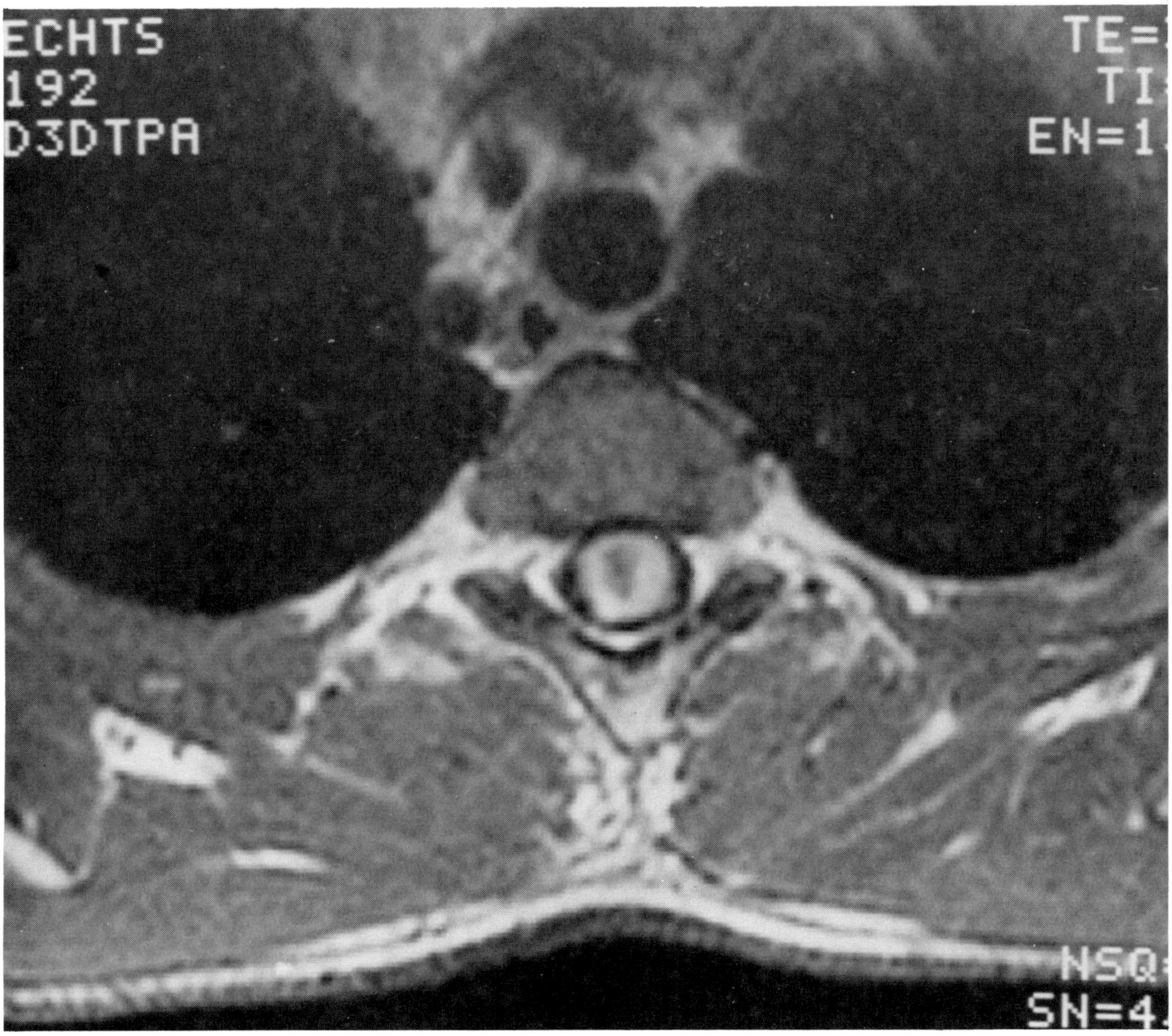

Figure 10.46

The intramedullary location of this process was confirmed by subsequent axial and coronal images (Figures 10.46 and 10.47). Conventional radiographs of the chest showed multifocal nodular lesions bilaterally, some of them contained small necrotic cavitations (arrow) (Figure 10.48). At this moment, a presumptive diagnosis of Wegener's granulomatosis was made, fine needle biopsy of a pulmonary nodule was done and the mass lesions were, in fact, due to lymphomatoid granulomatosis.

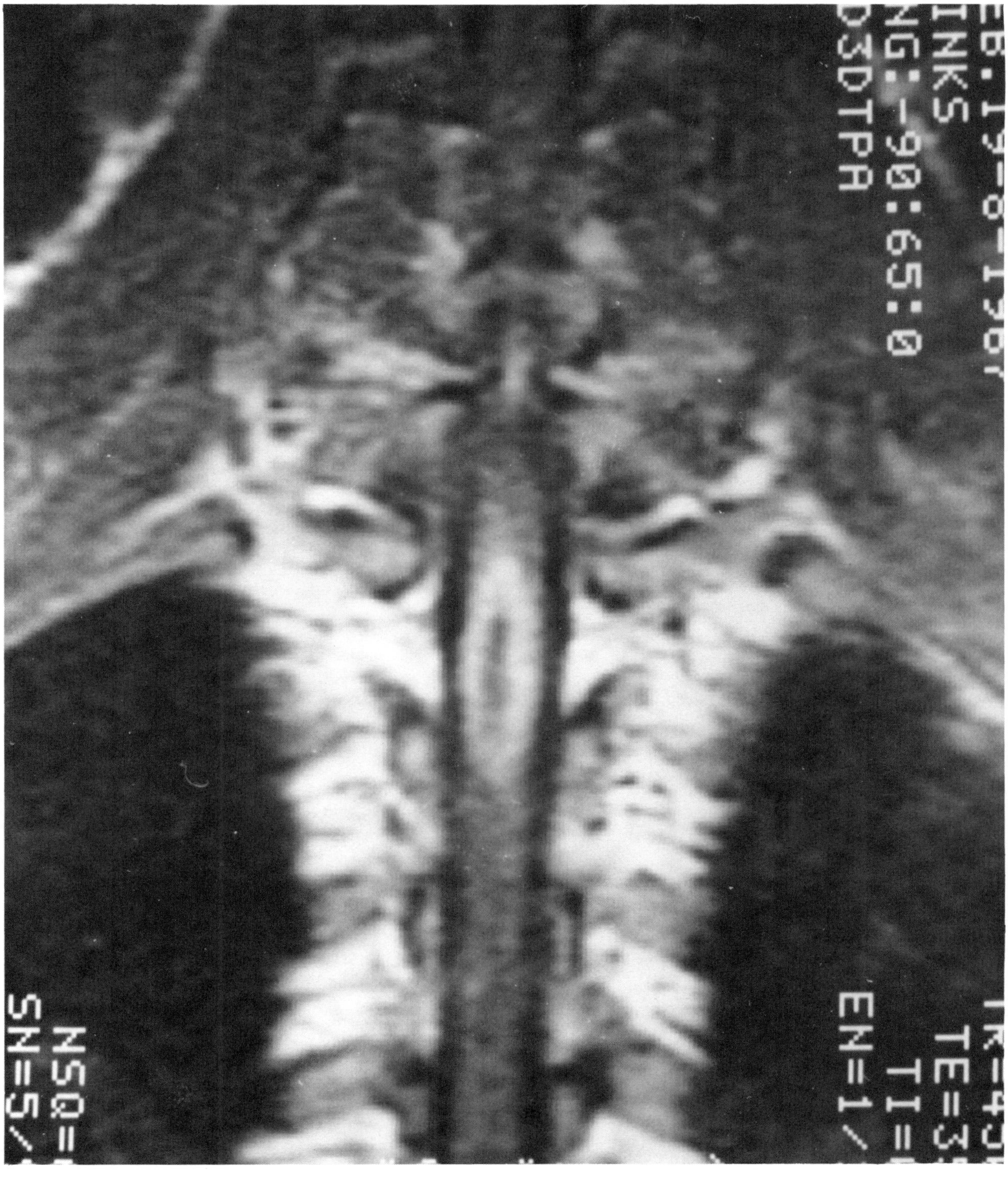

Figure 10.47

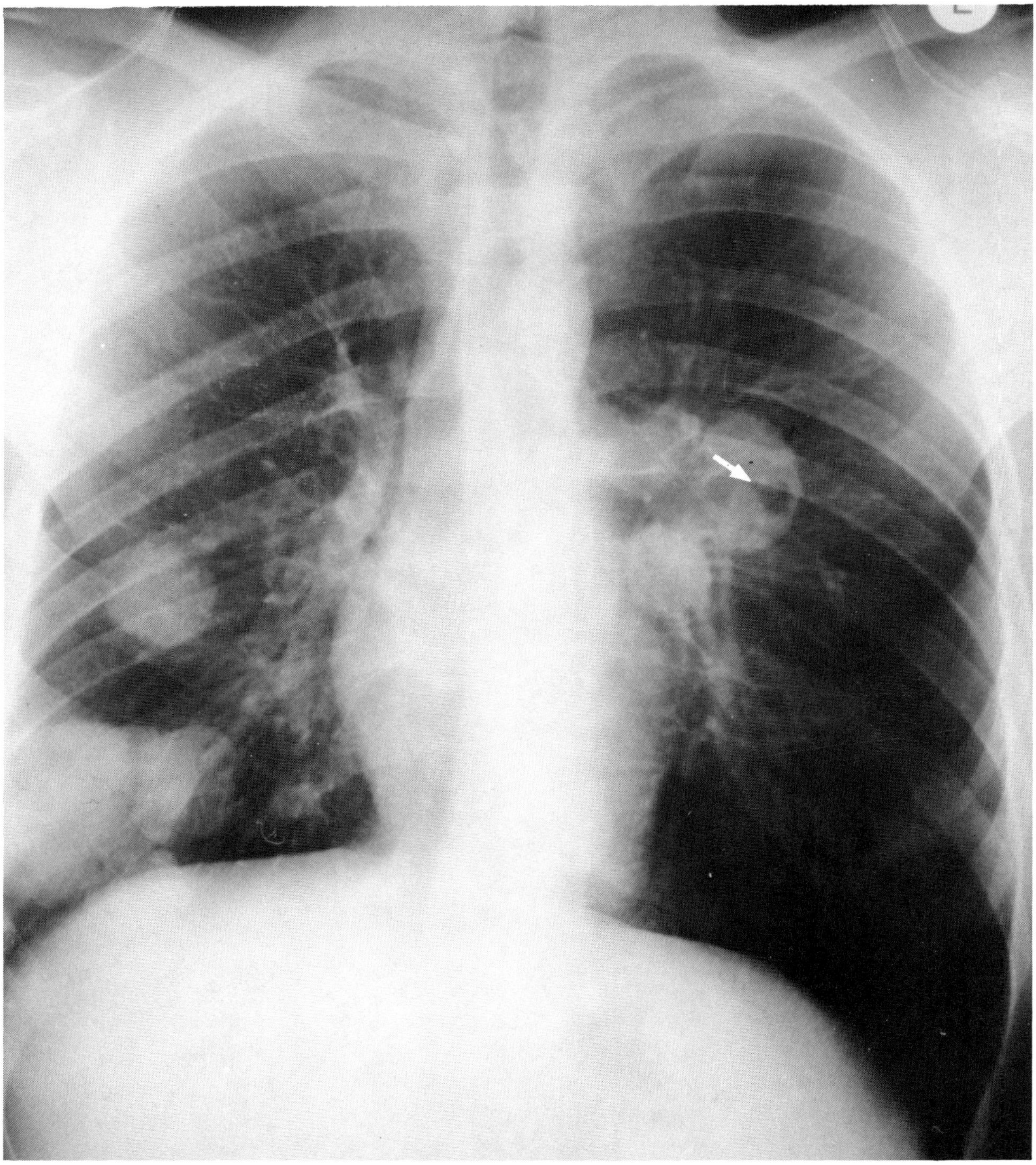

Figure 10.48

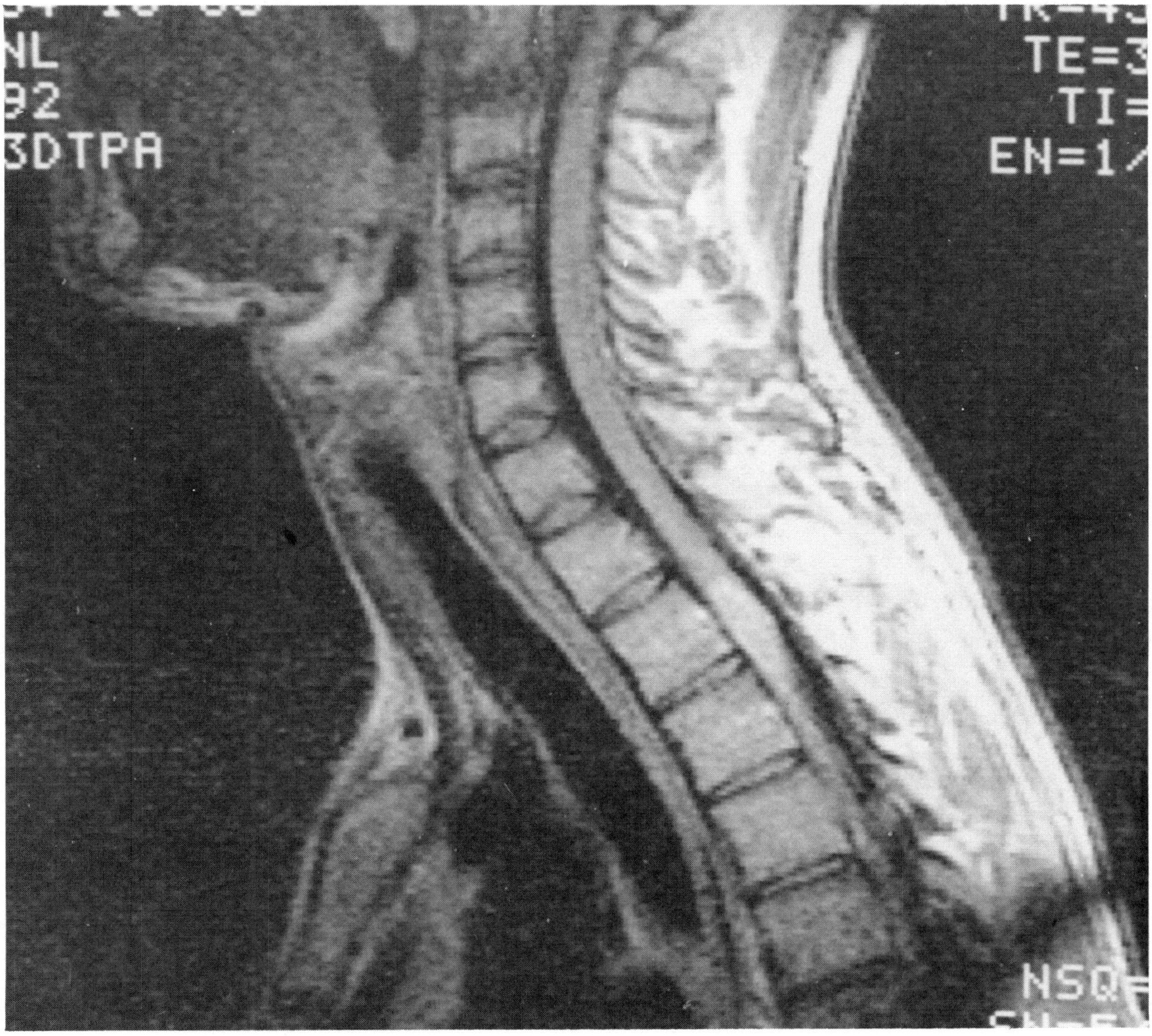

Figure 10.49

Corticosteroid treatment was initiated. The patient's clinical condition improved rapidly and two weeks after the first investigation, MRI was repeated and gadolinium injection was performed again. Sagittal images of the spine demonstrated that the intramedullary mass at the level D2 - D3 had significantly diminished in size, and that its enhancement after contrast administration was obviously less intense than on the previous MR scan (Figure 10.49). The central area of intermediate signal intensity had completely disappeared.

At this moment, a complementary MRI of the chest was done. The pulmonary nodules showed a similar appearance to the intramedullary lesion on the first MRI scan, i.e., a relatively high intensity rim surrounding a central area of intermediate signal

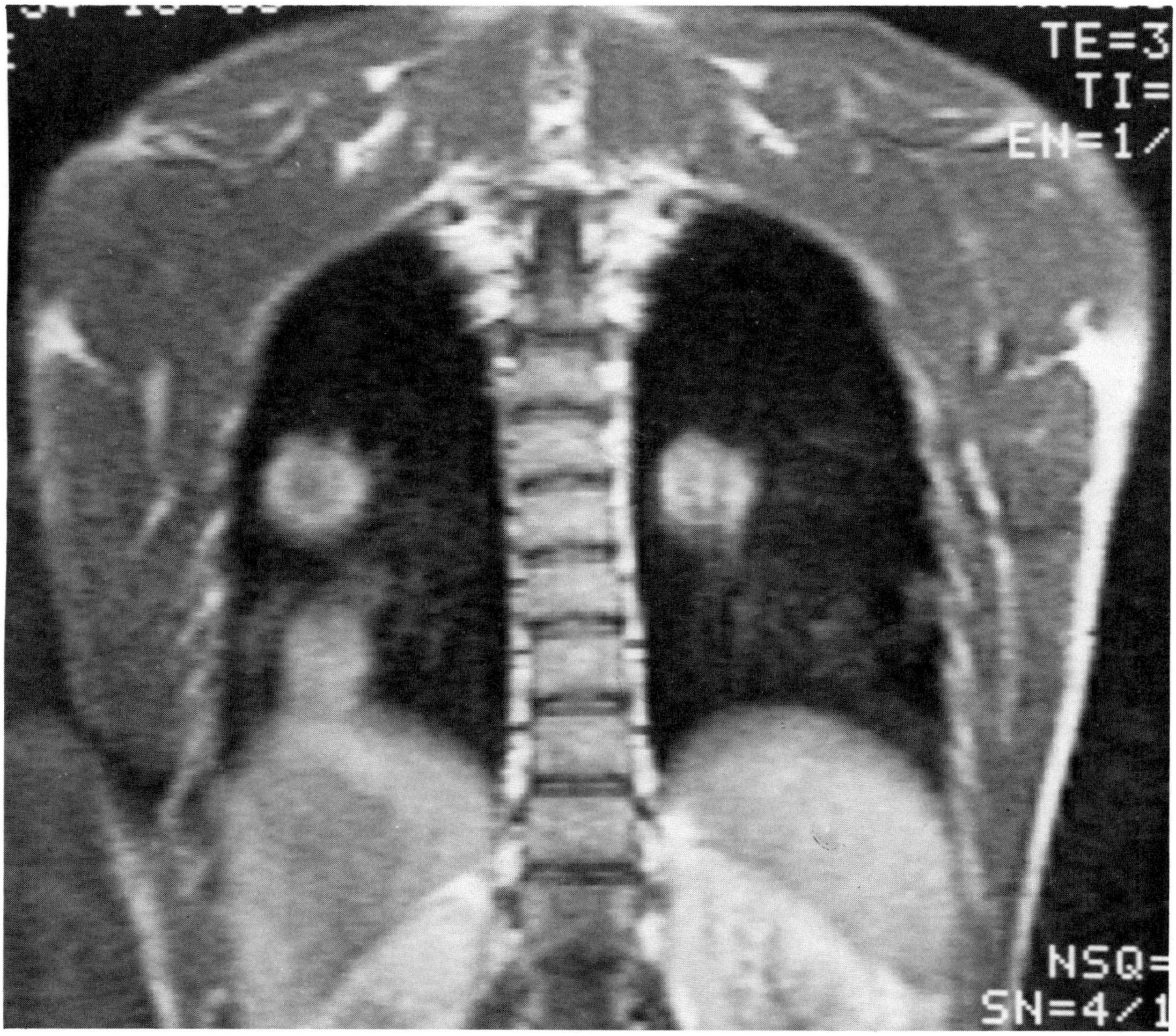

Figure 10.50

intensity (Figure 10.50). Some nodules presented small cavitations (arrowhead) and regional atelectasis was found on the right side (Figure 10.51).

Lymphomatoid granulomatosis has been described as an angiodestructive lymphoreticular proliferative and granulomatous disorder involving predominantly the lungs. Central nervous system (CNS) involvement occurs in approximately 20% of patients while Wegener's granulomatosis usually has no such tendency to involve the CNS. Lymphomatoid granulomatosis may progress to frank malignant lymphoma. Two different radiological patterns have been described:

1. reticulo-nodular infiltrates,
2. nodular parenchymal masses occur in 80% of patients.

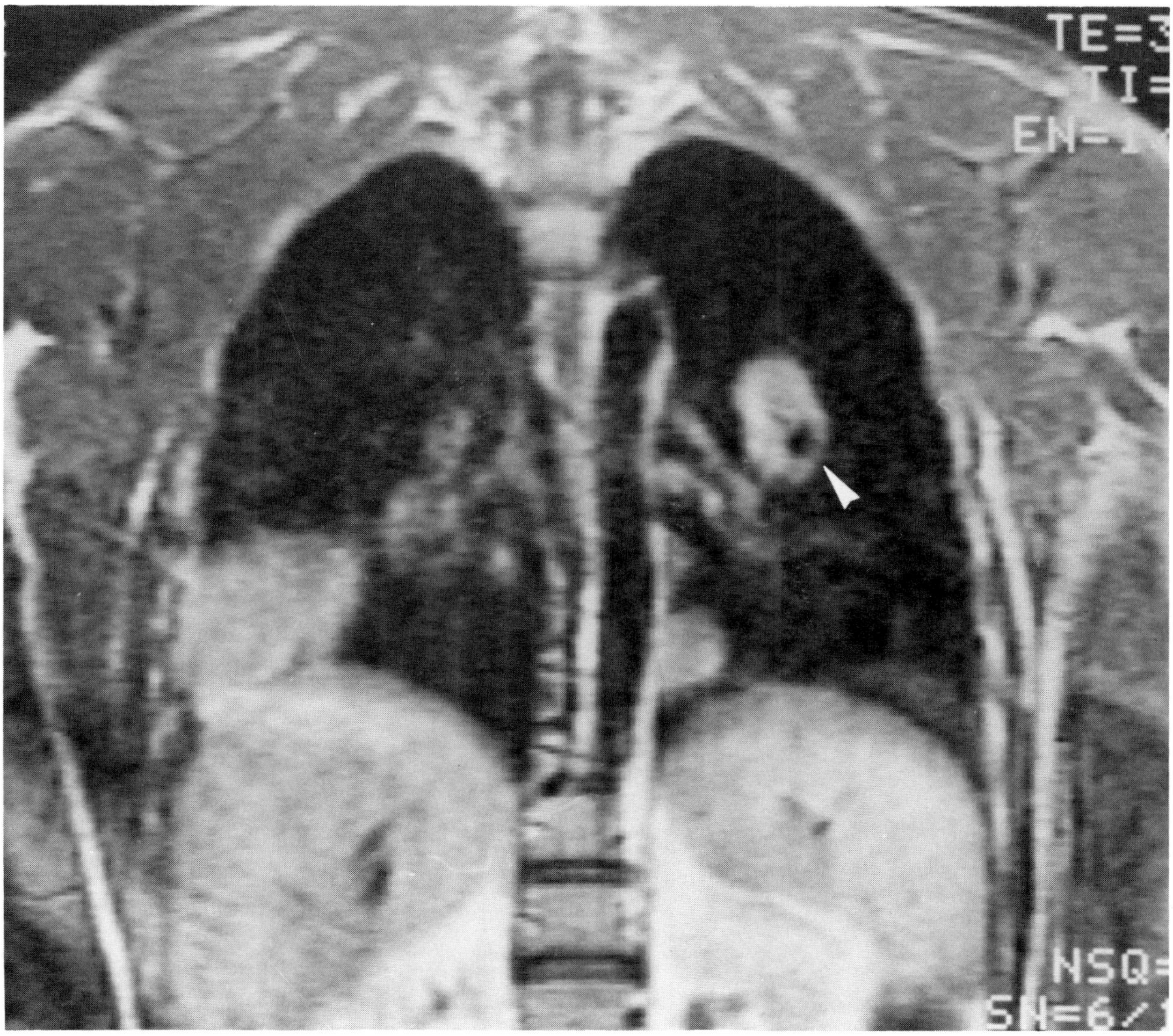

Figure 10.51

These lesions tend to be basal and may become confluent. Cavitation may be encountered as pulmonary infarction occurs, secondary to the angiodestructive nature of the lesion. Cavitation may be associated with life-threatening hemoptysis. In general, patients respond rather well to immunosuppressive and corticosteroid treatment, and complete resolution of the radiographic abnormalities may be seen. The two different radiological patterns may be determined by the varying degree of associated pulmonary infarction.

The lesions outlined by MRI of the spine and thorax correspond to regions in which vascular compromise (angiitis) and focal infarction have occurred. Acute and chronic inflammatory cellular changes are mixed among the necrotic tissue.

Notes

11

Current Status and Developing Technologies

When attempting to assess the value of MRI in the study of thoracic abnormalities with emphasis on the comparison with other existent diagnostic techniques, several factors have to be taken into consideration.

In the first place, the main qualities of MR imaging, which are superior contrast resolution and ability of multiplanar imaging, have to be clearly understood. Therefore, MRI is ideally suited for the study of abnormalities which are in prominent contrast with the normal broncho-vascular anatomy. Moreover, the lack of need of contrast material injection makes MRI the method of choice in the evaluation of vascular abnormalities even in patients in which injection of contrast material is not permitted.

There are almost no restrictions in what patient selection for an MRI examination of the thorax is concerned. Magnetic fields influence certain metallic implants and surgical clips. Although most surgical clips are non-ferromagnetic, caution has to be observed with clips which are located on vascular structures. Therefore, patients with aneurysm-clips, for example, and with pacemakers have to be excluded from MRI examinations. Orthopaedic appliances are occasionally encountered in patients with thoracic spine pathology and because of their incidental content of iron impurities may create disturbing artifacts

Clinical criteria for patient selection should take into consideration the ability of MRI to add information to less expensive and time consuming modalities the same as such individual patient characteristics as general condition or claustrophobia. In the acutely distressed patient, the same as in post-traumatic conditions, the prolonged scanning time may be a limiting factor.

The benefit of MRI investigations as shown by studies performed until now has been demonstrated in such clinical conditions as staging of bronchogenic carcinoma, cardiac and vascular abnormalities and mediastinal lesions. A large variety of clinical conditions have only been investigated in a limited manner and it is expected that the indications for MR imaging will increase with further experience. Improvements in MRI will also contribute to the enlargement of specific applications of MR. Such an improvement will include the reduction in scanning time due to expected shortening in the average scan time per body slice. Also more extensive clinical studies will enable a better understanding of the optimal pulse sequences to be used in specific clinical conditions. The quality of MR images is greatly dependent on the interference of respiratory and cardiovascular motion. ECG gating has already proved its efficiency whereas respiratory gating still needs further technical refinement. Future improvement of both gating techniques will permit the performance of MRI in patients with respiratory problems.

The use of contrast materials has brought the chance of significant improvement of MR imaging of the thorax. The most representative contrast agent is gadolinium-DTPA which has been shown to have low toxicity (1, 2) and being able to reduce T_1 and T_2 relaxation times while it enhances pathological processes. Under study are more sophisticated contrast agents as expected to concentrate in specific organs and/or pathological processes. Such a substance, for example metalloporphyrine, is liable to concentrate exclusively in tumoral lesions.

Surface coils placed close to various body surfaces produce a small field of view and an improved signal to noise ratio. Especially surface coil images using high field magnets (1, 5 - 2 Tesla) provide prominent increase in image quality and detail distinction (3). In the thorax the use of surface coils is recommended especially for the study of lesions in areas close to the thoracic spine.

MR images can be obtained in a single plane or there is a possibility of volume data acquisition. There is also the possibility to have a single or multiple slices obtained. The two-dimensional Fourier transformation (2 FDT) has been shown to allow an improved imaging speed and a better image quality (4). A three-dimensional technique is also available when data are acquired through a whole volume of tissue and can be reconstructed in various planes. This technique is especially valuable in the imaging of the heart when a process can be visualized during the same phase of the ECG cycle.

In an attempt to reduce prolonged examination times, efforts are being made to develop fast imaging techniques which permit examination in patients unable to remain still for prolonged periods of time. In the study of the mediastinum, for example, it seems that images obtained with short TR and TE together with heavy signal averaging succeed in eliminating both cardiac and respiratory motion artifacts. Fast scanning techniques permitting data acquisition for an image in 10 to 20 seconds are being introduced. Furthermore, the possibility exists of the development of echo-planar pulse sequences (real-time MRI) which allow image acquisition in 50 msec or less (5). In the study of the heart and related vascular structures, dynamic MRI has a special value when the in- and output volumes can be estimated.

MR spectroscopy has initially been developed for the analysis of chemical composition of various substances in the laboratory. Recently this technique has been applied to the study of compositions of cell cultures and isolated body organs. Moreover, in vivo experiments are increasingly being performed. The most studied paramagnetic ions are phosphorus 31, hydrogen 1, sodium 23, carbon 13 and fluorine 19. Among them, due to its great metabolic significance, phosphorus 31 is the one mainly studied in clinical practice. Major possible use of this non-invasive diagnostic modality can be the diagnosis and detection of neoplasms and the assessment of their metabolism (6, 7). A specific application of spectroscopy in the thorax could be the ability of identifying the relative composition of fluid collections. A different technique which makes use of spectroscopic analysis of hydrogen and not phosphorus is clinical shift imaging. The result in this case is not a spectroscopic graph, but an anatomical image and the major value of this method is to identify minimal amounts of fat in a given lesion. It is expected that even more sophisticated techniques will be developed in the ongoing process of MRI improvement.

REFERENCES

1. McNamara MT, Higgins CB, Ehman RL, Revel D, Sievers R, Brasch RC: NMR contrast enhancement of acute myocardial ischemia using the paramagnetic pharmaceutical complex gadolinium-DTPA. *Radiology, 153:*157-163, 1984.

2. Weinman HJ, Brasch RC, Press WR, Weshey GE: Characteristics of gadolinium-DTPA complex: A potential NMR contrast agent. *AJR, 142:* 619-624, 1984.

3. Berquist TH: Technical considerations in Magnetic Resonance Imaging. In: *MRI of the Musculoskeletal System.* Raven Press, 1987.

4. Davis PL, Kaufman L, Crooks LE: Tissue characterization. In: *Clinical Magnetic Resonance Imaging.* Radiology Research and Education Foundation, San Francisco, 1983.

5. Ogie PL: Fast scanning helps make abdominal MRI of more than academic interest. *Diag Imag Internat, 5:*35-41, 1986.

6. Newman RJ: Clinical applications of nuclear magnetic resonance spectroscopy: A review. *J R Soc Med, 77:*774-779, 1984.

7. Radda GK: Clinical studies by 31P NMR spectroscopy. Society of Magnetic Resonance in Medicine Scientific Program, New York, Society of Magnetic Resonance, 1984.

Index

N

O

P